PROBIOTICS AND PREBIOTICS IN HUMAN NUTRITION AND HEALTH

Edited by **Venketeshwer Rao**
and **Leticia G. Rao**

Probiotics and Prebiotics in Human Nutrition and Health
http://dx.doi.org/10.5772/61495
Edited by Venketeshwer Rao and Leticia G. Rao

Contributors

Sabina Fijan, Katarzyna Neffe-Skocińska, Karolina Maria Wójciak, Dorota Zielińska, Gabriela Tenea, Lucia Yépez, Zhongke Sun, Vengadesan Krishnan, Pedro De Oliva-Neto, Márcia Zilioli-Bellini, Estevão Zilioli, Sidmeire Santos-Oliveira, Amirreza Khalighi, Reza Behdani, Shabnam Kouhestani, Nditange Shigwedha, Li Jia, Shuang Zhang, Liubov Sichel, Penny Hiwilepo-Van Hal, Claudio Gonzalez, Danielle Kling, Guillermo Marcial, Dana Roberson, Graciela Lorca, Todd Callaway, Luis Tedeschi, William Smith, Francis Rouquette, Trisha Sheridan, Jennifer Adamski, Mario Cruz, Samuel Longoria, Ruth Belmares, Mildred Flores, Juan Contreras, Julio Montanez, Qing Gu, Ping Li, Silvia Marina González, Mariela Ramona Michel Michel, Rosa María Rodríguez Jasso, Cristobal Aguilar, Adriana Carolina Flores Gallegos, Raul Rodriguez-Herrera, Yasuhiko Komatsu, Yasuhiro Koga, Yuji Aiba, Yasuhiro Nakano, Lucia Pacifico, Caterina Anania, Francesca Olivero, Eugenia Olivero, José Luis Alonso, Beatriz Miguez, Belén Gómez, Patricia Gullón, Beatriz Gullon, Anna Forsberg, Michelle Peneluppi Silva, Rodnei Dennis Rossoni, Antonio Olavo Cardoso Jorge, Juliana Campos Junqueira

Published by InTech

Janeza Trdine 9, 51000 Rijeka, Croatia

Publishing Process Manager Dajana Pemac

Technical Editor SPi Global

Cover InTech Design team

First published July, 2016

Printed in Croatia

Additional hard copies can be obtained from orders@intechopen.com

Probiotics and Prebiotics in Human Nutrition and Health, Edited by Venketeshwer Rao and Leticia G. Rao

p. cm.

Print ISBN 978-953-51-2475-7

Online ISBN 978-953-51-2476-4

For EU product safety concerns:
IN TECH d.o.o., Prolaz Marije Krucifikse Kozulić 3, 51000 Rijeka, Croatia,
info@intechopen.com or visit our website at intechopen.com.

Meet the editors

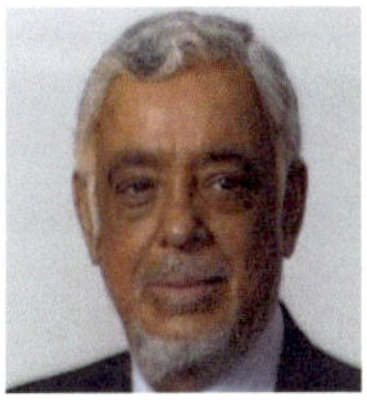

Dr. Rao, Professor Emeritus, Department of Nutritional Sciences, Faculty of Medicine, University of Toronto, has established a major focus in the area of diet, nutrition and health. His research has focused on the role of oxidative stress and antioxidant phytochemicals in the causation and prevention of chronic diseases, with particular emphasis on the role of carotenoids and polyphenols. His research interest also includes the role of prebiotics and probiotics in human health. He is recognized internationally for his contributions in this area. He has over 100 publications in scientific journals and several books and book chapters. He has a distinguished academic career spanning over 50 years. He is popularly sought by the international media to express his opinions on the subjects of nutrition, probiotics, prebiotics and antioxidant phytochemicals in human health.

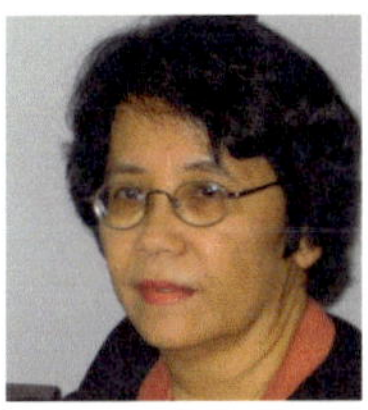

Dr. Leticia Rao is an adjunct professor of Medicine; a full member of the Graduate Faculty, Institute of Medical Science, at the University of Toronto; the director of the Calcium Research Laboratory, Department of Medicine; and a staff scientist at St. Michael's Hospital, Toronto, Ontario. She has a BSc Chemistry from the University of the Philippines, an MSc in Food Science and Technology from Oregon State University, and a PhD in Biochemistry from the University of Toronto. Her expertise is in the area of bone cell biology with the goal of finding the prevention of osteoporosis by studying bone cells in the laboratory and carrying out clinical studies of drugs and nutritional supplements in postmenopausal women. Her research has been presented to a number of symposia both nationally and internationally and published extensively in peer-reviewed scientific journals. She coauthored a book entitled 'Bone Building Solution' and coedited the book 'Phytochemicals: Isolation, Characterization and Role in Human Health'.

Contents

Preface

Human intestinal tract is colonised by several thousand species of bacteria. They represent both the beneficial bacteria as well as harmful ones. Beneficial bacteria are referred to as 'probiotics'. Predominance of probiotic bacteria is considered essential for the prevention of human diseases and maintenance of good health. Prebiotics are non-digestible food ingredients that selectively promote the growth of probiotics in the gastrointestinal tract. More recently, the concept of 'synbiotic' relationship between the probiotics and prebiotics is being used as an effective strategy to maintain the predominance of the probiotics in the gastrointestinal tract. Research over the years and more recent research have shown the beneficial effect of probiotics in the prevention and management of several human diseases including cancer, cardiovascular diseases, gastrointestinal disorders, osteoporosis and neurodegenerative diseases. The recent focus of research is to identify the specific species of probiotics, types of prebiotics, their interactions and mechanisms of action in providing health benefits. Recognition of the health benefits of probiotics and prebiotics has led to the marketing of several supplements. Government agencies are actively developing regulatory guidelines for the safety and efficacy of such supplements. In recognition of the importance of probiotics and prebiotics, the contents of the book include all the major concepts from their identification to clinical trials. The book has been carefully reviewed to include chapters that are relevant and representative of current research. We are confident that the readers of this book published by InTech publication that include researchers, health professionals, government regulatory agencies and industries will find it highly useful as a standard reference book.

Dr. L. G. Rao
Adjunct Professor and
Director Calcium Research Laboratory
St. Michael's Hospital
University of Toronto

Dr. A. Rao
Professor Emeritus
Department of Nutritional Sciences
Faculty of Medicine
University of Toronto

Chapter 1

Prebiotic and Probiotic Approaches to Improving Food Safety on the Farm and Their Implications on Human Health[1]

William B. Smith, Todd R. Callaway, Luis O. Tedeschi,
Francis M. Rouquette Jr., Trisha Sheridan and
Jennifer Adamski

Additional information is available at the end of the chapter

http://dx.doi.org/10.5772/63114

Abstract

Human health is a broad category that encompasses the entirety of the food production system. Livestock production practices have important effects on human health because livestock not only are a primary food source but also can be the source of pathogenic bacteria that may enter the food chain indirectly. As government regulation and public scrutiny restrict the prophylactic use of antibiotic and antimicrobial interventions, other techniques must be used to reduce the burden of animal-borne pathogenic bacteria entering the food system. Prebiotics (isolated compounds that enhance natural microflora and thereby decrease pathogens) and probiotics (live microbes that are administered to livestock to enhance microbial diversity and crowd out pathogens) represent two unique opportunities for alternative measures in pathogen reduction. This review addresses the link between animal production and human health, the agricultural sources of pathogenic organisms, and the probiotic and prebiotic approaches that have been evaluated in an effort to reduce carriage of foodborne pathogenic bacteria by livestock.

Keywords: food safety, livestock, prebiotic, preharvest intervention, probiotic

[1] Proprietary brand names are necessary to report factually on available data; however, the USDA neither guarantees nor warrants the standard of the product, and the use of the name by the USDA implies no approval of the product and/or exclusion of others that may be suitable.

1. Introduction: why is farm-based intervention of interest to human health?

This book is dedicated to the understanding and dissemination of knowledge surrounding prebiotic use in human health. Thus, it begs the following questions: When a reader finds this particular manuscript, what is the point? What is the objective of a farm-based perspective when the focus is on human health? While these may be valid questions to the casual observer, a full understanding of potential pathogens and intervention in the subject of human health must by rights include a discussion of the foodstuff at its source. Like all mammals, livestock harbor a diverse collection of bacteria [1]. In fact, the gastrointestinal tract of these animals can harbor in excess of 2000 bacterial species at concentrations of 10^{10} cells/g of digesta [2]. While the majority of these organisms are beneficial to the host and part of the stable native microflora of the gut [3], certain instances or conditions allow pathogenic bacteria to colonize within the animal. Some of these bacteria can make their way from the gut or the hide during processing [4], introducing pathogens into the abattoir (slaughter plant) at harvest that must then be dealt with in final food products. As noted in Reference [1], a great number of these pathogenic bacteria in the realm of human health are also of interest in that of livestock animal health and can commonly be traced back to those very animals. Since these pathogens are a threat to the well-being of both humans and livestock, one must then investigate intervention strategies by which the microbial burden may be reduced at the source so that these pathogenic organisms would never enter the human food chain.

Traditionally, farm-level or feeder/finisher-level control of pathogens has been achieved through prophylactic antibiotic and antimicrobial addition to feeds. The main source of prevention of pathogenic bacterial entry into the food system is through Hazard Analysis and Critical Control Point (HACCP) plans at the abattoir [5]. It should be noted that HACCP control measures are only effective to a certain point (i.e., they are not perfect), but any reduction of pathogen shedding prior to entry into the abattoir will reduce the burden and assist in the efficacy of in-plant HACCP-based controls [6]. In fact, with the subtherapeutic antibiotic use ban in the European Union [7,8] and increased public scrutiny of antibiotic use in livestock in the United States [9], alternative preharvest control strategies must be devised and implemented, especially given the direct correlation between live animals shedding foodborne pathogenic bacteria, such as *Escherichia coli* O157:H7, and the incidence of positive carcasses at the abattoir [5]. Thus, preharvest intervention strategies, such as use of probiotics and prebiotics, need to be viewed as an additional critical control measure that can be included in the food safety continuum.

So how then do preharvest interventions in animals work? Much of the efficacy of products that will be described in the present review can be loosely grouped under an umbrella concept known as a "competitive enhancement" approach to pathogen reduction [1,10–13]. The first facet is based upon the introduction of naturally-occurring microflora isolates from the gastrointestinal tract of an animal of the same species [1], occupying all available ecological niches in the gastrointestinal tract and thereby excluding pathogens [1,14]. When used in neonatal (or newly hatched) animals, this technique is known as "competitive exclusion" (CE), which reduces pathogen penetration of the naive and essentially sterile neonatal gastrointestinal tract [1,14]. Use of probiotics (also known in the animal industry as direct-fed microbials [DFMs]) is a slightly different approach in which existing gastrointestinal microbial populations can be diversified or modified/attenuated by daily inclusion of a bacterial or fungal population or end-product, and this may have an inhibitory effect on pathogenic bacteria, including foodborne pathogens [1,15]. A further competitive enhancement strategy is the addition of prebiotics, which are limiting nutrients or isolated compounds that are indigestible by the host but give specific innate microbes a competitive advantage that can have a deleterious effect on pathogenic bacteria, to the diet [1]. Furthermore, several of these approaches can be synergistically combined and are termed "synbiotics"; for example, a DFM dependent on the inclusion of prebiotics can be maintained in the gut and given a further competitive advantage to remain in the population to benefit host animal health and production or to improve food safety.

2. Pathogens: what are the sources?

As previously noted, the body , and especially the gut, of most food animals contains many microorganisms [2]. While the vast majority of these are beneficial (commensal) to the host, there are select species and serovars (e.g., *Salmonella*) that exhibit pathogenic or toxigenic effects in both humans and livestock. These pathogens are naturally occurring organisms that, given the opportunity, can colonize the environment of the innate gut microflora and take hold of niches in an otherwise healthy animal. This section provides a discussion of some of the more common pathogenic bacteria in livestock and how these microbes may become a problem in the safety and security of the food chain.

2.1. Campylobacter

Campylobacter has been identified as one of the most common foodborne pathogenic bacteria. Most commonly, *Campylobacter* has been linked to poultry products and linked to human cases of gastroenteritis in most cases as well as the Guillain-Barré syndrome, reactive arthritis, and irritable bowel syndrome or inflammatory bowel disease in the most severe cases [16,17]. *Campylobacter* is a major concern for infection in poultry production [16–18]. One route of contamination, also common to most other pathogens, is through livestock water sources [19]. In an area of intense livestock (dairy) production in England, *Campylobacter jejuni* was found in 14.3% of water sources sampled (predominantly in running water or troughs), *Campylobacter coli* was found in 18.5% (predominantly in stagnant water), and *Campylobacter lari* was identified in 4.2% [20]. In this same study, variables were regressed to show their impact on the prevalence of *Campylobacter* spp. In a multiple regression model, water source and soil type played the most significant role in determining the environmental prevalence of *Campylobacter*, with natural water sources and high clay content both increasing its prevalence [20].

2.2. Enterohemorrhagic *E. coli* (EHEC)

Enterohemorrhagic *E. coli* is a group of highly virulent foodborne pathogenic bacteria that is of great interest to human health. The well-known *E. coli* serotype O157:H7 was first identified in a clinical outbreak of undercooked hamburger patties at a commercial fast food chain in the United States [21]. In fact, this pathogenic serotype has been linked to one of the greatest foodborne pathogen outbreaks in American history [22,23]. In this landmark case, in which over 150 cases were reported and multiple deaths occurred [22], *E. coli* O157:H7 was isolated from ground beef patties and subsequently sourced to the abattoir in which meat was contaminated from pathogenically infected animals [23]. These human infections commonly resulted in postdiarrheal hemolytic uremic syndrome (HUS) and disproportionately affected the young and elderly [22]. While inoculation of the livestock host is generally achieved through fecal-oral contamination or contaminated drinking sources [19,24], this does not account for the transmission of pathogens from the live animal to the meat during processing. Much of the contamination in the plant, especially with regard to *E. coli* O157:H7, can be traced to contamination of the hide and interaction during hide removal and evisceration [25]. In a sampling of over 2500 cattle hides from across North America, researchers discovered that over half of the hides were contaminated with nearly 300 unique isolates of *E. coli* O157:H7 [4]. Additionally, the frequency of the unique isolates obtained from cattle hides was very similar to the prevalence of isolates identified in human clinical cases [4]. In a survey of high-throughput Midwestern United States abattoirs, 11% of all hides, 43% of pre-eviscerated carcasses, and 2% of postprocessed carcasses tested positive for EHEC O157:H7 [5]. This included positive tests for hides in 38% of introduced lots, pre-eviscerated carcasses in 87% of lots, and post-processed carcasses in 17% of lots [5]. While *E. coli* O157:H7 is the best known of the EHEC group, other members (e.g., O26, O111) also pose significant threats to the food supply around the world. Although *E. coli* O157:H7 was quickly categorized by the U.S. Food Safety Inspection Service as an adulterant [26], an additional six serotypes are now included in this important category [27] and thus carry an important public health and economic impact.

2.3. Salmonella

Salmonella is another bacterial pathogen of significant concern both as a foodborne pathogen and as a threat to animal health, having been identified in all vertebrates [28]. More than 2500 separate serotypes comprise *Salmonella enterica* [29], which is the most common species found in food animals. *Salmonella* accounted for 55% of the foodborne illness outbreaks in the United States from 1993 to 1997 [30] and 26% of the outbreaks from 1998 to 2008 [31], with one of the most massive outbreaks being from ice cream hauled in tanker trucks that had improperly handled raw eggs [30]. Although researchers identify *Salmonella* as a ubiquitous microbe, it has been noted that the primary reservoir for such a pathogen is the digestive tract of the animal (indicating fecal-oral transmission or accidental contamination at the abattoir) and conditions under intensive production where animals are in close contact with one another are favored [32]. It should be noted, however, that a common vehicle for *Salmonella* contamination in human food is not livestock per se but instead vine-stalk vegetables [31]. That said, in an evaluation of butcher shop poultry in Portugal, 60% of the products were found to be contaminated with *Salmonella* and the pathogen *S. enteritidis* was found to make up 44% of those cases [32].

2.4. Others of interest

While *Campylobacter, E. coli,* and *Salmonella* are all identified and targeted as the primary pathogens of interest for reduction in the human food system [19], there are other pathogens of importance that are far less commonly addressed in scientific research. *Clostridium,* like many other pathogens discussed herein, is a Gram-positive, spore-forming pathogenic bacterium [33]. *Clostridium difficile* infection is characterized by severe diarrhea and pseudomembranous colitis [33]. *C. difficile* is a known potential resident of the livestock intestinal tract and has been identified in up to 12% of sampled retail ground beef and ground pork in a Canadian study [34]. *Clostridium perfringens,* the leading cause of necrotic enteritis, can also become a human health issue and has been isolated as a portion of the natural microflora of the jejunum, cecum, and cloaca of poultry [35]. *Listeria monocytogenes* is a pathogen most commonly associated with dairy products [36]. At the time of their review, Skovgaard and Morgen [37] stated that most human cases of listeriosis are of unknown origin, although food was suspected, and recent high-profile outbreaks have definitely confirmed such suspicion [36]. Listeriosis has been linked to central nervous system infections, bacteremia, and endocarditis [37]. Listeria has been isolated from dairy feces as well as feedstuffs and attributed to mastitis in these animals [38]. *Staphylococcus aureus* has been associated with all livestock species [39]. It is an opportunistic pathogen that will colonize both livestock and humans in an infectious nature [40].In dairy cattle, the pathogen is known as one of the leading causes of mastitis, and mastitis is among the leading losses to the dairy industry [41]. In one study, 296 individual isolates of *S. aureus* of animal origin were discovered; while none of the isolates from cattle or swine were found to be common with human infection, a significant number of the poultry isolates were common with those found in the bloodstream of humans [40].

3. Probiotics/direct-fed microbials (DFMs)

A list of probiotics that have been used in food animals to reduce pathogenic bacteria is presented in **Table 1.** Probiotics used in animals are known as DFMs and defined as live, biologically active microbes (bacterial or fungal), or dead cultures that include the end-products of their fermentation, that are administered to an animal in hopes of enhancing the natural gastrointestinal ecosystem and occupying any niches in which pathogenic organisms may thrive [10,42]. Again, this concept is broadly categorized as competitive enhancement in which live, naturally occurring microbes are added to the host animal to enhance the innate population in the gut [10,15]. As noted in Reference [43], the concept of CE specifically originated with the application of mature broiler gastrointestinal contents for the reduction of *Salmonella* [44]. While addition of DFMs to mature animals yields mixed and often negative results, their administration to livestock early in life (as early as the day of hatch in broilers) has been shown to be effective in reducing pathogenic bacterial loads by kick-starting the natural succession of commensal bacterial colonization of the gastrointestinal microflora [18]. In addition to the direct addition of probiotics to neonatal diets, passive immunity may also be conveyed to the neonate through supplementation of the dam before birth [45].

In addition to the benefits to livestock and human health in terms of a reduction in colonization and shedding of pathogenic microbes, probiotics have also found a niche in the livestock market because of their added benefit of enhanced production performance. Because there are currently no economic incentives to implement food safety interventions in live animals, interventions should be able to "pay for themselves" by improving animal growth or production efficiency. Many studies report the beneficial effects of DFMs on production efficiency in cattle [9,46,47], swine [48], and poultry. The supplementation of feedlot cattle with a combination of *Lactobacillus acidophilus* NP45/NP51 and *Propionibacterium freudenreichii* NP24 resulted in an increase in the graded fat thickness of the animals at slaughter [9], indicative of improved gain and efficiency. The use of *Enterococcus faecium* in feedlot cattle was able to increase the energetic efficiency of the rumen by increasing the proportion of propionate (a glucogenic volatile fatty acid) produced through ruminal fermentation, but all other digestive and production traits were not altered although fecal coliform shedding was increased, potentially due to colonic acidification [46]. Feeding multiparous dairy cows a combination of *Saccharomyces cerevisiae* (Diamond V-XP, Diamond V, Cedar Rapids, IA) and *Propionibacterium* spp. P169 resulted in an increase in fat-corrected milk yield, percent lactose, and weight gain postpartum [47]. When nursery piglets were supplemented with a combination of *Bacillus subtilis* and *Bacillus amyloliquefaciens*, their average daily gain increased and gain-to-feed ratios decreased [48]. However, because the focus of this publication is on human health, the beneficial effects of probiotics on animal production will be disregarded in this review, although it is important to understand that the economic benefits may indeed pay for the inclusion of a food safety enhancement.

Product	Species	Effective against	Reported results	Source
Bacillus spp.	Broilers	*Campylobacter jejuni*	1 to 3 log reduction intracloacally	[17]
		Samonella Typhimurium[21]	Percentage reduction in the crop and ceca	[55]
B. subtilis	Swine	*Clostridium perfringens* *Escherichia coli*	Increased litter survival, weaning weights and *Lactobacillus* populations	[50]
Biofeed™ (*Bifidobacterium longhum, B. thermophylum, Lactobacillus acidophilus* and *Streptococcus faecium*)	Swine	- - -	Reduced pathogen load and incidence of diarrhea	[1]
Bovamine™ (*L. acidophilus* and *Propionibacterium freudenreichii*)	Beef cattle	*Escherichia coli*	Reduces populations of O157:H7	[1]
Enterococcus faecium	Swine	Swine influenza A	Up to 4 log reduction in virus titers	[59]

Product	Species	Effective against	Reported results	Source
			Enhancement in nitric oxide production	
Lactic acid bacteria	Cattle	Escherichia coli *Samonella* Typhimurium	High efficacy in reduction by two isolates Moderate efficacy by 12 isolates	[49]
L. acidophilus NPC 747	Cattle	*Escherichia coli*	49% reduction in fecal shedding	[45]
L. crispatus	Cattle (*in vitro*)	*Escherichia coli*	Reduction on agar spot plates, no antibiotic resistance, and survival in manure and rumen fluid	[46]
LiveBac^{TM}	Dairy cattle	-	Pathogenic protection agent	[1]
Pedicoccus acidilactici	Cattle (*in vitro*)	*Escherichia coli*	Effective inhibition on agar spots	[46]
Spiromac-C^{TM} (*Bacillus, Cellulomonas, Lactobacillus, Saccharomyces cerevisiae* and *Spirulina*)	Cattle	- - -	Reduced disease incidence	[1]

Table 1. Experimental results reported for selected probiotics for use in control of pathogenic bacteria in livestock species.

3.1. Cattle

In an evaluation of multiple potential candidates as probiotics for use in beef cattle, Brashears et al. [49] found several viable isolates from small and large intestinal and fecal samples *in vitro*, all of the lactic acid bacteria (LAB) family. Twenty-seven of the 86 isolates exhibited greater than 50% survival after 3 hours at pH 3; of these, 8 isolates that could withstand 3 hours in a bile solution with greater than or equal to 60% survival were identified [49]. Finally, LAB S7 and F30 had a high level of efficacy against *E. coli* ATCC 25923 and 80% of the isolates used in bile testing had moderate efficacy in *Salmonella* Typhimurium activity. When feedlot cattle were administered a combination of *L. acidophilus* NP51 and *P. freudenreichii* NP24, fecal shedding of *E. coli* O157 was reduced 1 week prior to and on the day of shipment to the abattoir [9]. However, the trend shifted in terms of hide contamination in which the highest reduction in pathogen incidence was found when a high concentration of *L. acidophilus* NP45 was added to the previously mentioned microbial cocktail [9].

The dietary addition of the DFM *L. acidophilus* NPC 747 reduced shedding of *E. coli* O157:H7 in feedlot cattle [50]. While this trend was observed in the feedlot, fecal shedding was not found to be different at the time of slaughter, mainly due to the overall shedding level to which the animals had been reduced (1.47% of treated animals). A decrease in shedding prevalence in the feedlot, however, was seen as a significant benefit given that the pathogen load at abattoir entry was highly reduced and the subsequent opportunity for contamination by transfer of *E. coli* O157:H7 from hides (1.66% infection) or the environment (in both the feedlot and the abattoir) was therefore not as great [50].

Brashears et al. [51] conducted a systematic review and meta-analysis of studies in which DFMs were used in the suppression of verotoxin-producing or Shiga toxin-producing *E. coli* O157. Their study found that there was an odds ratio of 0.46 (0.46 times as likely to exhibit presence) for the efficacy of DFMs on the suppression of *E. coli* O157 at the conclusion of an experiment, with over 50% of the variability in efficacy coming from the heterogeneity in experiments [51]. When looking at the combination effect of DFMs NP51 and NP24, there was an odds ratio of 0.43, with 58% of the variability due to heterogeneity. This effect somewhat changed, however, when the evaluation was made throughout the individual trial [51]. In this instance, the efficacy of DFMs exhibited an odds ratio of 0.55.

In an effort to isolate and identify LAB for *E. coli* control in cattle, Nurmi et al. [52] were able to identify several microbes with the characteristics necessary for introduction as probiotics. *Pediococcus acidilactici* was identified as having the most control of *E. coli* O157:H7 *in vitro*, exhibiting 129% of the spot plate inhibition of *L. acidophilus* [52]. However, *P. acidilactici* was shown to be resistant to common antibiotics and therefore dropped from the final selection of potential candidate organisms. Based on its lack of antibiotic resistance, effective inhibition of *E. coli*, and survival and efficacy in both manure and rumen fluid, *Lactobacillus crispatus* was recommended for further work as a probiotic for cattle feed inclusion to reduce *E. coli* O157:H7 [52].

3.2. Poultry

Competitive exclusion has its origins in poultry production. Following a severe *Salmonella* outbreak in Finland in 1971, researchers began administering obligate anaerobes to populate the gut of poultry, albeit with little success [44]. However, when natural microflora were taken from adult poultry and administered to newly hatched chicks, the results gave rise to the concept of CE (also known at that time as the Nurmi concept) by early population of intestinal microflora [53]. Stemming from this, most probiotic research studies dealing with CE have taken place in the poultry industry [54], given that poultry production is riddled with concerns surrounding *Salmonella* and *Campylobacter*, the production setting lends itself to immediate inoculation of naive hatchlings, and poultry have a very short growth phase (approximately 42 days from hatch to processing) [1].

The efficacy of probiotics is impacted by the ability of bacteria or isolates to pass through the harsh conditions of the gastric stomach (or proventriculus) to make it to the lower intestine, where conditions are favorable for microbial growth. In an investigation of the administration of *Bacillus* spp. isolated from broiler ceca, oral administration was only able to reduce *C. jejuni* populations in the cecum by 1 log in 1 of 10 instances, whereas intracloacal administration reduced *C. jejuni* populations by 1 to 3 $\log_{10}$ [17]. This was attributed to the inability of the *Bacillus* spp. to survive the conditions of the proventriculus for colonization of the lower gut. It should be noted that this is not a practical route of administration in a commercial setting and thus only demonstrates a need for probiotic survival to demonstrate proof of concept for product efficacy. The results of this trial are supported by the work of Arsi et al. [18], who reported that certain isolates of *Bacillus* spp. and *Lactobacillus* spp. reduced *Campylobacter* colonization *in vitro* by 1 to 2 log. However, when tested *in vivo*, these same isolates were ineffective in reducing *Campylobacter* populations, demonstrating the inconsistency of probiotic intervention with pathogen colonization of poultry [18]. However, an *in vitro* evaluation of *Bacillus* spp. isolates revealed that three strains (AM 0902, AM1109A, and B2) were able to tolerate pH 2 for up to 4 hours, with an additional two strains (NP122 and RW41) able to tolerate this pH for up to 2 hours, indicating a potential to survive the proventriculus [55]. It was further deduced that NP122 could reduce *Salmonella* Typhimurium concentrations in the crop by 16% and in the ceca by 50%, with AM1109A/B exhibiting a slight reduction in both locations in young broilers [55].

3.3. Swine

While most research studies are directed toward establishing an innate microbial population in neonatal livestock, other work has shown positive results with administration of DFMs to mature animals. *Bacillus* species are Gram-positive bacteria that, in the spore stage, are resistant to acidic conditions (due to the enhanced spore coat that protects the bacteria through the stomach [56]) and have been shown to reduce pathogenic clostridial strains, such as *C. difficile* and *C. perfringens* [45,57]. When *B. subtilis* was administered to mature sows, nursing piglets at 3 days of age were shown to have increased ileal concentrations and piglets at 10 days of age were shown to have increased colonic concentrations of *Lactobacillus gasseri* or *Lactobacillus johnsonii* as well as decreased incidence of *E. coli* and *C. perfringens* [57]. These benefits were linked to a decrease in pathogen shedding in the sows and a more rapid gastrointestinal colonization of commensal bacteria in piglets. A preliminary study demonstrated that when piglets were treated with a porcine-derived bacterial culture at farrowing and weaning, they exhibited decreased *Salmonella* serovar Choleraesuis shedding from 65% to 70% postweaning as well as decreased colonization in both the colon and the cecum [58].

Enterococcus faecium NCIMB 10415 is a recognized probiotic approved by the European Union and has been evaluated for its efficacy in reducing swine influenza virus (SwIV), specifically H1N1 and H3N2 [59]. *E. faecium* was shown to increase cell survivability (40-80%) and reduce viral titers (up to 4 log) of both SwIV strains in two media [59]. In this publication, it was hypothesized and demonstrated that *E. faecium* operates through the adsorption of viral particles as well as the stimulation of nitric oxide production, which in itself has antiviral properties.

The link between livestock production and human health exists not only in their direct relationship through the food chain but also in the coexistence of the species in close proximity to human housing. Puphan et al. [48] reported a reduction in fecal ammonia and hydrogen sulfide, both highly noxious gases, from swine that were supplemented orally with a combination of *B. subtilis* and *B. amyloliquefaciens*. Furthermore, when a combination of *B. subtilis* and *Bacillus licheniformis* was administered to growing pigs, manure from the pens dispersed more quickly, meaning that pens could be cleaned and manure solubilized more quickly for a less noxious waste product [60]. These data indicate that a positive impact on humans that goes far beyond the direct health/non-health dichotomy can be mediated by probiotics.

4. Prebiotics

Prebiotic treatment involves the inclusion of non-host-digestible compounds (often oligosaccharides) in diets to provide a competitive advantage to a segment of the microbial population. Unfortunately, prebiotics have previously not been a common adjunct in livestock production settings, largely due to their cost and the narrow profit margins associated with agricultural production. The use of prebiotics is most often seen coupled with a complementary probiotic (often described as "synbiotics"), and recent research has demonstrated the benefits that may exist with the coordinated use of such a complementary intervention. A list of the prebiotics identified for pathogen reduction in the literature is presented in **Table 2**.

Product	Species	Effective against	Reported results	Source
Avigaurd™ (freeze-dried extract from healthy poultry)	poultry	*Clostridium* *Escherichia coli* *Salmonella*	- - -	[1]
Chitosan	broilers	*Campylobacter jejuni*	1 log reduction with 0.5% *in vitro* and *in vivo*	[16]
FOS	broilers	*Escherichia coli* *Clostridium perfringens*	B cell reduction; increased IgM and IgG titers >Reduced population Reduced population	[7] [8]
Mannan-oligosaccharides (MOS)	broilers	*Escherichia coli* *Clostridium perfringens*	Reduced population Reduced population	[8]
Tasco-14/EX® (brown seaweed; *Ascophyllum nodosum*)	cattle	*Escherichia coli* *Salmonella*	79% reduction in fecal O157:H7 Reduction in shedding	[58] [53]

Table 2. Experimental results reported for selected prebiotics for use in control of pathogenic bacteria in livestock species.

As previously discussed, *Campylobacter* is among the leading foodborne pathogenic bacteria found in livestock and the majority of bacteria are introduced into the human food chain via poultry [16,17]. In an evaluation of *Campylobacter* colonization in hatchling chicks, chitosan (a compound from the chitinous shells of crabs and shrimp) was shown to reduce the population of *C. jejuni* both *in vitro* and *in vivo* when added to the feed [16]. This reduction of colonization was attributed to a down-regulation of *fliA*, *motA*, *motB*, and *CadF* genes, which are all involved in the synthesis and function of the flagella used in cellular function and movement [16].

Fructooligosaccharides (FOSs) and mannan-oligosaccharides (MOSs) have been evaluated for oral administration in broiler chickens in hopes of reducing the colonization of *C. jejuni* [7,8,18]. When used in isolation, neither of these substances was effective in reducing pathogen colonization in broiler chicks. However, the synergistic combination of *Bacillus* spp., *Lactobacillus* spp., and MOSs reduced *Campylobacter* colonization. As an added benefit, FOSs were demonstrated to induce weight gain in broiler chicks both alone and in combination with probiotics [18]. This is in contrast to the work of Janardhana et al. [7] and Kim et al. [8], with both groups having examined FOSs and MOSs for prebiotic addition to the feed of broiler chicks. The dietary addition of FOSs has been shown to reduce B cells and increase IgM and IgG titers in broiler chicks, both indicators of an enhancement of gastrointestinal immune function [7]. Likewise, FOSs were shown to decrease the incidence of *C. perfringens* and *E. coli* at 0.25% inclusion as well as bolster the population of *Lactobacillus* spp. [8]. This same reduction in *C. perfringens* and *E. coli* was achieved with 0.05% inclusion of MOSs [8].

Essential oils and polyphenolics have also been tested in relation to the reduction of pathogen spread from livestock [61]. Noted essential oil components that have been tested include carvacrol (from savory), curcumin (from turmeric), eugenol (from allspice, betel pepper, and cloves), piperin (from black pepper), and thymol (from thyme) [35,62]. Fecal shedding of *C. perfringens* was reduced up to 30 days following supplementation with two essential oil blends [35]. Intestinal concentrations of *C. perfringens* were reduced for up to 21 days with essential oil administration, but this effect was negated by day 30 [35]. Tedeschi et al. [63] demonstrated that purified coumaric and cinnamic acids, both components of lignin, were able to reduce *E. coli* survival by 10- to 20-fold when mixed with feces, although diets containing forage rich in such compounds had no such effect. Berard et al. [62] also noted that catechol and pyrogallol (hydroxylated phenols) have toxic effects in the presence of microorganisms, mainly through substrate deprivation. Callaway et al. [64] discussed the concept that saponins (natural plant-based detergents) may have an antimicrobial effect by binding cholesterol, thereby disrupting the microbial membrane, in addition to tannins, which may act in substrate deprivation by binding protein and essential cations. Orange peel, a source of essential oils in the citrus family, has been shown to reduce cecal and rectal populations of *E. coli* O157:H7 with 5% and 10% dietary inclusion in sheep 96 hours following inoculation, but fecal shedding was only reduced at 10% inclusion [65]. Inclusion of orange peel at 10% of the diet was also shown to reduce *Salmonella* populations, although diet palatability issues were detected in excess of 10% inclusion [66].

Brown seaweed (*Ascophyllum nodosum*) is another prebiotic additive that has been noted for both its production and antimicrobial characteristics [61,67]. The use of Tasco-14® increased the marbling in carcasses from supplemented animals [67] and reduced fecal shedding of *E. coli* O157:H7 from 34% of the population to 7% of the population with supplementation [68], but there was no effect in *Salmonella*. However, unpublished data from the Callaway laboratory at USDA-ARS in College Station, Texas, demonstrate a small reduction in both *E. coli* O157:H7 and *Salmonella* populations *in vitro*.

5. Conclusions

The gastrointestinal tracts of humans and animals are living ecosystems teeming with diversity, and harnessing that ecology is a vital step toward a full understanding and appreciation of both livestock and human health. As was stated in the beginning, an understanding of the human-animal interface is crucial to the homogeny of food safety protocols and health concerns. While most prebiotic and probiotic innovations in livestock production have sought to increase performance characteristics for maximization of potential, these ventures have often led to the discovery of novel avenues in the improvement of food safety. These new approaches to health and safety come at a crucial time when governmental regulation and public scrutiny necessitate an alteration in current practices in animal health and management. It is through the use of novel and innovative techniques that we will enhance our knowledge of the ecosystem in which we live and will forge new paths in scientific discovery and healthy living.

Author details

William B. Smith[1], Todd R. Callaway[2*], Luis O. Tedeschi[3], Francis M. Rouquette Jr.[1], Trisha Sheridan[4] and Jennifer Adamski[4]

*Address all correspondence to: todd.callaway@ars.usda.gov

1 Department of Soil and Crop Sciences, Texas A&M AgriLife Research, Overton, TX, USA

2 Food and Feed Safety Research Unit, Southern Plains Agricultural Center, Agricultural Research Service, USDA, College Station, TX, USA

3 Department of Animal Science, Texas A&M University, College Station, TX, USA

4 Nell Hodgson Woodruff School of Nursing, Emory University, Atlanta, GA, USA

References

[1] Callaway T.R., Edrington T.S., Anderson R.C., Harvey R.B., Genovese K.J., Kennedy C.N., et al. Probiotics, prebiotics and competitive exclusion for prophylaxis against bacterial disease. Animal Health Research and Reviews. 2008;9:217-225.

[2] Hungate R.E. The Rumen and Its Microbes. New York, NY: Academic Press; 1966. 533 pp.

[3] Lu J., Idris U., Harmon B., Hofacre C., Maurer J.J., Lee M.D. Diversity and succession of the intestinal bacterial community of the maturing broiler chicken. Applied and Environmental Microbiology. 2003;69:6816-6824.

[4] Arthur T.M., Bosilevac J.M., Nou X., Shackelford S.D., Wheeler T.L., Koohmaraie M. Comparison of the molecular genotypes of *Escherichia coli* O157:H7 for the hides of beef

cattle in different regions of North America. Journal of Food Protection. 2007;70(7): 1622-1626.

[5] Elder R.O., Keen J.E., Siragusa G.R., Barkocy-Gallagher G.A., Koohmarie M., Lagreid W.W. Correlation of enterohemorrhagic *Escherichia coli* O157:H7 prevalence in feces, hides, and carcasses of beef cattle during processing. Proceedings of the National Academy of Science (USA). 2000;97(7):2999-3003.

[6] Sargeant J.M., Amezcua M.R., Rajic A., Waddell L. Pre-harvest interventions to reduce the shedding of *E. coli* O157 in the faeces of weaned domestic ruminants: A systematic review. Zoonoses and Public Health. 2007;54:260-277.

[7] Janardhana V., Broadway M.M., Bruce M.P., Lowenthal J.W., Geier M.S., Hughes R.J., et al. Prebiotics modulate immune responses in the gut-associated lymphoid tissue of chickens. Journal of Nutrition. 2009;139:1404-1409.

[8] Kim G.-B., Seo Y.M., Kim C.H., Paik I.K. Effect of dietary prebiotic supplementation on the performance, intestinal microflora, and immune response of broilers. Poultry Science. 2011;90:75-82.

[9] Elam N.A., Gleghorn J.F., Rivera J.D., Galyean M.L., Defoor P.J., Brashears M.M., et al. Effects of live cultures of *Lactobacillus acidophilus* (strains NP45 and NP51) and *Propionibacterium freudenreichii* on performance, carcass, and intestinal characteristics, and *Escherichia coli* strain O157 shedding of finishing beef steers. Journal of Animal Science. 2003;81:2686-2698.

[10] Callaway T.R., Edrington T.S., Anderson R.C., Byrd J.A., Kogut M.H., Harvey R.B., et al. Using antimicrobial cultures, bacteriocins and bacteriophages to reduce carriage of foodborne pathogens in cattle and swine. In: LaCroix C., editor. Protective Cultures, Antimicrobial Metabolites and Bacteriophages for Food and Beverage Biopreservation. Oxford, UK: Woodhead Publishing; 2011. pp. 204-224.

[11] Callaway T.R., Edrington T.S., Loneragan G.H., Carr M.A., Nisbet D.J. Current and near-market intervention strategies for reducing Shiga-toxin producing *Escherichia coli* (STEC) shedding in cattle. Agriculture, Food and Analytical Bacteriology. 2013;3:103-120.

[12] Callaway T.R., Anderson R.C., Edrington T.S., Genovese K.J., Harvey R.B., Poole T.L., et al. Novel methods for pathogen control in livestock preharvest: An update. In: Sofos J.N., editor. Advances in Microbial Food Safety. Oxford, UK: Woodhead Publishing; 2013. pp. 275-304.

[13] Callaway, T.R., Edrington T.S., Nisbet D.J. Ecological and dietary impactors of food-borne pathogen prevalence and methods to reduce colonization in cattle. Journal of Animal Science. 2014;92:7308-7342.

[14] Steer T., Carpenter H., Tuohy K., Gibson G.R. Perspective on the role of the human gut microbiota and its modulation by pro- and prebiotics. Nutrition Research Reviews. 2000;13(2):229-254. DOI: 10.1079/095442200108729089

[15] Collins D.M., Gibson G.R. Probiotics, prebiotics, and synbiotics: Approaches for modulating the microbial ecology of the gut. American Journal of Clinical Nutrition. 1999;69:1052S-1057S.

[16] Arambel H.R., Donoghue A.M., Arsi K., Upadhyay A., Woo-Ming A., Blore P.J., et al. Chitosan supplementation reduces enteric colonization of *Campylobacter jejuni* in broiler chickens and down-regulates expression of colonization genes. Advances in Food Technology and Nutritional Sciences Open Journal. 2015;1(5):104-111.

[17] Arsi K., Donoghue A.M., Woo-Ming A., Blore P.J., Donoghue D.J. Intercloacal inoculation, an effective screening method for determining the efficacy of probiotic bacterial isolates against *Campylobacter* colonization in broiler chickens. Journal of Food Protection. 2015;78(1):209-213. DOI: 10.4315/0362-028X.JFP-14-326

[18] Arsi K., Donoghue A.M., Woo-Ming A., Blore P.J., Donoghue D.J. The efficacy of selected probiotic and prebiotic combinations in reducing *Campylobacter* colonization in broiler chickens. Journal of Applied Poultry Science. 2005;pfv032. DOI: 10.3382/japr/pfv032

[19] Doyle M.P., Erickson M.C. Reducing the carriage of foodborne pathogens in livestock and poultry. Poultry Science. 2006;85:960-973.

[20] Kemp R., Leatherbarrow A.J.H., Williams N.J., Hart C.A., Clough H.E., Turner J., et al. Prevalence and genetic diversity of *Campylobacter* spp. in environmental water samples from a 100-square-kilometer predominately dairy farming area. Applied and Environmental Microbiology. 2005;71(4):1876-1882. DOI: 10.1128/AEM.71.4.1876-1882.2005

[21] Riley L.W., Remis R.S., Helgerson S.D., McGee H.B., Wells J.G., Davis B.R. Hemorrhagic colitis associated with a rare *Escherichia coli* serotype. The New England Journal of Medicine. 1983;308(12):681-685.

[22] Bell B.P., Goldoft M., Griffin P.M., Davis M.A., Gordon D.C., Tarr P.I., et al. A multistate outbreak of *Escherichia coli* O157:H7 — Associated bloody diarrhea and hemolytic uremic syndrome from hamburgers: The Washington experience. Journal of the American Medical Association. 1994;272(17):1349-1353.

[23] Tuttle J., Gomez T., Doyle M.P., Wells J.G., Zhao T., Tauxe R.V., et al. Lessons from a large outbreak of *Escherichia coli* O157:H7 infections: Insights into the infectious dose and method of widespread contamination of hamburger patties. Epidemiology and Infection. 1999;122:185-192.

[24] LeJeune J.T., Besser T.E., Hancock D.D. Cattle water troughs as reservoirs of *Escherichia coli* O157. Applied and Environmental Microbiology. 2001;67(7):3053-3057. DOI: 10.1128/AEM.67.7.3053-3057.2001

[25] Nou, X., Rivera-Betancourt M., Bosilevac J.M., Wheeler T.L., Shackelford S.D., Gwartney B.L., et al. Effect of chemical dehairing on the prevalence of *Escherichia coli* O157:H7 and the levels of aerobic bacteria and Enterobacteriaceae on carcasses in a commercial beef processing plant. Journal of Food Protection. 2003;66(11):2005-2009.

[26] FSIS. FSIS Policy on Non-intact Raw Beef Products Contaminated with E. coli O157:H7 [Internet]. January 1999 [Updated: 17 February 1999]. Available from: http://www.fsis.usda.gov/Oa/background/O157policy.htm [Accessed: 28 April 2016]

[27] USDA/FSIS. Shiga toxin-producing *Escherichia coli* in certain raw beef products. In: FSIS, editor. Federal Register. 2012.

[28] Genovese K.J., Anderson R.C., Harvey R.B., Callaway T.R., Poole D.H., Edrington T.S., et al. Competitive exclusion of *Salmonella* from the gut of neonatal and weaned pigs. Journal of Food Protection. 2003;66(8):1353-1359.

[29] Popoff M.Y., Bockemuhl J., Gheesling L.L. Supplement 2002 (no. 46) to the Kauffman-White scheme. Research in Microbiology. 2004;155:568-570.

[30] Olsen S.J., MacKinon L.C., Goulding J.S., Bean N.H., Slutsker L. Surveillance for foodborne disease outbreak — United States, 1993-1997. Morbidity and Mortality Weekly Report. 2000;49(SS01):1-51.

[31] Gould, L.H., Walsh K.A., Vieira A.R., Herman K., Williams I.T., Hall A.J., et al. Surveillance for foodborne disease outbreaks — United States, 1998-2008. Morbidity and Mortality Weekly Report. 2013;62(SS02):1-34.

[32] Antunes P., Reu C., Sousa J.C., Peixe L., Pestana N. Incidence of *Salmonella* from poultry products and their susceptibility to antimicrobial agents. International Journal of Food Microbiology. 2003;82(2):97-103. DOI: 10.1016/S0168-1605(02)00251-9

[33] CDC. Severe *Clostridium difficile*-associated disease in populations previously at low risk — Four states, 2005. Morbidity and Mortality Weekly Report. 2005;54(47): 1201-1205.

[34] Weese J.S., Avery B.P., Rousseau J., Reid-Smith R. Detection and enumeration of *Clostridium difficile* spores in retail beef and pork. Applied and Environmental Microbiology. 2009;75(15):5009-5011. DOI: 10.1128/AEM.00480-09

[35] Mitsch P., Zitterl-Eglseer K., Kohler B., Gabler C., Losa R., Zimpernik I. The effect of two different blends of essential oil components on the proliferation of *Clostridium perfringens* in the intestines of broiler chickens. Poultry Science. 2004;83(4):669-675. DOI: 10.1093/pa/83.4.669

[36] CDC. Multistate outbreak of listeriosis linked to Blue Bell Creameries products (final update) [Internet]. [Updated: 10 June 2015]. Available from http://www.cdc.gov/listeria/outbreaks/ice-cream-03-15/ [Accessed: 31 January 2016]

[37] Farber J. M., Peterkin P.I. *Listeria monocytogenes*, a food-borne pathogen. Microbiology and Molecular Biology Review. 1991;55(3):476-511.

[38] Skovgaard N., Morgen C.-A. Detection of *Listeria* spp. in faeces from animals, in feeds, and in raw foods of animal origin. International Journal of Food Microbiology. 1988;6(3):229-242. DOI: 10.1046/0168-1605(88)90015-3

[39] Deiters C., Gunnewig V., Friedrich A.W., Mellmann A., Kock R. Are cases of methicillin-resistant *Staphylococcus aureus* clonal complex (CC) 398 among humans still livestock-associated? International Journal of Medical Microbiology. 2015;305:110-113.

[40] Hasman H., Moodley A., Guardabassi L., Stegger M., Skov R.L., Aarestrup F.M. *spa* type distribution in *Staphylococcus aureus* originating from pigs, cattle and poultry. Veterinary Microbiology. 2010;141(3-4):326-331. DOI: 10.1016/j.vetmic.2009.09.025

[41] Barkema H.W., Schukken Y.H., Zadoks R.N. Invited review: The role of cow, pathogen, and treatment regimen in the therapeutic success of bovine *Staphylococcus aureus* mastitis. Journal of Dairy Science. 2006;89(6):1877-1895. DOI: 10.3168/jds.S0022-0302(06)72256-1

[42] Fuller R. Probiotics in man and animals. Journal of Applied Bacteriology. 1989;66:365-378.

[43] Bielke L.R., Elwood A.L., Donoghue A.M., Newberry L.A., Neighbor N.K., Hargis B.M. Approach for selection of individual enteric bacteria for competitive exclusion in turkey poults. Poultry Science. 2003;82:1378-1382.

[44] Nurmi E., Rantala M. New aspects of *Salmonella* infection in broiler production. Nature. 1973;241:210-211.

[45] Baker A.A., Davis E., Rehberger T., Rosener D. Prevalence and diversity of toxigenic *Clostridium perfringens* and *Clostridium difficile* among swine herds in the Midwest. Applied and Environmental Microbiology. 2010;76:2961-2967.

[46] Beauchemin K.A., Yang W.Z., Morgavi D.P., Ghorbani G.R., Kautz W., Leedle J.A.Z. Effects of bacterial direct-fed microbials and yeast on site and extent of digestion, blood chemistry, and subclinical ruminal acidosis in feedlot cattle. Journal of Animal Science. 2003;81:1628-1640.

[47] Lehloenya K.V., Stein D.R., Allen D.T., Selk G.E., Jones D.A., Aleman M.M., et al. Effects of feeding yeast and propionibacteria to dairy cows on milk yield and components, and reproduction. Journal of Animal Physiology and Animal Nutrition. 2007;92:190-202. DOI: 10.1111/j.1439-0396.2007.00726.x

[48] Cai L., Indrakumar S., Kiarie E., Kim I.H. Effects of a multi-strain *Bacillus* species-based direct-fed microbial on growth performance, nutrient digestibility, blood profile, and gut health in nursery pigs fed corn-soybean meal-based diets. Journal of Animal Science. 2015;93:4336-4342. DOI: 10.2527/jas2015-9056

[49] Puphan K., Sornplang P., Uriyapongson S., Navanukraw C. Screening of lactic acid bacteria as potential probiotics in beef cattle. Pakistan Journal of Nutrition. 2015;14(8): 474-479.

[50] Brashears M.M., Galyean M.L., Loneragan G.H., Mann J.E., Killinger-Mann K. Prevalence of *Escherichia coli* O157:H7 and performance by beef feedlot cattle given *Lactobacillus* direct-fed microbials. Journal of Food Protection. 2003;66:748-754.

[51] Wisener L.V., Sargeant J.M., O'Connor A.M., Faires M.C., Glass-Kaastra S.K. The use of direct-fed microbials to reduce shedding of *Escherichia coli* O157 in beef cattle: A systematic review and meta-analysis. Zoonoses and Public Health. 2014;62:75-89. DOI: 10.1111/zph.12112

[52] Brashears M.M., Jaroni D., Trimble J. Isolation, selection, and characterization of lactic acid bacteria for a competitive exclusion product to reduce shedding of *Escherichia coli* O157:H7 in cattle. Journal of Food Protection. 2003;66(3):355-363.

[53] Nurmi E., Nuotio L., Schneitz C. The competitive exclusion concept: Development and future. International Journal of Food Microbiology. 1992;15(3-4):237-240. DOI: 10.1016/0168-1605(92)90054-7

[54] Nava G.M., Bielke L.R., Callaway T.R., Castaneda M.P. Probiotic alternatives to reduce gastrointestinal infections: The poultry experience. Animal Health Research Reviews. 2005;6(1):105-118. DOI: 10.1079/AHR2005103

[55] Menconi A., Morgan M.J., Pumford N.R., Hargis B.M., Tellez G. Physiological properties and *Salmonella* growth inhibition of probiotic *Bacillus* strains isolated from environmental and poultry sources. International Journal of Bacteriology. 2013;958408:1-8. DOI: http://dx.doi.org/10.1155/2013/958408

[56] Hong H.A., Duc L.H., Cutting S.M. The use of bacterial spore formers as probiotics. FEMS Microbiology Review. 2005;29:813-835.

[57] Baker A.A., Davis E., Spencer J.D., Moser R., Rehberger T. The effect of a *Bacillus*-based direct-fed microbial supplemented to sows on the gastrointestinal microbiota of their neonatal piglets. Journal of Animal Science. 2013;91:3390-3399. DOI: 10.2527/jas2012-5821

[58] Anderson R.C., Stanker L.H., Young C.R., Buckley S.A., Genovese K.J., Harvey R.B., et al. Effect of competitive exclusion treatment on colonization of early-weaned pigs by *Salmonella* serovar Choleraesuis. Swine Health and Production. 1999;7(4):155-160.

[59] Wang Z., Chai W., Burwinkel M., Twardziok S., Wrede P., Palissa C., et al. Inhibitory influence of *Enterococcus faecium* on the propagation of Swine Influenza A virus *in vitro*. PLoS One. 2013;8(1):e54043. DOI: 10.1371/journal.pone.0053043

[60] Davis M.E., Parrott T., Brown D.C., de Rodas B.Z., Johnson Z.B., Maxwell C.V., et al. Effect of a *Bacillus*-based direct-fed microbial feed supplement on growth performance

and pen cleaning characteristics of growing-finishing pigs. Journal of Animal Science. 2008;86:1459-1467. DOI: 10.2527/jas.2007-0603

[61] Crossland W.L., Callaway T.R., Tedeschi L.O. Shiga toxin-producing *E. coli* and ruminant diets: A match made in heaven? In: Ricke S.C., Donaldson J.R., Phillips C.A, editors. Food safety: Emerging issues, technologies and systems. London, UK: Elsevier; 2015. pp. 185-213.

[62] Cowan M.M. Plant products as antimicrobial agents. Clinical Microbiological Reviews. 1999;12(4):564-582. DOI: 0893-8512/99/$04.00+0

[63] Berard N.C., Holley R.A., McAllister T.A., Ominski K.H., Wittenberg K.M., Bouchard K.S., et al. Potential to reduce *Escherichia coli* shedding in cattle feces by using sainfoin (*Onobrychis viciifolia*) forage, tested in vitro and in vivo. Applied and Environmental Microbiology. 2009;75(4):1074-1079. DOI: 10.1128/AEM.00983-08

[64] Tedeschi L.O., Callaway T.R., Muir J.P., Anderson R.C. Potential environmental benefits of feed additives and other strategies for ruminant production. Revista Brasileira de Zootecnia. 2011;40:291-309.

[65] Callaway T.R., Carroll J.A., Arthington J.D., Edrington T.S., Rossman M.L., Carr M.A., et al. *Escherichia coli* O157:H7 populations in ruminants can be reduced by orange peel product feeding. Journal of Food Protection. 2011;74(11):1917-1921.

[66] Callaway T.R., Carroll J.A., Arthington J.D., Edrington T.S., Anderson R.C., Rossman M.L., et al. Orange peel products can reduce *Salmonella* populations in ruminants. Foodborne Pathogens and Disease. 2011;8(10):1071-1075.

[67] Anderson M.J., Blanton Jr. J.R., Gleghorn J., Kim S.W., Johnson J.W. *Ascophyllum nodosum* supplementation strategies that improve overall carcass merit of implanted English crossbred cattle. Asian-Australasian Journal of Animal Science. 2006;19(10): 1514-1518. DOI: 10.5713/ajas.2006.1514

[68] Braden K.W., Blanton Jr. J.R., Allen V.G., Pond K.R., Miller M.F. *Ascophyllum nodosum* supplementation: A preharvest intervention for reducing *Escherichia coli* O157:H7 and *Salmonella* spp. in feedlot steers. Journal of Food Protection. 2004;67(9):1824-1828.

Chapter 2

Probiotics: A Comprehensive Review of Their Classification, Mode of Action and Role in Human Nutrition

Amirreza Khalighi, Reza Behdani and
Shabnam Kouhestani

Additional information is available at the end of the chapter

http://dx.doi.org/10.5772/63646

Abstract

Probiotics are live microorganisms that live in gastrointestinal (GI) tract and are beneficial for their hosts and prevent certain diseases. In this chapter, after a complete introduction to probiotics, definition, mechanism of action, and their classification, currently used organisms will be discussed in detail. Moreover, different kinds of nutritional synthetic products of probiotics along with their safety and drug interaction will be noticed. This chapter mentions all clinical trial studies that have been done to evaluate probiotic efficacy with a focus on gastrointestinal diseases.

In the end, findings of our pilot study regarding the effect of probiotic on Small Intestinal Bacterial Overgrowth (SIBO) will be presented. The nutritional effects of Probiotics on a host's health will be collected and their usage criteria will be discussed. Some suggestions for the Probiotics daily consumption will be presented and the follow-up for their new adverse reaction will be emphasized, if any.

Keywords: probiotics, gastrointestinal (GI) tract, nutrition, related disorders, probiotic products

1. Introduction to probiotics

The term probiotic is derived from Greek and literally means "for life." It was first coined in 1965 by Lilley and Stillwell to describe substances secreted by one microorganism that stimulate the growth of another [1, 2]. In 1974, Parker modified this definition to "...organisms and substances which contribute to intestinal microbial balance" [1, 3]. The current definition of probiotics by Food and Agriculture Organization of the United Nations (FAO) and the World Health Organization (WHO) is "live microorganisms which when administered in adequate amounts confer a health benefit to the host" [4–6]. Probiotic organisms require certain characteristics to enable them to exert maximum therapeutic effects. Of these characteristics, there are some that are considered almost essential for a probiotic to have therapeutic effects, including gastric acid and bile salt stability, ability to adhere to the intestinal mucosa, and ability to colonize the intestinal tract [1, 7].

2. Mechanism of action

The exact mechanisms by which probiotics accomplish their beneficial actions have not been well documented. However, there are several postulated mechanisms that explain many of their favorable effects [8] (**Figure 1**).

One of such mechanisms is a competition for adhesion sites, which means probiotics fight for cellular attachments. Many pathogenic organisms must associate with the GI tract epithelium to colonize effectively [9]. However, some strains of bifidobacteria and lactobacilli can adhere to the epithelium and act as "colonization barriers" by preventing pathogens from adhering to the mucosa [1, 10]. This effect was demonstrated with the *Lactobacillus rhamnosus* strain GG and *Lactobacillus plantarum* 299v. Both of these organisms showed the ability to inhibit attachment of *Escherichia coli* to human colon cells [1, 11].

Another possible mechanism of action is the modification of the microbial flora through the synthesis of antimicrobial compounds [12]. Many types of lactobacilli and bifidobacteria produce bacteriocinsor and other antimicrobial compounds. Bacteriocins are defined as "compounds produced by bacteria that have a biologically active protein moiety and a bactericidal action" [1, 13]. Other biologically active compounds produced by lactic acid bacteria include hydrogen peroxide, diacetyl, and short-chain fatty acids. The release of these compounds by probiotic organisms results in a beneficial modification of the microflora [1, 14]. However, not all strains of lactobacilli or bifidobacteria produce antimicrobial compounds, and some produce compounds that are fairly nonspecific in their activity, so that beneficial bacteria, as well as pathogenic organisms, may be negatively affected [1].

It has also been observed that probiotics can stimulate the immune response [15]. This immune response may take the form of increased secretion of immunoglobulin-A (IgA) [1, 16], elevated numbers of natural killer cells, or enhanced phagocytic activity of macrophages [1, 17]. Increased secretion of IgA may decrease numbers of pathogenic organisms in the gut, thus improving the composition of the microflora [1, 10]. Due to these immunomodulating effects, some researchers think probiotics might not only fight intestinal and urogenital pathogens, but might also be helpful for conditions, such as inflammatory bowel disease (IBD), pouchitis, food allergy, and for use as an adjuvant to vaccination [18–22]. Probiotics may also compete for nutrients that would otherwise be utilized by pathogens [1, 23]. This situation occurs with *Clostridium difficile*, a potentially pathogenic organism that is dependent upon monosaccharides for its growth. Probiotic organisms in sufficient numbers can utilize most of the available monosaccharides, which results in the inhibition of *C. difficile* [1, 24].

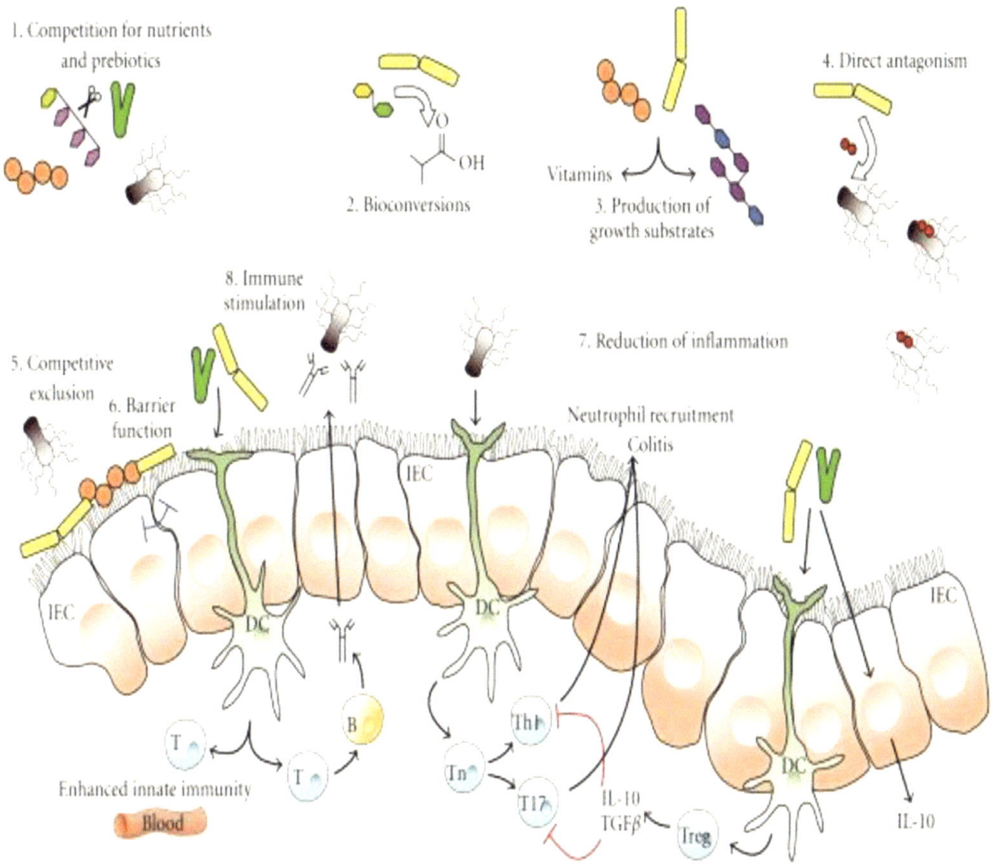

Figure 1. Schematic diagram illustrating potential or known mechanisms whereby probiotic bacteria might impact on the microbiota. These mechanisms include (1) competition for dietary ingredients as growth substrates, (2) bioconversion of, for example, sugars into fermentation products with inhibitory properties, (3) production of growth substrates, for example, EPS or vitamins, for other bacteria, (4)direct antagonism by bacteriocins, (5) competitive exclusion for binding sites, (6) improved barrier function, (7) reduction of inflammation, thus altering intestinal properties for colonization and persistence within, and (8) stimulation of innate immune response (by unknown mechanisms). IEC : intra epithelial cells, DC: dendritic cells, T:T-cells.

3. Classification

There are many different microorganisms currently used as probiotics [1, 20, 25] (**Table 1**). To better understand how bacteria are named and classified, the following discussion may be helpful. Genus is the first name of a bacterium (e.g., *Lactobacillus*). It is somewhat general and refers to a grouping of organisms based on similarity of qualities, such as physical characteristics, metabolic needs, and metabolic end products.

Species is a bacterium's second name (e.g., *acidophilus*). It is a much more narrow classification based on shared common characteristics that distinguish them from other species. Strain is an even more specific classification that divides members of the same species into subgroups based on several properties that these bacteria have in common that are distinct from other members of the species (e.g., strain LA5) [1, 26].

Lactobacillus spp.	acidophilus
	plantarum
	rhamnosus
	paracasei
	fermentum
	reuteri
	johnsonii
	brevis
	casei
	lactis
	delbrueckii gasseri
Bifidobacterium spp.	Breve
	infantis
	longum
	bifidum
	thermophilum
	adolescentis
	animalis
	lactis
Bacillus spp.	coagulans
Streptococcus spp.	thermophilus
Enterococcus spp.	faecium
Saccharomyces spp.	cerevisiae

Table 1. Common probiotic microorganisms.

3.1. Lactobacillus species

Lactobacillus refers to a group of lactic acid–producing Gram-positive rods that are obligate and facultative anaerobes in the human gastrointestinal and genitourinary tracts [27, 29–32]. The name lactobacillus refers to the bacterium's ability to produce lactic acid, not to the ability to digest lactose [28]. Lactobacilli are used therapeutically as probiotics, the opposite of antibiotics. They are considered "friendly" bacteria and are taken for the purpose of recolonizing areas of the body to provide nutritional benefits including inducing growth factors and increasing the bioavailability of minerals [32]. Lactobacilli also stabilize the mucosal barrier and decrease intestinal permeability [33].

Altering the normal flora allows for potential colonization by pathogenic organisms [34], which can result in side effects, such as diarrhea, cramping, and less commonly pseudomembranous colitis (PMC), caused by *C. difficile*. The theory is that taking lactobacillus probiotics during antibiotic treatment can prevent or minimize normal flora depletion and pathogenic bacteria colonization. There is some evidence to support this theory [35, 36]. Hydrogen peroxide–producing lactobacilli are bactericidal to the vaginal pathogen *Gardnerella vaginalis*, and their presence in the vagina has been associated with decreased frequencies of bacterial vaginosis and trichomoniasis [37]. In the vagina, lactic acid from lactobacilli lowers vaginal pH, which can prevent pathogen growth.

There is some preliminary evidence that lactobacilli and other probiotics might help protect against cancer. In animal models, lactobacillus has been shown to bind dietary carcinogens [38] and decrease development of tumors in the colon after carcinogen challenge [39, 40]. Preliminary research also suggests that lactobacilli, especially *L. plantarum*, can reduce the severity of chemotherapy-induced enterocolitis [41]. According to other research studies, *Lactobacillus bulgaricus* and *Lactobacillus sporogenes* might have hypolipidemic and antiatherosclerotic effects. Limited clinical evidence suggests that it can reduce total and low-density lipoprotein (LDL) cholesterol with no effect on high-density lipoprotein (HDL) [42, 43]. Fermented dairy products, such as yogurt and acidophilus milk, also seem to have a beneficial effect on cholesterol. Lactobacilli and other probiotic bacteria seem to bind bile acids to cholesterol. They also seem to increase fatty acid production in the intestine, which decreases circulatory fatty acid concentrations either by inhibiting hepatic cholesterol synthesis or redistributing cholesterol from the plasma to the liver.

Most researchers agree that the effectiveness of lactobacilli and other probiotics for all indications depends on their ability to colonize an area of tissue. To do this, lactobacillus preparations must contain live and viable organisms. Products stored for long periods of time or stored improperly may contain few live and active organisms. For oral preparations, bacteria must also remain viable after passing through the gut, and then they must be able to latch on to the intestinal epithelium. Lactobacilli strains might vary in their effectiveness due to differences in their ability to adhere to the epithelial cells by host factors such as hormone levels [30, 44, 45]. This ability can change during a woman's menstrual cycle in response to changing hormone levels. In postmenopausal women, correcting low estrogen levels can help restore lactobacillus colonization without supplementation [29, 30].

3.2. Bifidobacterium species

Bifidobacterium is an anaerobic, Gram-positive, nonspore-forming, pleomorphic rod. Bacteria in the *Bifidobacterium* genus produce lactic and acetic acids as by-products of glucose utilization. BB536 is a type of probiotic bacteria, which, according to secondary sources, was first isolated from the intestinal tract of healthy infants. Bifidobacteria, in combination with *Lactobacillus* species and the probiotic yeast *Saccharomyces boulardii*, seem to reduce the adverse effects of *Helicobacter therapy*, but do not seem to improve compliance [46]. In addition,

Bifidobacterium infantis in combination with *Lactobacillus acidophilus* seems to reduce the incidence of NEC and NEC-associated mortality in critically ill neonates [47].

3.3. Bacillus species

Bacillus coagulans is a Gram-positive rod, which produces lactic acid, and therefore is often misclassified as lactic acid bacteria, such as lactobacillus. In fact, some commercial products containing *B. coagulans* are marketed as *Lactobacillus sporogenes* or "spore-forming lactic acid bacterium." It forms spores, which is an important factor in differentiating these species. *B. coagulans* is used therapeutically in a similar manner as other probiotics such as lactobacillus and bifidobacterium; however, *B. coagulans* is not a component of the normal human flora. In order to be effective for restoring normal flora and prevent pathogenic colonization, probiotics must have the ability to persist and colonize in the intestinal mucosa. When the Bacillus spore is ingested by humans, it is unknown what happens to the spore. It is unknown if the Bacillus spore is capable of germinating in the intestinal tract or if colonization occurs [48].

B. coagulans might reduce pathogenic bacteria colonization through several mechanisms. *B. coagulans* produces coagulin and lactic acid, which have antibacterial activity and might reduce pathogenic bacteria growth through this mechanism [29, 49, 50]. Animal model research also suggests that ingesting bacillus spores increases immune response [48]. Proponents of *B. coagulans* suggest that this species of probiotics offers advantages over others such as lactobacillus because Bacillus species can be stored indefinitely in desiccated forms [48]. Bacillus spores are also resistant to high temperatures and to acid.

3.4. *Saccharomyces* spp.

S. boulardii, also known as *Saccharomyces cerevisiae*, is a nonpathogenic yeast strain that has been used for the treatment and prevention of diarrhea resulting from multiple etiologies. *S. boulardii* has been isolated from the skins of tropical fruits found in Indochina. The indigenous population of Indochina has long used these fruit skins to prevent and treat diarrhea [51].

S. boulardii is prepared by lyophylization (freeze drying) of live yeast organisms and encapsulation using lactose in the preparation. *S. boulardii* cannot be distinguished from other *S. cerevisiae* strains by phenotypic criteria, so identification of these infections requires molecular typing. Comparative molecular studies show that *S. boulardii* is genetically very close or nearly identical to *S. cerevisiae* [52]. Results suggest that microsatellite polymorphism analysis of the YKL139w and YLR177w genes and the analysis by Ty917 hybridization are the most useful tools for the correct identification of *S. boulardii* strains [53]. However, metabolically and physiologically, *S. boulardii* shows a very different behavior than *S. cerevisiae*, particularly in relation to growth yield and resistance to temperature and acidic stresses, which are important characteristics for a microorganism to be used as a probiotic. The German Commission E monograph lists *S. boulardii* as *S. cerevisiae* Hansen CBS 5926.

4. Commercial forms

There are two main forms in which probiotic organisms can be ingested—fermented foods and supplements. Fermented foods can be of both dairy and vegetable origin, with the most commonly known of each being yogurt and sauerkraut, respectively. Probiotic supplements consist of freeze-dried (lyophilized) bacteria in powder, capsule, or tablet form. Regardless of the form in which the microorganisms are consumed, for clinical efficacy, products containing probiotic organisms must provide live organisms in sufficient numbers to exert therapeutic effects. Both types of fermented foods and supplements are able to do this. Pros (advantage) and cons (disadvantage) of common probiotic delivery systems are compared [1] (**Table 2**).

Delivery system	Pros	Cons
Fermented dairy	-Affordability and easy Availability -Ease of incorporation into daily patterns -Additional nutritional benefits -Enhanced bacterial survival through upper GI tract (100× less bacteria can be given per dose) -Effective in the upper GI tract	-Contains dairy proteins and lactose -Taste can be issue -Not suitable when travelling -Not suitable for vegans
Capsules	-Ease of administration -Contain no binders	-Not therapeutic in upper GI tract (unless opened or chewed) -May contain allergenic excipients -Higher cost
Tablets	-Ease of administration -Effective in the upper GI tract	-May contain allergenic or otherwise problematic binders and excipients (e.g., gluten) -Higher cost
Powders	-Effective in the upper GI tract -Dosages can be easily adjusted -Can be incorporated into foods or drinks -Contain no binders	

Table 2. The pros and cons of different probiotic delivery systems.

4.1. Using the right strain

To achieve successful and reproducible clinical outcomes, it is imperative to use the exact probiotic strain that has been proven to have the specific therapeutic action that is desired. For example, *L. rhamnosus* GG was found to prevent viral gastroenteritis [1, 54] and maintain ulcerative colitis in remission [1, 55]. Other strains of *L. rhamnosus* cannot be assumed to act in a similar manner. The clinician who chooses to use the exact strain that had the effects in clinical trials can be confident of similar results. Using another closely related strain may or may not have any effect. Whenever possible, use the exact strain used in research, as other strains, even closely related ones, may not have the same effects [1].

4.2. Dosage

The dosage of probiotic foods and supplements is based solely upon the number of live organisms present in the product. Successful results have been attained in clinical trials using between $10^7$and 10^{11} viable bacteria per day [1, 56, 57]. Interestingly, it appears that 100 times fewer viable bacteria need to be given in a dairy medium than in a freeze-dried supplement to achieve similar numbers of live bacteria in the lower bowel [1, 58]. Dairy appears to work as an ideal transport medium for the bacteria, enhancing their survival through the upper GI tract [1, 59].

4.2. Safety and adverse reactions

While probiotics are used widely and adverse effects are uncommon, there is no systematic reporting system for probiotics. Most studies did not report a statistically significant increase in adverse events compared with controls, but it has been questioned if probiotics are safe in immunosuppressed individuals [60]. There are isolated case reports of bacteremia with Lactobacillus and fungemia with *S. boulardii.* A case-review study found sepsis, liver abscess, and endocarditis from *Lactobacillus GG* to occur mostly in patients with severe illness [61]. The same paper reviewed *S. boulardii* fungemia and found numerous cases, some related to ingestion of *S. boulardii,* but others resulting from suspected contamination of central lines when the product capsules were opened, and the lyophilized yeast was allowed to become airborne. Again, most, but not all, cases were in immunosuppressed individuals [60, 62]. Two systematic reviews and an Agency for Healthcare Research and Quality study have evaluated the safety of probiotics and concluded that adverse effects are uncommon, but serious infections with *Lactobacilli or S. boulardii* can occur [63, 64]. Given this conclusion, it is prudent to avoid probiotics in individuals who are immunosuppressed or severely ill.

4.3. Drug interaction

Lactobacilli and bifidobacteria are negatively affected by alcohol and antibiotics [1, 65]. Although there is no evidence that the organism interferes with the activity of most antibiotics, the metabolism of sulfasalazine, chloramphenicol palmitate, and phthalylsulfathiazole may be affected by some strains of *L. acidophilus* [1, 66].

4.4. Clinical studies of probiotics

Table 3 lists conditions for which probiotics have been studied in more than 800 randomized, controlled clinical trials (RCT) [4]. It is notable that there has been at least one clinical trial in a variety of clinical conditions. GI tract conditions, such as inflammatory illnesses (e.g., inflammatory bowel diseases or necrotizing enterocolitis in neonates) or enteric infections, have been studied most often [4, 67].

http://dx.doi.org/10.5772/63646

Abdominal conditions	
Acute amebiasis	
Acute pancreatitis	
Alcoholic liver injury	
Collagenous colitis	
Constipation	
Colorectal neoplasia prevention	
Diverticular colonic disease	
Gas and bloating	
Gastrointestinal transit time and gastric emptying	
Gastrointestinal symptoms after loop ileostomy reversal	
Helicobacter pylori infection	
Hematochezia in breastfed infants and in presumed infant allergic colitis	
Hepatic encephalopathy	
Infant colic	
Inflammatory bowel diseases (Crohn's disease, ulcerative colitis, pouchitis)	
Irritable bowel syndrome (IBS)	
Lactose intolerance	
Nonalcoholic steatohepatitis	
NSAID-induced small bowel injury	
Prevention and treatment of pediatric cow's milk allergy	
Prevention and treatment of diarrheal diseases (infectious and noninfectious)	
Prevention of antibiotic-associated diarrhea (AAD)	
Prevention of necrotizing enterocolitis (NEC)	
Primary sclerosing cholangitis (PSC) in patients with IBD	
Small intestinal bacterial overgrowth (SIBO)	
Tolerance of enteral feeds in ICU patients	
Viral shedding	
Oral and respiratory tract conditions	
Gingivitis	

Dental caries

Halitosis

Prevention of upper respiratory tract infections (URTI)

Pulmonary exacerbations in cystic fibrosis (CF)

Urinary and reproductive tract conditions

Prevention and treatment of bacterial vaginosis and fungal vulvovaginosis

Prevention of preterm deliveries associated with bacterial vaginosis

Recurrent urinary tract infections (UTI)

Recurrent bladder cancer

Allergic or skin conditions

Atopic dermatitis

Allergic rhinitis and rhinosinusitis

Allergic asthma

Cutaneous viral warts

Prevention and treatment of pediatric eczema

Skin burns

Other

Acute otitis media

Chronic kidney disease

Effect on infant mortality in preterm infants

Effect on CD4 count in patients with HIV

Estrogen metabolism

Fasting glucose, insulin sensitivity, and glucose control in diabetic patients

Hyperlipidemia

Hypertension

Infant blood pressure and metabolic profile from mothers treated with probiotics

Inhibition of nasal, oral, or fecal colonization with pathogenic bacteria

Markers of metabolic syndrome and cardiovascular disease

Mastitis

Pediatric otitis media

http://dx.doi.org/10.5772/63646

Pregnancy after *in vitro* fertilization (IVF)
Prevention and treatment of gestational diabetes
Prevention of type-1 diabetes mellitus
Prevention of infections in preterm infants, infants, and young children
Prevention of nosocomial infections in ICUs
Prevention of infections in the postoperative setting
Prevention of skeletal muscle damage under oxidative stress
Psychological distress, mood, and cognition
Reduction of biologically active aflatoxin
Rheumatoid arthritis (RA)
Spondyloarthropathy
Urinary oxalate excretion (risk factor for nephrolithiasis)
Vaccine-specific antibody development
Waist circumference and obesity

Table 3. Clinical conditions or settings studied in randomized, controlled clinical trials to evaluate probiotic efficacy.

Indication	Efficacy and quality of evidence
Infectious diarrhea	
Prevention	Moderate
Treatment	High
Traveler's diarrhea prevention	Moderate
Antibiotic-associated diarrhea prevention	High
Clostridium difficile infection (CDI)	
Prevention	Moderate
Treatment	None
Recurrent CDI treatment	Low to moderate
IBD	
UC treatment	Moderate
Pouchitis treatment and prevention	High
Crohn's disease treatment	Low
IBS treatment	Moderate

Table 4. Indications, efficacy, and quality of evidence for probiotics in GI diseases.

4.5. Efficacy in GI diseases

An ambitious meta-analysis of 11 species of probiotics evaluated their efficacy in the prevention and/or treatment of eight major GI tract diseases and concluded that there was efficacy in treatment of infectious diarrhea, antibiotic-associated diarrhea (AAD), *C. difficile* infection (CDI), *Helicobacter pylori* eradication, IBS, and pouchitis; there was a lack of efficacy for traveler's diarrhea (TD) and necrotizing enterocolitis (NEC) [60, 68]. Some of these results conflict with meta-analyses of individual diseases, and results of all studies should be interpreted with caution. Rigorous blinded RCTs of specific probiotics are needed to provide robust data on efficacy, adverse events, and cost benefit before widespread use can be recommended for many products on an evidence-based approach (**Table 4**);despite the lack of data, these products are widely used [60].

5. A pilot study to evaluate the efficacy of probiotic on treatment in patients with small intestinal bacterial overgrowth (SIBO)

Generally, small intestinal bacterial overgrowth (SIBO) can be the result of a change in the clinical condition which has altered the pH and the bowel movements. In addition, immune deficiency and malnutrition are the other risk factors accompanying it [69, 70]. SIBO can leads to steatorrhea, vitamin B12-absorptive impairment, injury to the small intestinal microvilli, which itself causes malabsorption, coma, neurological deficit, and acidosis-induced shock [70]. SIBO has also been proposed to be a common causative factor in the pathogenesis of irritable bowel syndrome (IBS) [71]. The diagnosis of this syndrome is made by hydrogen breath test (HBT) [71, 72].

This study was performed on the patients with chronic stomach pain and discomfort or changes in their defecation, who were referred to the Infectious and Internal Diseases Clinics of Quaem Hospital, Mashhad, Iran, from May 2010 to October 2011 [73]. The study protocol was approved by the Research Council Ethics Committee of Mashhad University of Medical Sciences. Accordingly, the diagnosis was confirmed by hydrogen breath test (HBT) after obtaining informed written consent. Thirty consecutive cases with a positive test result were included in the study and were randomized in a double-blind manner into two groups: probiotic drug user and control group. After an initial 3-week aggressive therapy with broad-spectrum antibiotics, a 15-day maintenance antibiotic therapy with minocycline, 100 mg twice a day, and 15 days with a probiotic (named Lactol), including *Bacillus coagulan* spores and fructo-oligosaccharides (Bioplus Life Sciences Pvt. Ltd., India), twice a day after meals, were administered for the study group, and the same regimen without probiotic for the control group. After 6 months, the HBT result and the GI symptoms were analyzed and compared between the two groups.

As presented in the following tables, the number of patients with complaints of bloating, belching and diarrhea was remarkably less in the patients receiving a probiotic in comparison to controls (**Tables 5** and **6**). In spite of the aggressive and maintenance treatments administered for all the cases, 93.3% patients showed negative result of the HBT at the end of treatment in the study group compared to 66.7% in the control group, showing the effectiveness of the probiotic treatment. As an additional finding, 33.3% patients of the study group and 53.3% of the controls had a Bachelor degree or higher education, with no significant difference [75–79].

Parameter	Study group	Control group	Total
Gender(M/F)			
Male	8 (53.3)	7 (46.7)	15(50.0)
Female	7 (46.7)	8 (53.3)	15(50.0)
Age (years)	34.60 ± 10.68	42.86 ± 16.61	38.73 ± 14.35
Location of pain			
Epigastric	8 (53.3)	5 (33.3)	13 (43.3)
Umbilical	6 (40.0)	6 (40.0)	12 (40.0)
Other sites	1 (6.7)	4 (26.7)	5 (16.7)
Flatulence			
Yes	6 (40.0)	11 (73.3)	17 (56.7)
No	9 (60.0)	4 (26.7)	13 (43.3)
Belching			
Yes	9 (60.0)	10 (66.7)	19 (63.3)
No	6 (40.0)	5 (33.3)	11 (36.7)
Nausea			
Yes	3 (20.0)	3(20.0)	6 (20.0)
No	12 (80.0)	12(80.0)	24 (80.0)
Vomiting			
Yes	4 (26.7)	3 (20.0)	7 (23.3)
No	11 (73.3)	12(80.0)	23 (77.7)
Constipation			
Yes	9 (60.0)	3 (20.0)	12 (40.0)
No	6 (40.0)	12 (80.0)	18 (60.0)
Diarrhea			
Yes	2 (13.3)	8 (53.3)	10 (33.3)
No	13 (86.7)	7 (46.7)	20 (66.7)
Loss of appetite			
Yes	6(40.0)	5 (33.3)	11 (36.7)
No	9(60.0)	10 (66.7)	19 (63.3)

Table 5. Clinical characteristics of subjects at baseline (values in parentheses are percentages).

In conclusion, the results of this pilot study showed that addition of a probiotic to the maintenance regimen may improve the GI tract symptoms and prevent the probable complications in patients with SIBO. Therefore, based on low side effects of the probiotics, it seems that their long-term prescription in SIBO, considering the recurrence favor of this syndrome, is desirable (e.g., probiotic containing dairy products or supplement daily drugs).

Parameter	Study group	Control group	Total	P value
Location of pain				
Epigastric	0 (0.0)	3 (20.0)	3 (10.0)	0.002
Umbilical	0 (0.0)	3 (20.0)	3 (10.0)	
Other sites	0 (0.0)	2 (13.3)	2 (6.7)	
Without pain	15 (100.0)	7 (46.7)	22 (73.3)	
Flatulence				
Yes	2 (13.3)	8 (53.3)	10 (33.3)	0.049
No	13 (86.7)	7 (46.7)	20 (66.7)	
Belching				
Yes	3 (20.0)	9 (60.0)	12 (40.0)	0.025
No	12 (80.0)	6 (40.0)	18 (60.0)	
Nausea				
Yes	0 (0.0)	1 (6.7)	1 (3.3)	0.999
No	15 (100.0)	14 (93.3)	29 (96.7)	
Vomiting				
Yes	1 (6.7)	1 (6.7)	2(6.7)	0.999
No	14 (93.3)	14 (93.3)	28 (93.3)	
Constipation				
Yes	1 (6.7)	2 (13.3)	3 (10.0)	0.999
No	14 (93.3)	13 (86.7)	27 (90.0)	
Diarrhea				
Yes	1 (6.7)	8 (53.3)	9 (30.0)	0.014
No	14 (93.3)	7 (46.7)	21 (70.0)	
Loss of appetite				
Yes	1 (6.7)	4 (26.7)	5 (16.7)	0.330
No	14 (93.3)	11 (73.3)	25 (83.3)	
Hydrogen breath test				
Positive	1 (6.7)	5 (33.3)	6 (20.0)	0.169
Negative	14 (93.3)	10 (66.7)	24 (80.0)	

Table 6. Clinical characteristics data of subjects after 6 months of treatment (values in parentheses are percentages).

http://dx.doi.org/10.5772/63646

Author details

Amirreza Khalighi[1*], Reza Behdani[2] and Shabnam Kouhestani[3]

*Address all correspondence to: dr_a_khalighi@yahoo.com, a.khalighi@razavihospital.com

1 Infectious diseases Specialist, Head of Infectious Diseases Ward & Infection Prevention & Control (IPC) coordinator, Razavi Hospital, Mashhad, Iran

2 GP, Volunteer Research Assistant, Hepatology Research Department, Toronto General Hospital, University Health Network (UHN), Toronto, Canada

3 Internist, Internal Medicine & Nutritional Consultant, Medical Council of Iran/Mashhad branch, Mashhad, Iran

References

[1] Hawrelak J, BNat(Hons). Probiotics. In: Pizzorno JE, Murray MT, editors. Textbook of Natural Medicine. 4th ed. St. Louis, Missouri: Churchill Livingstone Elsevier; 2013. p. 979–94.

[2] Lilly DM, Stillwell RH. Probotics: growth-promoting factors produced by microorganisms. Science (New York, NY). 1965;147(3659):747–8.

[3] Parker R. Probiotics, the other half of the antibiotic story. Animal Nutrition and Health. 1974;29:4–8.

[4] Chen LA, Sears CL. Prebiotics, Probiotics, and Synbiotics. In: Bennett JE, Dolin R, Blaser MJ, editors. Mandell, Douglas, and Bennett's Principles and Practice of Infectious Diseases. 8th ed. Philadelphia, PA: Saunders Elsevier; 2015. p. 19–25.e1.

[5] Sanders ME. Probiotics: definition, sources, selection, and uses. Clinical Infectious Diseases: An Official Publication of the Infectious Diseases Society of America. 2008;46 Suppl 2:S58–61; discussion S144–51.

[6] Guarner F, Schaafsma GJ. Probiotics. International Journal of Food Microbiology. 1998;39(3):237–8.

[7] Dunne C, O'Mahony L, Murphy L, Thornton G, Morrissey D, O'Halloran S, et al. In vitro selection criteria for probiotic bacteria of human origin: correlation with in vivo findings. The American Journal of Clinical Nutrition. 2001;73(2 Suppl):386s–92s.

[8] O'Toole PW, Cooney JC. Probiotic bacteria influence the composition and function of the intestinal microbiota. Interdisciplinary Perspectives on Infectious Diseases. 2008; 2008:175285.

[9] Fuller R. Probiotics in human medicine. Gut. 1991;32(4):439–42.

[10] Fuller R, Gibson GR. Modification of the intestinal microflora using probiotics and prebiotics. Scandinavian Journal of Gastroenterology Supplement. 1997;222:28–31.

[11] Mack DR, Michail S, Wei S, McDougall L, Hollingsworth MA. Probiotics inhibit enteropathogenic *E. coli* adherence in vitro by inducing intestinal mucin gene expression. The American Journal of Physiology. 1999;276(4 Pt 1):G941–50.

[12] Rolfe RD. The role of probiotic cultures in the control of gastrointestinal health. The Journal of Nutrition. 2000;130(2S Suppl):396s–402s.

[13] Juven BJ, Meinersmann RJ, Stern NJ. Antagonistic effects of lactobacilli and pediococci to control intestinal colonization by human enteropathogens in live poultry. The Journal of Applied Bacteriology. 1991;70(2):95–103.

[14] Mishra C, Lambert J. Production of anti-microbial substances by probiotics. Asia Pacific Journal of Clinical Nutrition. 1996;5(1):20–4.

[15] Perdigon G, Alvarez S, Rachid M, Aguero G, Gobbato N. Immune system stimulation by probiotics. Journal of Dairy Science. 1995;78(7):1597–606.

[16] Link-Amster H, Rochat F, Saudan KY, Mignot O, Aeschlimann JM. Modulation of a specific humoral immune response and changes in intestinal flora mediated through fermented milk intake. FEMS Immunology and Medical Microbiology. 1994;10(1):55–63.

[17] Schiffrin EJ, Rochat F, Link-Amster H, Aeschlimann JM, Donnet-Hughes A. Immunomodulation of human blood cells following the ingestion of lactic acid bacteria. Journal of Dairy Science. 1995;78(3):491–7.

[18] Schultz M, Sartor RB. Probiotics and inflammatory bowel diseases. The American Journal of Gastroenterology. 2000;95(1 Suppl):S19–21.

[19] Sutas Y, Hurme M, Isolauri E. Down-regulation of anti-CD3 antibody-induced IL-4 production by bovine caseins hydrolysed with Lactobacillus GG-derived enzymes. Scandinavian Journal of Immunology. 1996;43(6):687–9.

[20] Goldin BR. Health benefits of probiotics. The British Journal of Nutrition. 1998;80(4):S203–7.

[21] Pelto L, Isolauri E, Lilius EM, Nuutila J, Salminen S. Probiotic bacteria down-regulate the milk-induced inflammatory response in milk-hypersensitive subjects but have an immunostimulatory effect in healthy subjects. Clinical and Experimental Allergy: Journal of the British Society for Allergy and Clinical Immunology. 1998;28(12):1474–9.

[22] Miele E, Pascarella F, Giannetti E, Quaglietta L, Baldassano RN, Staiano A. Effect of a probiotic preparation (VSL#3) on induction and maintenance of remission in children with ulcerative colitis. The American Journal of Gastroenterology. 2009;104(2):437–43.

[23] Vanderhoof JA, Young RJ. Use of probiotics in childhood gastrointestinal disorders. Journal of Pediatric Gastroenterology and Nutrition. 1998;27(3):323–32.

[24] Wilson KH, Perini F. Role of competition for nutrients in suppression of Clostridium difficile by the colonic microflora. Infection and Immunity. 1988;56(10):2610–4.

[25] Macfarlane GT, Cummings JH. Probiotics and prebiotics: can regulating the activities of intestinal bacteria benefit health? BMJ (Clinical Research ed). 1999;318(7189):999–1003.

[26] McKane L, Kandel J, eds. Microbiology: Essentials and Applications. New York: McGraw-Hill; 1986.

[27] Fujisawa T, Benno Y, Yaeshima T, Mitsuoka T. Taxonomic study of the *Lactobacillus acidophilus* group, with recognition of *Lactobacillus gallinarum* sp. nov. and *Lactobacillus johnsonii* sp. nov. and synonymy of *Lactobacillus acidophilus* group A3 (Johnson et al. 1980) with the type strain of *Lactobacillus amylovorus* (Nakamura 1981). International Journal of Systematic Bacteriology. 1992;42(3):487–91.

[28] Vanderhoof JA, Young RJ. Current and potential uses of probiotics. Annals of Allergy, Asthma & Immunology: Official Publication of the American College of Allergy, Asthma, & Immunology. 2004;93(5 Suppl 3):S33–7.

[29] McGroarty JA. Probiotic use of lactobacilli in the human female urogenital tract. FEMS Immunology and Medical Microbiology. 1993;6(4):251–64.

[30] Bruce AW, Reid G. Intravaginal instillation of lactobacilli for prevention of recurrent urinary tract infections. Canadian Journal of Microbiology. 1988;34(3):339–43.

[31] Gupta K, Stapleton AE, Hooton TM, Roberts PL, Fennell CL, Stamm WE. Inverse association of H2O2-producing lactobacilli and vaginal *Escherichia coli* colonization in women with recurrent urinary tract infections. The Journal of Infectious Diseases. 1998;178(2):446–50.

[32] Madsen KL, Doyle JS, Jewell LD, Tavernini MM, Fedorak RN. Lactobacillus species prevents colitis in interleukin 10 gene-deficient mice. Gastroenterology. 1999;116(5): 1107–14.

[33] Shornikova AV, Casas IA, Isolauri E, Mykkanen H, Vesikari T. Lactobacillus reuteri as a therapeutic agent in acute diarrhea in young children. Journal of Pediatric Gastroenterology and Nutrition. 1997;24(4):399–404.

[34] Reid G, Bruce AW, Cook RL, Llano M. Effect on urogenital flora of antibiotic therapy for urinary tract infection. Scandinavian Journal of Infectious Diseases. 1990;22(1):43–7.

[35] Alander M, Satokari R, Korpela R, Saxelin M, Vilpponen-Salmela T, Mattila-Sandholm T, et al. Persistence of colonization of human colonic mucosa by a probiotic strain,

Lactobacillus rhamnosus GG, after oral consumption. Applied and Environmental Microbiology. 1999;65(1):351–4.

[36] Sullivan A, Barkholt L, Nord CE. *Lactobacillus acidophilus, Bifidobacterium lactis* and Lactobacillus F19 prevent antibiotic-associated ecological disturbances of *Bacteroides fragilis* in the intestine. The Journal of Antimicrobial Chemotherapy. 2003;52(2):308–11.

[37] Maggi L, Mastromarino P, Macchia S, Brigidi P, Pirovano F, Matteuzzi D, et al. Technological and biological evaluation of tablets containing different strains of lactobacilli for vaginal administration. European Journal of Pharmaceutics and Biopharmaceutics: official journal of Arbeitsgemeinschaft fur Pharmazeutische Verfahrenstechnik eV. 2000;50(3):389–95.

[38] El-Nezami H, Kankaanpaa P, Salminen S, Ahokas J. Ability of dairy strains of lactic acid bacteria to bind a common food carcinogen, aflatoxin B1. Food and chemical toxicology: an international journal published for the British Industrial Biological Research Association. 1998;36(4):321–6.

[39] Goldin BR, Gualtieri LJ, Moore RP. The effect of Lactobacillus GG on the initiation and promotion of DMH-induced intestinal tumors in the rat. Nutrition and Cancer. 1996;25(2):197–204.

[40] McIntosh GH, Royle PJ, Playne MJ. A probiotic strain of *L. acidophilus* reduces DMH-induced large intestinal tumors in male Sprague-Dawley rats. Nutrition and Cancer. 1999;35(2):153–9.

[41] Mao Y, Nobaek S, Kasravi B, Adawi D, Stenram U, Molin G, et al. The effects of Lactobacillus strains and oat fiber on methotrexate-induced enterocolitis in rats. Gastroenterology. 1996;111(2):334–44.

[42] Doncheva NI, Antov GP, Softova EB, Nyagolov YP. Experimental and clinical study on the hypolipidemic and antisclerotic effect of *Lactobacillus Bulgaricus* strain GB N 1 (48). Nutrition Research. 2002;22(4):393–403.

[43] Losada MA, Olleros T. Towards a healthier diet for the colon: the influence of fructooligosaccharides and lactobacilli on intestinal health. Nutrition Research. 2002;22(1):71–84.

[44] Oberhelman RA, Gilman RH, Sheen P, Taylor DN, Black RE, Cabrera L, et al. A placebo-controlled trial of Lactobacillus GG to prevent diarrhea in undernourished Peruvian children. The Journal of Pediatrics. 1999;134(1):15–20.

[45] Reid G, Cook RL, Bruce AW. Examination of strains of lactobacilli for properties that may influence bacterial interference in the urinary tract. The Journal of Urology. 1987;138(2):330–5.

[46] Cremonini F, Di Caro S, Covino M, Armuzzi A, Gabrielli M, Santarelli L, et al. Effect of different probiotic preparations on anti-Helicobacter pylori therapy-related side

effects: a parallel group, triple blind, placebo-controlled study. The American Journal of Gastroenterology. 2002;97(11):2744–9.

[47] Hoyos AB. Reduced incidence of necrotizing enterocolitis associated with enteral administration of *Lactobacillus acidophilus* and *Bifidobacterium infantis* to neonates in an intensive care unit. International Journal of Infectious Diseases: IJID: official publication of the International Society for Infectious Diseases. 1999;3(4):197–202.

[48] Duc le H, Hong HA, Barbosa TM, Henriques AO, Cutting SM. Characterization of Bacillus probiotics available for human use. Applied and Environmental Microbiology. 2004;70(4):2161–71.

[49] Velraeds MM, van der Mei HC, Reid G, Busscher HJ. Inhibition of initial adhesion of uropathogenic *Enterococcus faecalis* by biosurfactants from Lactobacillus isolates. Applied and Environmental Microbiology. 1996;62(6):1958–63.

[50] Hyronimus B, Le Marrec C, Urdaci MC. Coagulin, a bacteriocin-like inhibitory substance produced by *Bacillus coagulans* I4. Journal of Applied Microbiology. 1998;85(1):42–50.

[51] Buts JP. [Lyophilized *Saccharomyces boulardii*: example of a probiotic medicine]. Revista de gastroenterologia del Peru: organo oficial de la Sociedad de Gastroenterologia del Peru. 2005;25(2):176–88.

[52] Fietto JL, Araujo RS, Valadao FN, Fietto LG, Brandao RL, Neves MJ, et al. Molecular and physiological comparisons between *Saccharomyces cerevisiae* and *Saccharomyces boulardii*. Canadian Journal of Microbiology. 2004;50(8):615–21.

[53] Posteraro B, Sanguinetti M, Romano L, Torelli R, Novarese L, Fadda G. Molecular tools for differentiating probiotic and clinical strains of *Saccharomyces cerevisiae*. International Journal of Food Microbiology. 2005;103(3):295–304.

[54] Szajewska H, Kotowska M, Mrukowicz JZ, Armanska M, Mikolajczyk W. Efficacy of Lactobacillus GG in prevention of nosocomial diarrhea in infants. The Journal of Pediatrics. 2001;138(3):361–5.

[55] Zocco MA, dal Verme LZ, Cremonini F, Piscaglia AC, Nista EC, Candelli M, et al. Efficacy of Lactobacillus GG in maintaining remission of ulcerative colitis. Alimentary Pharmacology & Therapeutics. 2006;23(11):1567–74.

[56] Hatakka K, Savilahti E, Ponka A, Meurman JH, Poussa T, Nase L, et al. Effect of long term consumption of probiotic milk on infections in children attending day care centres: double blind, randomised trial. BMJ (Clinical research ed). 2001;322(7298):1327.

[57] Shornikova AV, Casas IA, Mykkanen H, Salo E, Vesikari T. Bacteriotherapy with *Lactobacillus reuteri* in rotavirus gastroenteritis. The Pediatric Infectious Disease Journal. 1997;16(12):1103–7.

[58] Saxelin M. Colonization of the human gastrointestinal tract by probiotic bacteria. Nutrition Today. 1996;31(6):9S.

[59] Kailasapathy K, Chin J. Survival and therapeutic potential of probiotic organisms with reference to *Lactobacillus acidophilus* and Bifidobacterium spp. Immunology and Cell Biology. 2000;78(1):80–8.

[60] Surawicz CM, Brandt LJ. Probiotics and Fecal Microbiota Transplantation. In: Feldman M, Friedman LS, Brandt LJ, editors. Sleisenger and Fordtran's Gastrointestinal and Liver Disease. 10th ed. Philadelphia, PA: Saunders Elsevier; 2016. p. 2339–43.e3.

[61] Segarra-Newnham M. Probiotics for Clostridium difficile-associated diarrhea: focus on Lactobacillus rhamnosus GG and Saccharomyces boulardii. The Annals of Pharmacotherapy. 2007;41(7):1212–21.

[62] Elahi B, Nikfar S, Derakhshani S, Vafaie M, Abdollahi M. On the benefit of probiotics in the management of pouchitis in patients underwent ileal pouch anal anastomosis: a meta-analysis of controlled clinical trials. Digestive Diseases and Sciences. 2008;53(5): 1278–84.

[63] Hempel S, Newberry S, Ruelaz A, Wang Z, Miles JN, Suttorp MJ, et al. Safety of probiotics used to reduce risk and prevent or treat disease. Evidence Report/Technology Assessment. 2011(200):1–645.

[64] Whelan K, Myers CE. Safety of probiotics in patients receiving nutritional support: a systematic review of case reports, randomized controlled trials, and nonrandomized trials. The American Journal of Clinical Nutrition. 2010;91(3):687–703.

[65] Finegold S, Mathisen G, George W. Changes in the Human Intestinal Flora Related to the Administration of Antimicrobial Agents. In: Hentges DJ, editor. Human Intestinal Microflora in Health and Disease. London: Academic Press; 1983. p. 355–448.

[66] Pradhan A, Majumdar MK. Metabolism of some drugs by intestinal lactobacilli and their toxicological considerations. Acta Pharmacologica et Toxicologica . 1986;58(1):11–5.

[67] Goldin BR, Gorbach SL. Clinical indications for probiotics: an overview. Clinical Infectious Diseases: An Official Publication of the Infectious Diseases Society of America. 2008;46 Suppl 2:S96–100; discussion S44–51.

[68] Ritchie ML, Romanuk TN. A meta-analysis of probiotic efficacy for gastrointestinal diseases. PLoS One. 2012;7(4):e34938.

[69] Binder H. Disorders of Absorption. In: Fauci A, Kasper D, Longo D, Braunwald E, Hauser S, Jameson J, editors. Harrison's Principles of Internal Medicine. 18th ed. New york: McGraw Hill; 2012. p. 2460–76.

[70] Kleigman R, Behrman R, Jenson H, Stanton B. Nelson Textbook of Pediatrics. 19th ed. Philadelphia, PA: Saunders; 2011.

[71] Quigley EM. Bacteria: a new player in gastrointestinal motility disorders – infections, bacterial overgrowth, and probiotics. Gastroenterology Clinics of North America. 2007;36(3):735–48, xi.

[72] O'Mahony S, Shanhan F. Enteric microbiota and small intestinal bacterial overgrowth. In: Feldman M, Friedman LS, Brandt LJ, editors. Sleisenger & Fordtran's Gastrointestinal & Liver Disease: Pathophysiology, Diagnosis, Management. 9th ed. Philadelphia: Saunders Elsevier; 2010. p. 1772–7.

[73] Khalighi AR, Khalighi MR, Behdani R, Jamali J, Khosravi A, Kouhestani S, et al. Evaluating the efficacy of probiotic on treatment in patients with small intestinal bacterial overgrowth (SIBO) – a pilot study. The Indian Journal of Medical Research. 2014;140(5):604–8.

[74] Soifer LO, Peralta D, Dima G, Besasso H. [Comparative clinical efficacy of a probiotic vs. an antibiotic in the treatment of patients with intestinal bacterial overgrowth and chronic abdominal functional distension: a pilot study]. Acta gastroenterologica Latinoamericana. 2010;40(4):323–7.

[75] Barrett JS, Canale KE, Gearry RB, Irving PM, Gibson PR. Probiotic effects on intestinal fermentation patterns in patients with irritable bowel syndrome. World Journal of Gastroenterology. 2008;14(32):5020–4.

[76] Jonkers D, Penders J, Masclee A, Pierik M. Probiotics in the management of inflammatory bowel disease: a systematic review of intervention studies in adult patients. Drugs. 2012;72(6):803–23.

[77] Rohde CL, Bartolini V, Jones N. The use of probiotics in the prevention and treatment of antibiotic-associated diarrhea with special interest in *Clostridium difficile*-associated diarrhea. Nutrition in Clinical Practice: Official Publication of the American Society for Parenteral and Enteral Nutrition. 2009;24(1):33–40.

[78] Bixquert Jimenez M. Treatment of irritable bowel syndrome with probiotics. An etiopathogenic approach at last? Revista espanola de enfermedades digestivas: organo oficial de la Sociedad Espanola de Patologia Digestiva. 2009;101(8):553–64.

Chapter 3

Prebiotics: Metabolism and Symbiotic Synergy with Probiotics in Promoting Health

Nditange Shigwedha, Penny Hiwilepo-Van Hal,
Li Jia, Liubov Sichel and Shuang Zhang

Additional information is available at the end of the chapter

http://dx.doi.org/10.5772/64091

Abstract

Prebiotics are non-digestible food ingredients that beneficially affect the host by selectively stimulating the growth and activity of probiotic bacteria in the colon. All dietary prebiotics and/or dietary fiber provide the physiological and beneficial effects and, therefore, are considered as essential nutrients. According to the Codex Alimentarius and the Canadian Bureau of Nutritional Sciences, dietary fiber consists of carbohydrates with a degree of polymerization (DP) of three or more that naturally occur in foods of plant origin and that are not digested and absorbed by the small intestine. The same definition goes well along with the term dietary prebiotics. Food and Drug Administration (FDA) | Institute of Medicine (IOM) states that dietary fiber only comes from plant foods and anything else is regarded as "added fiber" or "novel fiber." Dietary fiber and/dietary prebiotics can be industrially produced for a broad range of food applications. They can also be processed into capsules for the purpose of microencapsulating probiotics. In this chapter, the most recognized physiological and/or beneficial effects of the prebiotics are clarified. New evidence on the concentrations of the short-chain fatty acids (SCFAs) and their metabolic relationship with better health or disease prevention in the host is provided.

Keywords: Prebiotics, Probiotics, Synbiotic, Microencapsulation, SCFA (short-chain fatty acids)

1. Introduction

All dietary prebiotics have the physiological and/or beneficial effects in humans and, thus, are regarded as essential nutrients. According to the Codex Alimentarius, Canadian Bureau of

Nutritional Sciences, IOM, and American Association of Cereal Chemistry International (AACCI), dietary fibers are identified as the edible parts of plants or analogous carbohydrates that are resistant to digestion and absorption in the human small intestine with complete or partial fermentation in the large intestine. Dietary fiber includes polysaccharides, oligosaccharides, lignin, and associated plants substances. Dietary fibers promote beneficial physiological effects including laxation and/or blood cholesterol attenuation, and/or blood glucose attenuation [1]. Ordinarily, a prebiotic is defined as a non-digestible food ingredient that confers beneficial effects in the host by selectively stimulating the growth and/or activity of one or a limited number of bacteria in the colon and thus improves host health and well-being [2–4]. From those two descriptions, it is clear that "dietary fiber" and/or "prebiotics" are certainly a complex of many different plant sources, with different chemical and physiological properties. Collectively when ingested, they are a cohesive unit for essentiality. In the United States of America, the joint recommendation by FDA | IOM says that dietary fiber only comes from plant food (fruits, vegetables, or grains); and anything else was regarded as "added fiber" or "novel fiber." Interestingly, that FDA | IOM recommendation fits well with the terminology "dietary prebiotics". A dietary prebiotic is defined as a selectively fermented ingredient that results in specific changes in the composition and/or activity of the gastrointestinal microbiota, thus conferring benefit(s) upon host health [5]. Polymers and oligomers are the common types. Besides, a proof of the new oligomers and/or polymers about whether they confer the physiological, or beneficial effects would be required before being started to be used in the public.

The primary reason that the prebiotics transit through the stomach and small intestines undigested is because humans do not have the intestinal enzymes needed to digest them. They characteristically make their way intact to the colon, where they will be bacterially fermented, together with the unabsorbed nutrients [6]. The salivary and pancreatic α-amylases are the only enzymes needed for starch digestion. It is also necessary to emphasize here that all sources of dietary fiber are potential prebiotics, and every source of dietary prebiotics (with a few exceptions) is selectively fermented, thus mutually providing energy and simple sugars to the host through the gut microbiota. Therefore, due to similarities between these two terms, we will use the term "prebiotics" to refer to both the "dietary fiber and dietary prebiotics" throughout this chapter.

2. Whole grain, roughages, and prebiotics as essential nutrients: linked with probiotics for health

Whole grain and roughage are terms that have been easily confused with prebiotics in research and sometimes used interchangeably. Whole grains are cereal grains that consist of the intact, ground, cracked, or flaked kernel, which includes the bran, the germ, and the innermost part of the kernel or endosperm [7]. Apart from prebiotics alone, whole grains provide a variety of other nutrients too. Roughages are the coarse indigestible constituents of food or fodder, which provide bulk to the diet and promote normal bowel function. Hence, it has now become clear that where deficiency occurs, the whole-grain products can be enriched with the prebiotics or else roughages. This fortification would be necessary and may clarify some of the confusions among the consumers who still believe that whole grains and prebiotics are one and the same. In **Figure 1**, for example, it can be observed that the average intake of prebiotics among Americans (male and female) between 2009 and 2010 was around 18 g/day, which was far below the daily recommended intakes (DRIs). The optimum daily requirement for prebiotics is estimated to be between 35 and 50 g/day [8]. This quantity would be needed for proper intestinal functions and to adequately support the immune functions. Fascinatingly, an additional severe deficiency of the prebiotics in some foods linked to whole grain and non-whole grain can be witnessed in **Figure 2**. Yeast bread and breakfast cereals each seem to provide nearly 1/3rd of the whole-grain per serving. Others such as the grain-based snacks appear to offer about 1/5th in addition to <1/10th which appears to come from rice, pasta, quick breads, pastries, cakes, pies, cookies, and miscellaneous grains [9]. Research has further revealed that whole-grain consumers had significantly better nutrient profiles (including higher intakes of minerals and vitamins as percentages of 1989 Recommended Dietary Allowances and as nutrients per 1000 kcal, and lower intakes of total fat, saturated fat, and added sugars as % of food energy) than the nonconsumers. It was found that consumers were more likely to meet pyramid recommendations for the grain, fruit, and dairy food groups than the nonconsumers [9].

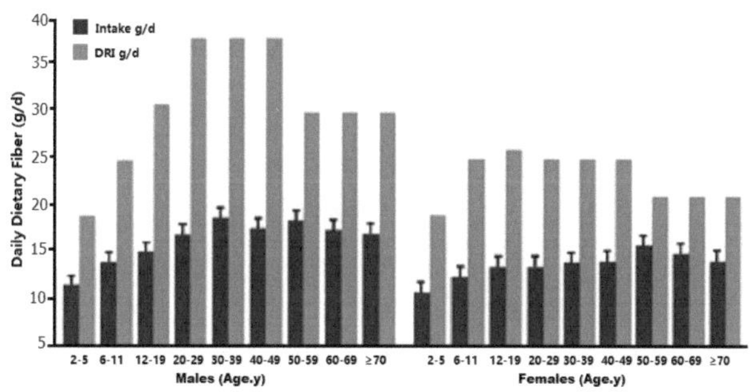

Figure 1. A parallel link of prebiotics made from the average intakes and projected daily recommended intakes or DRIs (g/day) among the American males and females, respectively. Source: Remade from Ref. [8].

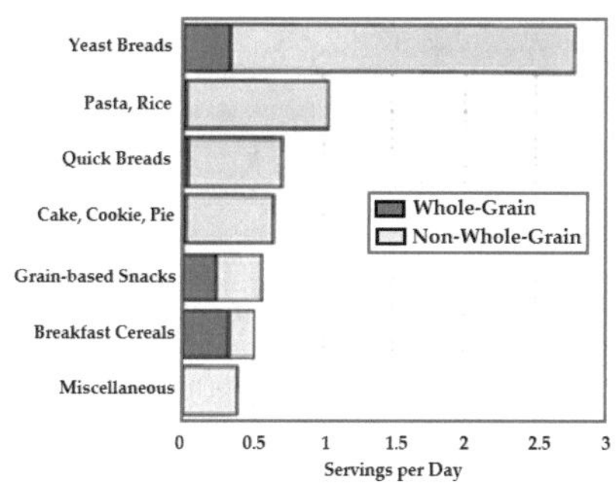

Figure 2. A comparison made between constituents of whole grain and non-whole grain as fiber representation in some common foods. Source: Modified from Ref. [9].

When the probiotic bacteria selectively ferment the prebiotics in the colon, a symbiotic synergy has been observed. During the metabolic process, that interdependent relationship exerts beneficial health effects to the host. For instance, probiotics selectively receive different prebiotics as nutrients from the host, initiate fermentation in the colon, provide the host with additional genetic and metabolic attributes, boost the immune system, and be able to harness nutrients that are otherwise inaccessible. Perceptibly, synbiotic is a mixture of both probiotics and prebiotics, which beneficially affect the host by improving the survival and implantation of live microbial dietary supplements in the gastrointestinal (GI) tract [2]. Therefore, prebiotics, probiotics, and synbiotics (combination of prebiotics and probiotics) can make up a distinct class of the essential functional ingredients in foods. Probiotics are defined as live microorganisms, which when administered in adequate amounts confer a health benefit on the host [10]. As a live microbial food supplement, probiotics have been linked to numerous beneficial effects of improving the intestinal microbial balance in humans. Naturally, the number of bacteria living in the human body and inside the gut is vast and is estimated to be 100 trillion bacteria [11, 12].

Besides commensal bacteria, probiotics, such as bifidobacteria, enterococci, streptococci, and lactobacilli, must co-exist with their host and must evade or endure the diversity of responses that the host has already developed to eliminate pathogenic bacteria while at the same time selectively ferment all the prebiotics. All these functions are mutually coordinated and provide a significant synergy to the host. An advancement of intestinal microbiota including bifidobacteria (representing some of the probiotic bacteria) in early childhood from birth to 24 months is being demonstrated in **Figure 3** [13]. In fact, an understanding on how the human immune system could differentiate between probiotics and harmful bacteria is no longer a serious challenge as it used to be in the past [12, 14].

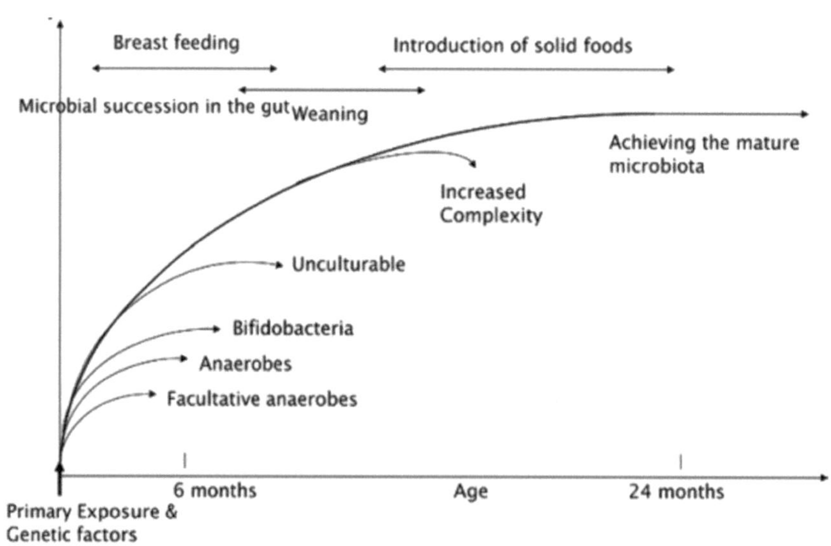

Figure 3. Succession flows of gut microbiota in a healthy infant from birth. Source: From Ref. [13].

http://dx.doi.org/10.5772/64091

3. The most quintessential beneficial effects of the prebiotics

The most recognized physiological and beneficial effects of the prebiotics are as follows: improving laxation or regularity by increasing stool bulk; reducing blood glucose and/or low-density lipoprotein (LDL)-cholesterol levels; increment of high-density lipoprotein (HDL)-cholesterol; reducing post-prandial blood glucose and/or insulin levels; providing energy-yielding metabolites through colonic fermentation; enhancing feeling of satiety; reducing energy intake (which results in weight management especially in combination with probiotics); having positive effects on immune system (e.g., less risk for allergy in both infants and adults especially in combination with probiotics), and others (see **Figure 4**). However, among those, only two quintessential properties of all prebiotics are historical and common, specifically to promote intestinal function (laxation), and to serve as the primary energy source of the gut microbiota. Both functions are synergistic and essential for the development of the immune system. Furthermore, these quintessential properties as "physiological and beneficial effects" of prebiotics are cumulative and also increase with a rise of prebiotics intake every day. However, an appropriate dose of probiotics in addition to the prebiotics would be required because bacterial overgrowth in the small intestine may lead to SIBO (small intestinal bacterial overgrowth) and, subsequently, a compromised immune system [11].

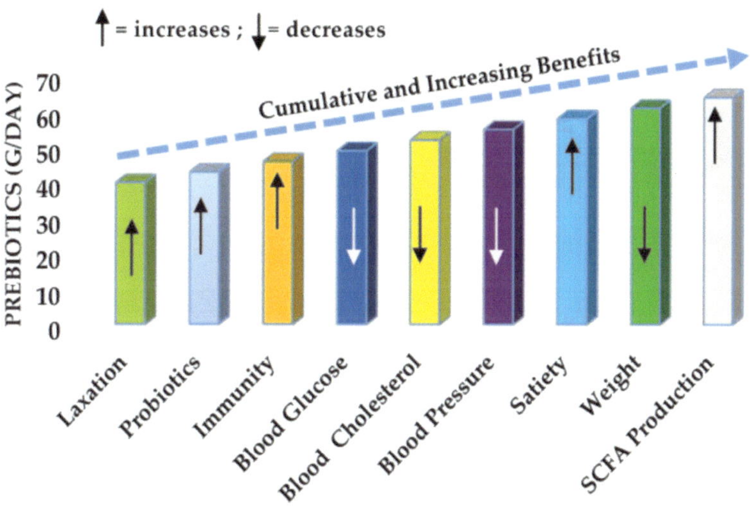

Figure 4. A classical model of the well-documented physiological and beneficial effects of adequate and continual intake of prebiotics in individuals.

Individual types of prebiotics, their beneficial roles, and additional characteristics are given in **Table 1**. Oligosaccharides (such as inulin and its derivatives), fructooligosaccharides (FOS), and others are some of the food ingredients recognized to meet the prebiotics' criteria. These low molecular weight carbohydrates naturally occur in artichokes, wheat, onions, chicory, garlic, leeks, and, to a lesser extent, in banana and cereals. Other oligosaccharides such as raffinose, stachyose, and verbascose are the major prebiotics in beans and peas. Interestingly, these simple molecules of soluble dietary fiber can be produced industrially, and more novel prebiotics continue to be developed as functional foods in the food industry (see **Table 2**). Various methods can be applied to produce prebiotics. These include an enzymatic method [e.g., galactooligosaccharides (GOS), FOS, and oligofructose]; extraction method (e.g., inulin and soy oligosaccharides from vegetable sources); chemical synthetic method (e.g., lactulose and polydextrose); and a combination of both chemical and enzymatic techniques (e.g., resistant maltodextrin). Inulin, GOS, and FOS, for instance, have been increasingly added to foods in many parts of the world. The practice started in Japan and some European countries a few decades ago. In Canada, pulses, peas, and others are acceptable in foods as "added fibers" and more ways to put prebiotics in different kinds of diets keep emerging with new technology.

Prebiotics	**Fermen tability**	**Primary source**	**Beneficial role‡**
Cellulose/hemicellulose/lignin/ waxes	Low	Plant foods	Laxation
Guar gum	High	Guar bean (legume)	Viscofier, blood lipid lowering, attenuates blood glucose response
Inulin/oligofructose/FOS	High	Chicory root, wheat, Jerusalem artichoke, banana, onions, leeks, garlic, can be synthesized from simple sugars	Prebiotic effects, calcium absorption, attenuates total cholesterol Rises HDL-cholesterol
Chitooligosaccharides (COS)	Low	Derivative of chitin	Rises HDL-cholesterol, attenuates total cholesterol
Galactooligosaccharide (GOS)	High	Human and cow's milk, synthesized from lactose	Prebiotic effects, calcium absorption, lipid profiles improvement
Xylooligosaccharides (XOS)	High	Corn cobs, rice hulls, straws, bagasse, malt cakes, and bran	Blood lipid lowering
Soybean oligosaccharides	High	Soybean	Blood lipid lowering, attenuates total cholesterol
β-Glucan and oat bran	High	Oats and barley	Blood lipid lowering, attenuates blood glucose response
Pectin, gums	High	Plant foods	Blood lipid lowering, attenuates blood glucose response, emulsifier, thickener
Polydextrose	High	Synthesized from dextrose (glucose)	Laxation, bulking agent, prebiotic effects
Psyllium	High	Psyllium husk (plant)	Laxation, blood lipid lowering

Prebiotics	Fermen tability	Primary source	Beneficial role[‡]
Resistant dextrin	High	Corn and wheat	Blood lipid lowering, attenuates blood glucose response
Resistant starch	Intermediate[†]	Plant foods	Laxation/fermentation
Soluble corn fiber	High	Corn	Laxation
Sialyllactoses (SLs)	High	Human milk	SCFA production, bifidogenic effect

† Most of the beneficial roles have been repeatedly confirmed by many authors in the literature and as the results of that, the references were neglected; † The classification of resistant starch has been a challenging task because it seems to be the only prebiotics that differs in individuals especially by means of the regulatory body controls (such as its mobility and amount of enzymes required) and, inhibitors also varied greatly. The source of resistant starch plays a significant role in its characterization as well.

Table 1. Individual prebiotics, their sources, and other properties.

Prebiotics	Manufacturer	Product name	Flavor and/or application
Inulin	Kraft	Cottage cheese	Plain, pineapple, mixed berry
Inulin	Attune	Wellness bars	Chocolate crisp, cool mint chocolate, blueberry vanilla, yogurt and granola strawberry bliss, yogurt and granola wild berry, and yogurt and granola lemon crème
Inulin	General mills	Yo-Plus yogurt	Strawberry, cherry, vanilla, peach
Inulin	Sensus, NL	Frutafit®	Applied in beverages, infant foods, confectionaries, ice creams, bakery products, and others
Inulin	Cosucra, B	Fibruline®	Tasteless, odorless, can be applied in beverages, confectionaries, bakery products, breakfast cereals, and others
Inulin	Orafti, B	Beneo®	Can be applied from beverages to baby food, from dairy to bakery, from confectionary to cereals and from soups to sauces
Oligo fructose	Sensus, NL	Frutalose®	Can be applied in beverages, infant foods, confectionaries, ice creams, bakery products, and many more
Oligo	Cosucra, B	Fibrulose®	Can be applied from beverages to baby food,

Prebiotics	Manufacturer	Product name	Flavor and/or application
fructose			from dairy to bakery, from confectionary to cereals and from soups to sauces
Oligo fructose	Orafti, B	Beneo	Can be applied from beverages to baby food, from dairy to bakery, from confectionary to cereals and from soups to sauces
GOS	Friesland Campina	Vivinal® GOS	For dairy products

Table 2. Samples of some of the prebiotic-enhanced foods available in the international market.

The Food scientists appear to be on the verge of being capable of manipulating the gut situations by diet control, thus possibly increasing an individual's health. It is also known that diets consisting of different components that are fermentable by gut microbiota are substrates for various kinds of probiotic bacteria in the gut. Moreover, the fact that minerals absorption and vitamin synthesis have been observed in the host confirms the symbiotic synergy of the prebiotics with probiotics in promoting health and suggests the existence of a multifunctional metabolism that directly involve a collective participation of many systems.

4. Prebioticious materials for encapsulation

Various kinds of prebiotics today are being processed into capsules (thickness: μm—mm) for the purpose of microencapsulating live and/or lysate probiotic cells. If both probiotic cells and prebiotics are combined, then the product becomes a synbiotic. Microencapsulation is the process by which viable and/or lysate probiotic cells are packed within a wall (an outer packaging) material for the purpose of shielding them from the surrounding environment. The standard load capacity of viable cells in the encapsulation materials varies from product to product. Usually, the viable cells occur at the concentration of 10^7–10^{12} CFU/g, while lysate cells are being measured in milligrams (mg). Most of the commercial yogurts or probiotic supplements contain 1–9 registered probiotic strains. In the case of multiple strains, the proportion of each probiotic strain in a package varies from batch to batch too. It is important to emphasize here that different combinations of probiotics are more likely to ferment all the prebiotics selectively and provide the host with the most significant needs. To achieve constant probiotical colonization in human or animal colon, microencapsulation is so far the best approach. Microencapsulation protects probiotics against O_2 toxicity [15], stomach's acid [16], and bile in the small intestines [16].

So far, the prebiotics in the make include oligofructose-enriched inulin [17], pullulan/starch-blended edible-films [18], denatured whey protein–alginate [19], alginate/chitosan/carboxy-methyl chitosan [20], resistant starch, carrageenan, chitosan, alginate, cellulose acetate phthalate, gellan gum, pectin, gum arabic, xanthan gum, guar gum, locust bean [21–23], starch/

spherulites [24, 25], and many others. Interestingly, a comparison was made between cocoa butter (lipid) and starch encapsulation materials, and a lipid system was found to be more effective at protecting the probiotics [25]. Whether the prebiotics are blended or used individually, they are all made to be harmonious mediators of probiotical or synbiotical microencapsulation. The selected materials (either oligomers or polymers) may also be used for the formation of microcapsules and body weight control in humans and animals. Moreover, high survival rates of encapsulated probiotics have been found in Cheddar cheese (6 months of storage period) [26] and in yogurt (4 weeks of storage period at 4°C [27].

5. Body weight management

All prebiotics appear to have a tremendous impact on body weight control in both animal models and humans. It has been found that the body fat in rats fed with a diet high in prebiotics was significantly lowered than the ones fed with a diet high in protein and control diet [28]. In similar studies on humans, it has also been shown that the increase in prebiotics intake was associated with weight loss due to a decrease in energy intake [11, 29]. Also, none of the polyols or sugar substitutes (sweeteners) were shown to have exerted any negative effect on the viability of the starter or probiotic cultures in cheese [30]. Apart from microencapsulation, it has also been indicated that the fat in cottage cheese provides some protection to the probiotics as they strive to survive the gastric and intestinal transit to confer health benefits in the terminal ileum and colon of the human GI tract [31]. Therefore, the inclusion of the adequate amount of prebiotics in every meal would be effective in controlling the current epidemic of overweight and few other digestion problems.

Noticeably, the speedy solution of weight control seems to be more in the lower fermentable prebiotics (such as lignin, waxes, cellulose, and hemicellulose) in combination with the probiotic strains which selectively favor them. Resistant starches are somewhat characterized between the lower and higher fermentability as part of the prebiotics (see Table 1). The prebiotics permitted in Canada include acacia gum, barley bran, oat bran, corn bran, β-glucan, fructooligosaccharide, galactooligosaccharide, inulin, modified wheat starch, oat hull fiber, partially hydrolyzed guar, pea hull fiber, polysaccharide complex (glucomannan, xanthan gum, sodium alginate), psyllium seed husk, sieved barley meal, sugar beet fiber, wheat bran, edible parts of traditional fruits, veggies, legumes, resistant maltodextrin (Fibersol-2), and many others [32].

6. SCFAs and monosaccharides homeostasis

Probiotics have been recognized to hydrolyze and selectively ferment prebiotics to generate the SCFAs and monosaccharides which can be absorbed and utilized as energy by the host. The three predominant SCFAs in the human gut are acetate, propionate, and butyrate. These have been reported with high levels in the colon. Propionate and butyrate are respectively utilized by the liver and colon, whereas acetate enters the systemic circulation and reaches the peripheral tissues [33]. Further literature highlights that the vast influence of these SCFAs on the host physiological benefits is through the nutri- and immuno-modulatory functions [34]. For example, butyrate expresses its potential in improving immune functions, intestinal barrier, and oxidative stress through silencing the histone deacetylation of nuclear factor kappa B (NF-κB), interferon-γ, peroxisome proliferator-activated receptor-γ (PPARγ), and glutathione-*S*-transferase (GST) [35].

It is well documented that the two endogenous ligands, G-protein coupled receptor 41 (GPR-41) and GPR-43 mediate the signaling actions of the SCFAs [36]. GPR-41 and GPR-43 are known proteins from the GPRs superfamily within the mammalian genome. They are particularly expressed in the adipocytes and identified as receptors for the fatty acids [37]. Acetate, preferentially, activates GPR-43 in vitro, whereas butyrate is more selective for GPR-41. Ordinarily, propionate displays most of the potent effect on both GPR-41 and GPR-43 [38]. It is important to highlight that GRP-41 has been associated more with a strong influence on the body weight and glucose homeostasis through increasing the enteroendocrine cell hormone known as peptide YY (PYY). The literature reported PYY as actually a key factor involved in energy homeostasis as well as in glucose metabolism [39, 40].

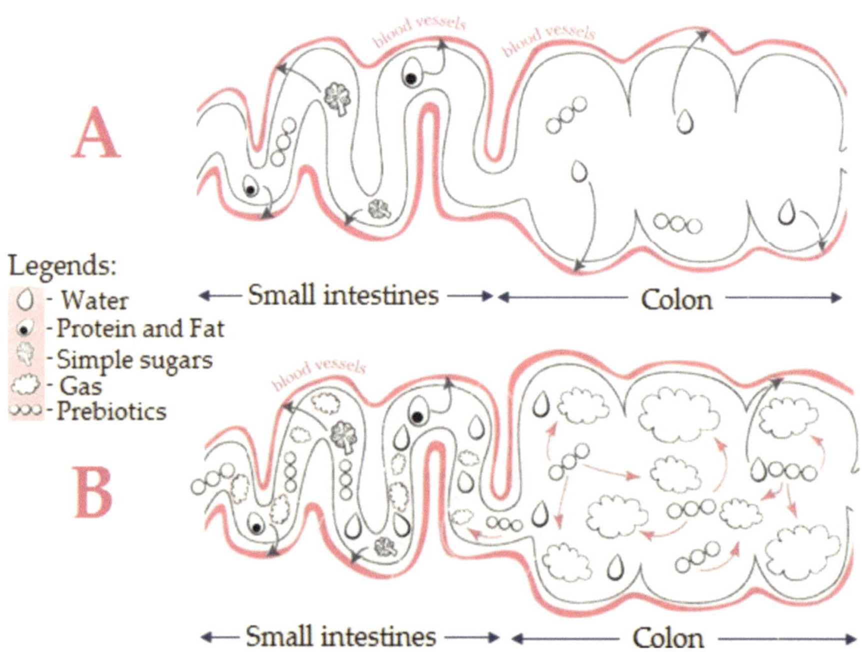

Figure 5. A represents a classical model of a normal digestion process; B represents a challenging digestion process due to an excessive intestinal fermentation of prebiotics. Source: Modified from Ref. [11].

Under a normal circumstance, the macronutrients are sensed in different parts of the small intestines. Also, the diverse types of gut hormones (such as PYY, cholecystokinin or CCK, and glucagon-like peptide-1 or GLP-1) control gastric emptying and the motility of food through the whole digestive tract. Gastric emptying is, in fact, the main controller of viscosity and the rate of nutrients delivery to the body. Up to now, no any in vitro technique can account for that sensation. A recent in vitro study revealed that some of the prebiotics (if not all) are slightly hydrolyzed—first in the stomach and small intestinal conditions—and then fermented in the colon [41]. In the same study, the SCFAs with lactate were synthesized and bifidobacterial population also significantly increased.

The GPR-43 as another sensor of metabolic homeostasis suppresses fat accumulation in the adipose tissue through insulin signaling pathway. Also, GPR-43 promotes the metabolism of unincorporated lipids and glucose in other tissues [40]. Apart from the amounts and proportions of those SCFAs during the fermentation stage of prebiotics, probiotics also simultaneously play other physiological benefits. Those include the balance of microbiological changes, locations of fermentation, and rates of fermentation for each prebiotic, locations of gas production, and pH changes throughout the digestion process. Naturally, all these parameters are difficult to measure in a real life situation. The batch systems which have been used in many experiments do not reflect the true interactions of a synbiotic community (combination of probiotics and prebiotics) in the host.

7. Implications of excessive bacteria and highly fermentable prebiotics in the small intestines

Probiotics too should be able to provide health benefits when administered in sufficient quantity. However, the recent data support that, beyond prebiotics being able to meet the nutritional benefits, options of food selection also may regulate various functions in the body and may play detrimental or beneficial roles in some diseases. For the prebiotics to meet the beneficial dietary effects, their fermentability status in the colon plays a significant role, especially to the commensal bacteria when all start to compete for nutrients. For example, flatulence is often a complaint when large doses of FOS are taken, which suggest that perhaps there is a tolerance limit for each prebiotics. Additionally, an overgrowth of bacteria in the small intestines (including those that for some reasons migrated from the colon) may cause digestion problems and poor overall health [11].

Figure 5(B) represents an example of excessive intestinal prebiotics fermentation. Here, it can be observed that the excess bacteria in the small intestines may result in the fermentation of undigested carbohydrates (starches and oligosaccharides) before being metabolized. Then again, some of the prebiotics may absorb much water from the rest of the body into the small intestine through osmosis, which can result in watery diarrhea. Fermentation of the undigested carbohydrates in the small intestine and an excessive fermentation of prebiotics in the colon create gas. When this happens, the pressure from an abnormal amount of gas inside the small intestine and colon, respectively, can cause bloating, abnormal pain, flatulence, diarrhea, or even constipation [11].

Unlike in the colon, excess gasses generated by excess bacteria in the small intestine cannot be easily expelled by passing it out and so the result is bloating. Apparently, if the excess bacteria produce methane (CH_3), this gas tells the intestines to move upwards, causing the content in the intestine to stall or to back up. In contrast, hydrogen (H_2) gas in the small intestines is associated with diarrhea. Furthermore, the unabsorbed monosaccharides in the small intestines can result in osmotic responses [11]. Another author has reported that about 84% of people with irritable bowel syndrome (IBS) have a bacterial overgrowth in the small intestine [42]. So, if this estimate is correct, people who complain of bloating, flatulence, diarrhea, or constipation are encouraged to take probiotics at appropriate doses to balance the intestinal bacterial structure, content viscosity, and to restore the beneficial and physiological activities in the intestines. Just like prebiotics, probiotics is as important as multi-vitamins and multi-minerals too, and all should be taken daily.

Figure 5(A) represents a normal process of digestion with balanced gut flora. Here, proteins, fats, and monosaccharides (such as glucose, fructose, and galactose) are absorbed from the small intestines, while water is absorbed from the colon into the bloodstream. The unabsorbed prebiotics (cellulose, hemicellulose, polyols, fructans, galactans, and others) do not cause any problem. Thus, diet control can be used to favor the growth of some selected gut inhabitants [43].

It is necessary to state here that the small intestines are a mysterious and largely inaccessible part of the body. Endoscopy tests are reported to have only shown about 60 cm of what is exactly happening inside of that part of the GI tract. Besides, a colonoscopy that goes through the rectum also shows extremely little of the other end of the small intestine. Therefore, it would be wise for individuals to ingest strong probiotic bacteria that survive and transit the stomach acid and bile salts during the digestion process. As discussed earlier on, the use of prebioticious materials for probiotic microencapsulation appears to be one of the best practices, and other similar kinds of materials continue to be developed. Usually, the probiotics that pass through the small intestine will meet on other extreme the commensal bacteria that migrated from the colon before they start prebiotic fermentation and compete for the nutrients (usually the monosaccharides) meant for assimilation by the host in a synergetic manner.

8. Conclusion

Prebiotics, either as occurring naturally in fruits, grain products, roughages, vegetables, legumes, soy, nuts, other foods or as added fibers, they all provide the physiological and/or beneficial effects in a symbiotic relationship with probiotics. Whole grains are not prebiotics. Both whole and refined grains need to be enriched with the prebiotics to meet the estimated daily requirement of 35–50 g/day. The benefits of dietary prebiotics are cumulative and increase with an increasing intake of the prebiotics in combination with the multi-vitamins, multi-minerals, and probiotic strains. While probiotic bacteria are easily found in capsules as dietary adjuncts, the consumers are also advised to opt for foods which provide more prebiotics for the overall health. Each prebiotic appears to have its tolerance limit. Beyond such a

http://dx.doi.org/10.5772/64091

tolerance limit, metabolism problems might occur. Diets consisting of different fermentable prebiotics are substrates for different probiotics in the gut. Furthermore, more evidence about the SCFAs to have a relationship with better health in the host has been provided. Extra care must also be taken into account when dealing probiotics and prebiotics relationship because the action of excess commensal bacteria in the small intestine may be detrimental in some disease. The involvement of excess anaerobic bacteria in the small intestine leads to prebiotic fermentation of which should only take place in the large intestines.

Acknowledgements

We are grateful to Ms. Dajana Pemac and the entire staff of InTech for helpful advice and the opportunity given to us to express our views. All the speakers on the Food, Health, & Nutrition Track at the Annual IFT Meetings, Chicago Ill., 2013 & 2015, are also gratefully acknowledged.

Author details

Nditange Shigwedha[1*], Penny Hiwilepo-Van Hal[2], Li Jia[3], Liubov Sichel[4] and Shuang Zhang[5]

*Address all correspondence to: nditange@gmail.com

1 School of Food Science and Engineering, Harbin Institute of Technology, Harbin, China

2 Department of Food Science and Technology, University of Namibia, Windhoek, Namibia

3 Wyeth-Nutrition, Suzhou, China

4 Pure Research Products LLC, Boulder, USA

5 Food College, Northeast Agricultural University, Harbin, China

References

[1] AACCI. The Definition of Dietary Fiber. 2001. Available from: http://www.aaccnet.org/initiatives/definitions/pages/dietaryfiber.aspx. [Accessed 2016-02-08]

[2] Gibson GR, McCartney AL. Modification of the gut flora by dietary means. Biochem. Soc. Trans. 1998;26(2):222–8. doi:10.1042/bst0260222

[3] Glenn GR, Roberfroid MB. Dietary modulation of the human colonic microbiota: introducing the concept of prebiotics. J. Nutr. 1995;125:1401–12.

[4] Gibson GR, Probert HM, Van Loo J, Rastall RA, Roberfroid MB. Dietary modulation of the human colonic microbiota: updating the concept of prebiotics. Nutr. Res. Rev. 2004;17(02):259–75. doi:10.1079/NRR200479

[5] Gibson GR, Scott KP, Rastall RA, Tuohy KM, Hotchkiss A, Dubert-Ferrandon A, Gareau M, Murphy EF, Saulnier D, Loh G, Macfarlane S. Dietary prebiotics: current status and new definition. Food Sci. Technol. Bull. Funct. Foods. 2010;7:1–9. doi:10.1616/1476-2137.15880

[6] Shigwedha N, Zhang L, Sichel L, Jia L, Gong P, Liu W, Wang S, Zhang S, Han X, Gao W. More than a few LAB alleviate common allergies: impact of paraprobiotics in comparison to probiotical live cells. J. Biosci. Med. 2014;2(03):56–64. doi:10.4236/jbm.2014.23008

[7] FDA. The Scoop on Whole Grains. 2009. http://www.fda.gov/ForConsumers/ConsumerUpdates/ucm151902.htm. Accessed 2016-02-08

[8] USDA/ARS. Food Surveys Research Group, NHANES 2009–2010. 2010. http://www.ars.usda.gov/research/projects/projects.htm?ACCN_NO=415257. Accessed 2016-02-08

[9] Cleveland LE, Moshfegh AJ, Albertson AM, Goldman JD. Dietary intake of whole grains. J. Am. Coll. Nutr. 2000;19(sup3):331S–8S.

[10] Jia L, Shigwedha N, Mwandemele OD. Use of D_{acid}-, D_{bile}-, z_{acid}-, and z_{bile}-values in evaluating bifidobacteria with regard to stomach pH and bile salt sensitivity. J. Food Sci. 2010;75(1):M14–8. doi:10.1111/j.1750-3841.2009.01398.x

[11] Jacob A. Digestive health with REAL food: a practical guide to an anti-inflammatory, nutrient dense diet for IBS and other digestive issues. In: Sylvester R, editor. Paleo Media Group, Bend; 2013. 396 p.

[12] Shigwedha N, Sichel L, Al-Shura AN, Zhang L, Jia L. Probiotics, paraprobiotics, and probiotical cell fragments (PCFs) as crisis management tools for important health problems. AASCIT J. Med. 2015;1(1):1–9. http://www.aascit.org/journal/archive2?journalId=979&paperId=1746

[13] Salminen S, Isolauri E. Intestinal colonization, microbiota, and probiotics. J. Pediatrics. 2006;149(5):S115–20. doi:10.1016/j.jpeds.2006.06.062

[14] Shigwedha N, Sichel L, Jia L, Zhang L. Probiotical cell fragments (PCFs) as "Novel Nutraceutical Ingredients". J. Biosci. Med. 2014;2(03):43–55. doi:10.4236/jbm.2014.23007

[15] Talwalkar A, Kailasapathy K. Effect of microencapsulation on oxygen toxicity in probiotic bacteria. Aust. J. Dairy Technol. 2003;58(1):36.

[16] Chandramouli V, Kailasapathy K, Peiris P, Jones M. An improved method of microencapsulation and its evaluation to protect *Lactobacillus* spp. in simulated gastric conditions. J. Microbiol. Methods. 2004;56(1):27–35. doi:10.1016/j.mimet.2003.09.002

[17] Fritzen-Freire CB, Prudêncio ES, Amboni RD, Pinto SS, Negrão-Murakami AN, Murakami FS. Microencapsulation of bifidobacteria by spray drying in the presence of prebiotics. Food Res. Int. 2012;45(1):306–12. doi:10.1016/j.foodres.2011.09.020

[18] Kanmani P, Lim ST. Development and characterization of novel probiotic-residing pullulan/starch edible films. Food Chem. 2013;141(2):1041–9. doi:10.1016/j.foodchem.2013.03.103

[19] Rajam R, Karthik P, Parthasarathi S, Joseph GS, Anandharamakrishnan C. Effect of whey protein–alginate wall systems on survival of microencapsulated *Lactobacillus plantarum* in simulated gastrointestinal conditions. J. Funct. Foods. 2012;4(4):891–8. doi:10.1016/j.jff.2012.06.006

[20] Li XY, Chen XG, Sun ZW, Park HJ, Cha DS. Preparation of alginate/chitosan/carboxymethyl chitosan complex microcapsules and application in *Lactobacillus casei* ATCC 393. Carbohydr Polymers. 2011;83(4):1479–85. doi:10.1016/j.carbpol.2010.09.053

[21] Wolfe LA. Encapsulation of probiotic bacteria in a water-in-solid-fat emulsion to promote acid resistance [Thesis]. The Pennsylvania State University, University Park, PA; 2012.

[22] Brinques GB, Ayub MA. Effect of microencapsulation on survival of *Lactobacillus plantarum* in simulated gastrointestinal conditions, refrigeration, and yogurt. J. Food Eng. 2011;103(2):123–8. doi:10.1016/j.jfoodeng.2010.10.006

[23] Ding WK, Shah NP. Acid, bile, and heat tolerance of free and microencapsulated probiotic bacteria. J. Food Sci. 2007;72(9):M446–50. doi:10.1111/j.1750-3841.2007.00565.x

[24] Chittiprolu S. Effect of starch spherulites on survival of bifidobacteria in the presence of acid or bile [Thesis]. The Pennsylvania State University, University Park, PA; 2009.

[25] Lahtinen SJ, Ouwehand AC, Salminen SJ, Forssell P, Myllärinen P. Effect of starch-and lipid-based encapsulation on the culturability of two *Bifidobacterium longum* strains. Lett. Appl. Microbiol. 2007;44(5):500–5. doi:10.1111/j.1472-765X.2007.02110.x

[26] Darukaradhya J. Enumeration and survival studies of free and encapsulated *Lactobacillus acidophilus* and *Bifidobacterium lactis* in Cheddar cheese [Thesis]. NSW: University of Western Sydney; 2005.

[27] Krasaekoopt W, Bhandari B, Deeth H. Survival of microencapsulated probiotics in high-solids yogurt from UHT milk. Aust. J. Dairy Technol. 2003;58(2):195.

[28] Reimer RA, Maurer AD, Eller LK, Hallam MC, Shaykhutdinov R, Vogel HJ, Weljie AM. Satiety hormone and metabolomic response to an intermittent high energy diet differs

in rats consuming long-term diets high in protein or prebiotic fiber. J. Proteome Res. 2012;11(8):4065–74. doi:10.1021/pr300487s

[29] Slavin J. Fiber and prebiotics: mechanisms and health benefits. Nutrients. 2013;5(4): 1417–35. doi:10.3390/nu5041417

[30] Esmerino EA, Cruz AG, Pereira EP, Rodrigues JB, Faria JA, Bolini HM. The influence of sweeteners in probiotic Petit Suisse cheese in concentrations equivalent to that of sucrose. J. Dairy Sci. 2013;96(9):5512–21. doi:10.3168/jds.2013-6616

[31] Abadía-García L, Cardador A, del Campo ST, Arvízu SM, Castaño-Tostado E, Regalado-González C, García-Almendarez B, Amaya-Llano SL. Influence of probiotic strains added to cottage cheese on generation of potentially antioxidant peptides, anti-listerial activity, and survival of probiotic microorganisms in simulated gastrointestinal conditions. Int. Dairy J. 2013;33(2):191–7. doi:10.1016/j.idairyj.2013.04.005

[32] Canadian Food Inspection Agency. Carbohydrates—elements within the nutrition facts table 2014. Available from: http://www.inspection.gc.ca. [Accessed 2016-02-08].

[33] Lin HV, Frassetto A, Kowalik Jr EJ, Nawrocki AR, Lu MM, Kosinski JR, Hubert JA, Szeto D, Yao X, Forrest G, Marsh DJ. Butyrate and propionate protect against diet-induced obesity and regulate gut hormones via free fatty acid receptor 3-independent mechanisms. PLoS One. 2012;7(4):e35240. doi:10.1371/journal.pone.0035240

[34] Sun Y, O'Riordan MX. Regulation of bacterial pathogenesis by intestinal short-chain fatty acids. Adv. Appl. Microbiol. 2013;85:93–118. doi:10.1016/B978-0-12-407672-3.00003-4

[35] Leonel AJ, Alvarez-Leite JI. Butyrate: implications for intestinal function. Curr. Opin. Clin. Nutr. Metab. Care. 2012;15(5):474–9. doi:10.1097/MCO.0b013e32835665fa

[36] Brown AJ, Goldsworthy SM, Barnes AA, Eilert MM, Tcheang L, Daniels D, Muir AI, Wigglesworth MJ, Kinghorn I, Fraser NJ, Pike NB. The Orphan G protein-coupled receptors GPR41 and GPR43 are activated by propionate and other short chain carboxylic acids. J. Biol. Chem. 2003;278(13):11312–9. doi:10.1074/jbc.M211609200

[37] Ge H, Li X, Weiszmann J, Wang P, Baribault H, Chen JL, Tian H, Li Y. Activation of G protein-coupled receptor 43 in adipocytes leads to inhibition of lipolysis and suppression of plasma free fatty acids. Endocrinology. 2008;149(9):4519–26. doi:10.1210/en.2008-0059

[38] Le Poul E, Loison C, Struyf S, Springael JY, Lannoy V, Decobecq ME, Brezillon S, Dupriez V, Vassart G, Van Damme J, Parmentier M. Functional characterization of human receptors for short chain fatty acids and their role in polymorphonuclear cell activation. J. Biol. Chem. 2003;278(28):25481–9. doi:10.1074/jbc.M301403200

[39] Samuel BS, Shaito A, Motoike T, Rey FE, Backhed F, Manchester JK, Hammer RE, Williams SC, Crowley J, Yanagisawa M, Gordon JI. Effects of the gut microbiota on host adiposity are modulated by the short-chain fatty-acid binding G protein-coupled

receptor, Gpr41. Proc. Natl. Acad. Sci. 2008;105(43):16767–72. doi:10.1073/pnas.0808567105

[40] Kimura I, Ozawa K, Inoue D, Imamura T, Kimura K, Maeda T, Terasawa K, Kashihara D, Hirano K, Tani T, Takahashi T. The gut microbiota suppresses insulin-mediated fat accumulation via the short-chain fatty acid receptor GPR43. Nat. Commun. 2013;4:1829. doi:10.1038/ncomms2852

[41] Moon JS, Joo W, Ling L, Choi HS, Han NS. In vitro digestion and fermentation of sialyllactoses by infant gut microflora. J. Funct. Foods. 2016;21:497–506. doi:10.1016/j.jff.2015.12.002

[42] Pimentel M. A New IBS Solution. 2005. http://anewibssolution.com. Accessed 2016-02-08

[43] Umu ÖC, Oostindjer M, Pope PB, Svihus B, Egelandsdal B, Nes IF, Diep DB. Potential applications of gut microbiota to control human physiology. Antonie Van Leeuwenhoek. 2013;104(5):609–18. doi:10.1007/s10482-013-0008-0

Chapter 4

Lactobacillus reuteri, Infant Allergy Prevention and Childhood Immune Maturation

Anna Forsberg

Additional information is available at the end of the chapter

http://dx.doi.org/10.5772/63120

Abstract

The increasing allergy prevalence in affluent countries may be caused by reduced microbial stimulation, resulting in an abnormal postnatal immune maturation. This chapter concerns the theories behind the use of probiotics in randomized prevention trials, and how this supplementation affects the immunity of pregnant women, the immune development in their children, and possibly preventing allergic diseases. Most studies investigating the underlying mechanisms have focused on postnatal microbial exposure. An increasing body of evidence from studies suggests that the maternal microbial environment during pregnancy can program the immune development of the child. In human allergy intervention studies, probiotic supplementation to the mother during pregnancy, as well as to her baby postnatally, may be important for preventive effects. Also, prenatal environmental exposures may alter gene expression via epigenetic mechanisms, aiming to induce physiological adaptations to the anticipated postnatal environment. The maternal microbial environment during pregnancy may program the immune development of the child.

Keywords: allergy, immune maturation, *Lactobacillus reuteri*, probiotics, allergy prevention, allergens, TLRs, cytokines, chemokines

1. Probiotics in allergy prevention

Different probiotic strains have been used in allergy prevention trials with successful and unsuccessful results. Why use probiotics to try and prevent childhood allergic diseases then? The increasing allergy prevalence in affluent countries may be caused by reduced microbial stimulation, reflecting an abnormal postnatal immune maturation [1], resulting in allergic diseases in children. Of course, this is a multifactorial problem where changing climate, living conditions, and urbanization have led to a biodiversity loss. Studies show altered microbiota and general microbial deprivation which characterize people living in urban affluent environments. Consequently, this seems to be a risk factor for immune dysregulation and impaired immune tolerance. It is further enhanced by physical inactivity and a western diet poor in fresh fruit and vegetables, which may act in synergy with dysbiosis of the gut flora [2]. Probiotics may be one way to increase microbial stimulation, enrich the gut flora and balance a skewed immune system, which will be discussed later.

2. A brief introduction to childhood allergic diseases

The cost of allergic diseases is burdening the society; reduced life quality and increased sick leave are common, asthma in children is one of the most common chronic diseases affecting children at an early age. About 20% of the population is affected by allergic disease such as atopic dermatitis, food allergy, asthma, allergic rhinitis, and conjunctivitis [3]. Furthermore, the "atopic march," as commonly referred to, is an age-associated variation in allergy-related symptoms in childhood. The first allergy-related symptoms are often eczema and food allergy at a young age, later followed by asthma and rhinoconjunctivitis in school-aged children. In addition to the age variation in allergic diseases, there seems to be a gender issue as well. Boys early in life have a higher incidence of allergic diseases than girls [4–6] and are also more susceptible to infections maybe due to the more Th2-deviated immunity [4, 5]. Females are characterized by increased inflammatory responses and infections clearance, possibly reflecting the stronger Th1 immunity observed in girls [4, 5]. Of course, this has its pros and cons. This results not only in a better protection against infection but also in increased susceptibility to autoimmunity later in life. Allergy-related sex differences diminish at puberty; at adult age, no clear sex differences concerning allergy can be found [7].

3. The importance of the environment and the discovery of the beneficial effect of exposure to microbes

In the beginning, when elucidating the mechanism behind the increasing rates of allergic diseases, the focus was on living conditions. In 1989, a researcher named Strachan discovered that there was an association between siblings, family size, and hay fever [8]. This led to discoveries that children born in a farm had less allergies than children born in urban areas. The step after that was to focus on postnatal microbial exposure [9–12]. How infants are prepared for life outside the uterus, and how can the maternal environment be protective against allergic development in the offspring? The maternal microbial environment has been proposed to be able to program the immune development of the child, during pregnancy [13]. Especially, if the mother is exposed to farm environment, in particular during pregnancy, development of allergic diseases seems to be attenuated. Interestingly, research has showed that exposure later in life, after pregnancy and later, seems to have a weaker effect [14, 15] which opens up several other questions. For example, is it possible to program the development of immunity in the child? When is the "window of opportunity"? Can we manipulate this and protect the child against the development of diseases? How can this be done? Numerous studies show that exposure to farm environments during infancy and even in fetal life [16, 17] reduces the incidence of allergic diseases. Furthermore, a recent report in Sweden presents data that contact with farm animals or dogs during childhood may protect against asthma development [18]. Exposures to farming areas and also consumption of raw milk have been associated with the upregulation of certain receptors associated with innate immunity. In the Protection Against Allergy: Study in Rural Environments (PASTURE) birth cohort study, 1133 pregnant women were recruited in rural areas of Austria, Finland, France, Germany, and Switzerland and showed that farming-related exposures, such as raw farm milk consumption, that were previously reported to decrease the risk for allergic outcomes, were associated with a change in gene expression of innate immunity receptors in early life. Raw milk of course includes many Lactobacilli strains among others. Therefore, it is believed that microbial exposure in early life educates the developing immune system, driving postnatal maturation of immune regulation as discussed in [19]. The author also suggests that the theory should be referred to as "microbial deprivation hypothesis" since the exposure to a wealth of commensal, non-pathogenic microorganisms early in life is of benefit. The epidemiological studies are supported by animal models, demonstrating that microbial exposure during gestation can prevent allergic responses in the offspring [20, 21].

3.1. Animal models show the benefit of microbial exposure during gestation

The beneficial effect of exposure to microbes have been further explored, primarily in animal models, to try to pinpoint what the mechanism on immune tolerance and protection of allergic disease might be. Of importance is the maternal environment, suggesting that maternal immunity may be transferred or at least influence the offspring. In experimental murine models, the mother is treated with lipopolysaccharide which attenuated allergic disease and associated inflammation in offspring [22–24]. One study explored the effect of LPS on female BALB/c mice before conception and during pregnancy. Several weeks after birth offspring were sensitized to ovalbumin (OVA) followed by aerosol allergen challenges. LPS may operate in prenatal life in order to modulate the development of allergies in the offspring since LPS exposure prenatally enhanced Th1-associated IFN-gamma in offspring. OVA sensitization was followed with a reduction in anti-OVA IgG1 and IgE as well as unchanged IgG2a antibody responses, accompanied by a significant decrease in Th2-associated cytokine levels. This was followed by a reduction of eosinophils and macrophages in bronchoalveolar lavage fluids, which are often increased in allergic airways. However, clinical manifestations such as airway hyper-responsiveness, a hallmark of bronchial asthma, were not affected [22]. Another study also investigated the effect of LPS on pregnant mice and further explored the effect of LPS on the offspring before allergen sensitization with OVA. Prenatal and postnatal LPS exposure suppressed allergen-specific IgE production, eosinophilic airway inflammation and *in vivo* airway reactivity in response to methacholine. The suppression of allergen-mediated inflammatory responses was associated with an increased shift toward Th1 responses in culture (spleen cells) and may be mediated via Toll-like receptor (TLR) and T-bet expression by lung tissues [23]. Another group used a rat model and investigated the effect of prenatal LPS exposure on postnatal T cell differentiation and experimental allergic airway disease. The expression of T cell-related transcription factors and cytokines was quantified in the lung, and airway hyper responsiveness was measured. Prenatal LPS exposure induced a Th1 immune milieu in the offspring of rats and also reduced OVA-induced airway inflammation, eosinophilia, and airway responsiveness [21].

The next step was to use the commensal *Acinetobacter lwoffii* [20]. *Acinetobacter lwoffii* is derived from cow shed and is non-pathogenic. The strain was used in an experimental allergic airway inflammation mouse model. Maternal intranasal exposure to *A. lwoffi* F78 protected the offspring from development of allergic disease and resulted in an induction of proinflammatory cytokines and upregulation of TLRs. On the contrary, suppression of TLRs was observed in placental tissue. To investigate if TLRs were of importance, a knockout mice was used (TLR2/3/4/7/9(-/-). In that model, the asthma-preventive effect was completely eliminated. Additionally, the mild local and systemic inflammatory response was also absent in these *A. lwoffii* F78-exposed mothers. Therefore, it is believed that there is a direct relationship between maternal bacterial exposures, functional maternal TLR signaling and asthma protection in the progeny. The main receptors for bacterial products are the TLRs. Farm studies have also shown that these receptors can be upregulated in neonates after maternal contact with farm animals and after farm-related exposures [14, 25, 26]. One study investigated both atopic sensitization and the gene expression of receptors of innate immunity (TLRs), and how they were related to maternal exposure to stables during pregnancy. A dose-response relation was found between the upregulation of these genes and the number of different farm animal species the mother had encountered during pregnancy. Interestingly, it seemed like each additional farm animal species increased the expression of TLR2, TLR4, and CD14 [14]. In another study, it was also shown that gene expression of innate immunity receptors in cord blood was overall higher in neonates of farmers, significantly so for TLR7 and TLR8. The study further enhanced the fact that farming-related exposures, such as raw farm milk consumption, that were previously reported to decrease the risk for allergic outcomes was associated with a change in gene expression of innate immunity receptors in early life [26].

3.1.1. Toll-like receptors in the immune system

TLRs are included in the innate immune system and belong to the group of pattern recognition receptors (PRRs) which recognize the so-called pathogen-associated molecular patterns (PAMPs). These are evolutionarily conserved structures from bacteria, viruses, parasites and fungi. The PRRs are expressed on a wide variety of immune cells as well as mucosal and epithelial cells. Some subgroups of the PRRs include TLRs, NOD-like receptors (NLRs), RIG-1-like receptors (RLRs), β-glucan receptors, and other C-type lectins.

3.2. Microbial exposure to counteract the Th2 skewing in allergic diseases?

Continued enhanced postnatal microbial exposure may be required for optimal allergy protection, however [15]. A reduced microbial pressure could result in insufficient induction of T cells with regulatory and/or Th1-like properties which counteract allergy-inducing Th2 responses [16, 17, 27, 28]. Farm exposures during pregnancy increase the number and function of cord blood Treg cells associated with lower Th2 cytokine secretion and lymphocyte

http://dx.doi.org/10.5772/63120

proliferation. Cord blood Treg cell counts were increased, with maternal farming exposures and associated with higher FOXP3 and higher lymphocyte activation gene 3 (Ppg) expressions. Furthermore, Treg cell function was more efficient, and FOXP3 demethylation in offspring of mothers with farm milk exposure was increased, possibly reflecting an increased immune regulatory capacity [17]. Also, failure to upregulate the interferon gamma (IFNγ) response during infancy is an important determinant of the risk of allergic disease. Early life exposure has also been associated with decreased IFNγ gene expression of naïve T cells [28]. Allergic diseases are known to be dependent on Th2 responses to allergens, and microbial stimulation may be one way to deviate a skewed Th2-associated immunity to a more Th1/Treg-associated response. The immune system is generally divided into the innate and adaptive arm. The first line of defense is the innate immunity which responds rapidly to common components of bacteria, viruses, parasites and fungi, structures preserved through evolution, such as pathogen-associated molecular patterns (PAMPs). The innate immune system includes physical barriers of the mucosa, the epithelial cell layer, as well as cell responding immediately with phagocytosis of microorganisms, extinction of infected cells, and cooperation with adaptive immunity. The PRRs are expressed on various cells of the immune system such as monocytes, macrophages, DC, natural killer cells, innate lymphoid cells as well as mucosal epithelial and endothelial cells. The adaptive immune system requires longer time to develop but is more specific and can develop memory to encounter antigens. The adaptive part, on the contrary, consists of T and B lymphocytes and a rich and specific antibody repertoire.

The key players in adaptive immunity may be the CD4+ T helper (Th) cells that have a central role by orchestrating immune responses to pathogens. As naïve cells they exit the thymus. Th cells may differentiate into four major effector subsets, Th1, Th2, Th17, and Treg cells. Microbial stimulation of DC leads to secretion of cytokines, such as IL-10 and the proinflammatory IL-12 as well as upregulation of co-stimulatory molecules. It has been suggested that different species of Lactobacillus exert very different DC activation patterns and, furthermore, at least one species may be capable of inhibiting activities of other species in the genus [29]. DCs are also able to attract cells via secretion of chemokines, for example, Th2 cells are attracted by the secretion of CCL17 and CCL18 and CCL22. There are two major DC populations in blood, mainly characterized by their different TLR receptor expression and different function, the myeloid-derived DCs and the plasmacytoid DCs. Surface expression of CD antigens also distinguish them from each other, both subtypes lack the common lineage markers but express HLA-DR for antigen presentation [30].

4. Probiotics and immune regulation

Probiotics have been defined as "live microorganisms which when ingested in adequate amounts confer a beneficial effect on the host" [31]. Probiotics to prevent allergic disease have gained much attention. Contacts with microbial organisms from the environment [8] and at mucosal sites, such as the gut [32, 33], may be essential in the induction of T regulatory cells after birth and have a beneficial effect on infant gut flora. The intestinal flora may vary between allergic and non-allergic infants. Also, allergic disease among children may be associated with differences in their intestinal microflora as evident in two countries with a low (Estonia) and a high (Sweden) prevalence of allergy. Differences in the indigenous intestinal flora might affect the development and priming of the immune system in early childhood. In one study [33], feces samples were diluted and cultured and the allergic. The allergic children in Estonia and Sweden were less often colonized with lactobacilli. When comparing allergic and non-allergic infants in Sweden, it was shown that there were differences in the composition of the gut microbiota before clinical manifestations. In comparison with healthy infants, babies who developed allergy were less often colonized with enterococci during the first month of life and with bifidobacteria during the first year of life. Furthermore, allergic infants had higher counts of clostridia at 3 months, *Staphylococcus aureus* at 6 months, whereas the counts of Bacteroides were lower at 12 months [32]. Possibly probiotics and prebiotics may modulate the composition of the gut flora in a healthy way.

It has also been suggested that certain strains of probiotic bacteria can induce immunoregulation by modulating dendritic cells and induce Tregs [12, 34–36]. A mixture of probiotics (a combination, or selectively, of *L. acidophilus, L. casei, Lactobacillus reuteri, Bifidobacterium bifidium,* and *Streptococcus thermophilus)* was found to upregulate $CD4^{+}Foxp3^{+}$ regulatory T cells (Tregs). The administration of the probiotics mixture in mice models induced both T cell and B cell hyporesponsiveness and downregulated Th1, Th2, and Th17 cytokines and generated Tregs with increased suppressor activity [12]. In another study [34], BALB/c mice were treated daily with *L. reuteri* by gavage which also increased Tregs with a great capacity to supress T effector cells [34]. O´Mahony and colleagues showed that ingestion with a probiotic strain enhanced the clearance of pathogens via the generation and function of Tregs that control excessive NFκB [35]. Lactobacilli species may have different properties to induce Tregs [36]. The intestine provides a unique environment for the development of both immunity and tolerance, and the initiated immune response is dependent on DC type and state of activation. The probiotic supplementation during pregnancy and early childhood could possibly provide microbial stimulation needed for normal development of immunoregulatory capacity, providing a source of TLR-ligand exposure [37, 38].

4.1. Treg cells in immunity

In addition to conventional Th cells, CD4+ T cells can also differentiate into T regulatory cells (Tregs) that are not only essential for the regulation of inflammatory responses to pathogens but also for peripheral tolerance and the protection against autoimmune diseases. There are two main types of Treg cells, thymic Tregs (also called natural) are generated in the thymus and are believed to protect against self-reactive immune responses, and peripheral Treg cells (also called inducible) that are generated in peripheral tissues and may have specificity to self- and foreign antigens. FoxP3 is a key transcription factor for the development and function of natural CD4+ regulatory T cells. As other cells, different subpopulations can be defined within the FoxP3-positive cells. The first definition of Treg cells is the CD4dimCD25hiFoxP3+ Treg cells, described in [39]. Later on, CD45RA+FoxP3lo resting Treg cells (rTreg cells) and CD45RA-FoxP3hi-activated Treg cells (aTreg cells) were discovered; both subtypes seem to be suppressive in vitro. In company of these subsets, the cytokine-secreting CD45RA-FoxP3lo non-suppressive T cells were defined. Terminally differentiated aTreg cells rapidly died, whereas rTreg cells proliferated and converted into aTreg cells in vitro and in vivo. Taken together, the dissection of FoxP3+ cells into subsets enables one to analyze Treg cell differentiation dynamics and interactions in normal and disease states, and to control immune responses through manipulating particular FoxP3+ subpopulations [40].

In allergic diseases, the Th1/Th2 paradigm is useful, but it is obviously a simplification. Treg cells are important in the suppression of allergen-specific responses in several ways [41].

5. *Lactobacillus reuteri*

Lactobacillus reuteri is an obligate heterofermative [42] Gram positive rod that has been isolated from the GI tract in several mammals, including humans, as well as from different food products [43, 44]. In addition to glycerol, *L. reuteri* produce the antimicrobial metabolite reuterin during anaerobic conditions [45]. The strain *L. reuteri* ATCC 55730 is considered to be safe, and in the USA, probiotics has started getting regulated in a similar way as pharmaceuticals [46].

6. Probiotics in human allergy prevention trials

Probiotics have been used in intervention studies with preventive effects on eczema during infancy with varying results. [47–52]. Different study design, probiotic strain, duration of follow up, etc. have resulted in different outcomes. However, there seems to be a benefit in supplementing with probiotics in prevention of childhood eczema. Randomized placebo controlled trial to prevent childhood eczema have been conducted since the first study in 2001 [53]. One of the main questions to answer is to whom you may supplement. Studies have been conducted with different modes of supplementation, supplementing only mothers during gestation, only mothers during breastfeeding, only infants after delivery or both mothers during gestation and infants after delivery [54]. Probiotic supplementation to the mother during pregnancy, as well as to her baby postnatally, may be important for preventive effects on childhood allergic disease [55]. Thus, a preventive effect on atopic eczema, the most common allergic disease at this age, has primarily been demonstrated in studies where probiotics were given both pre- and postnatally [48, 49, 56–59], whereas two studies with postnatal supplementation only failed to prevent allergic disease [60, 61].

6.1. Supplementation with *Lactobacillus reuteri* to prevent childhood IgE-associated eczema

Furthermore, in human allergy intervention studies, our study, using *Lactobacillus reuteri* supplementation, had the most clear effect on infant sensitization to allergens at 2 years of age [17]. *L reuteri* ATCC 55730 (1 x 10^8 colony forming units) was given to pregnant women daily from pregnancy week 36 until delivery. The infants continued with the same product to 12 months of age and were followed up until 24 months. Primary outcome was allergic disease, with or without positive skin prick test or circulating IgE to food allergens. The study was designed to have enough power to detect true differences between the probiotic-supplemented group and the placebo group, which was based on a 40% anticipated allergic disease risk at 2 years. The aim was a 50% reduction in frequency of allergic disease which could be detected at a 5% level of significance with 80% power. The study was also designed to allow a dropout frequency of 20%. Further considerations were done with differences in living environment and other possible confounding factors since the study was a randomized placebo-controlled multicenter trial. To achieve high-quality result study, participants were monitored regularly. At 2 years of age, children were examined by a pediatrician, 1 year after the termination of treatment. The *L. reuteri*-supplemented infants had less IgE-associated eczema during the second year, 8% versus 20% ($P = .02$). Skin prick test reactivity was also less common in the treated than in the placebo group, significantly so for infants with mothers with allergies, 14% versus 31% ($P = .02$). Wheeze and other potentially allergic diseases were not affected. A total of 184 completed a 7-year follow-up. The primary outcomes at 7 year of age were allergic disease and skin prick test reactivity. The prevalence of asthma (15% in the probiotic vs. 16% in placebo group), allergic rhinoconjunctivitis (27% vs. 20%), eczema (21% vs. 19%) and skin prick test reactivity (29% vs. 26%) was similar in the probiotic and placebo groups. No severe adverse events were reported [62]. Our study is one that has resulted in less IgE-associated eczema at 2 years of age and is one where both mother and child received the product, the mother from gestational week 32 and the child from birth to 1 year of age. If prenatal microbial exposure is vital for the preventive effect, starting supplementation already from the second trimester of pregnancy, when circulating fetal T cells have developed [63], may have a more powerful preventive effect on allergy development.

6.1.1. The importance of study design in probiotic trials

There have been implications that besides the design of the study the importance of the probiotic strain has been highlighted. To exemplify this, probiotics that are being used in trials to prevent childhood allergic disease, are also used to prevent necrotizing enterocolitis. The great importance of strain has been shown recently. Necrotizing enterocolitis is one of the most devastating diseases encountered in premature infants [64].

7. Clinical investigations and sample collection

In vitro studies examining responses to common allergens and determining the cytokine and chemokine patterns are a way to explore the effect of probiotic supplementation on immune status in infants. In vitro studies are a good complement to clinical studies in pinpointing the exact mechanism of probiotic supplementation in clinical trials. One way is to collect cord and peripheral blood from the infants included in the study at the different follow-up meetings with research nurses or doctors. From the blood, it is relatively simple to collect cells using gradient centrifugation and to store these cells for later use in liquid nitrogen. One of the benefits with this system is that you are able to analyze all samples during a limited time period instead of analyzing them over years, which is the usual time period for this kind of clinical trials. After thawing, counting, and stimulation of cells, it is important to incubate them with a proper media and in a time period that is optimal for your experiment. To have in mind is that when you investigate innate responses they are designed to respond rather immediately, whereas adaptive responses may need antigen presentation first and then start to produce the cytokines and chemokines associated with that type of response. Commonly thought, antigen presentation and production of allergen-associated biomolecules may take 6 days to reach levels of optimal detection.

7.1. Detection of biomolecules in serum and plasma, a way to determine immune status

To be able to investigate effects that are not obvious clinically one rather convenient way is to measure biomolecules in serum and plasma. Serum and plasma are quite easily collected; venous blood samples are centrifuged and aliquoted to several small tubes that are kept in the freezer at −20 or −70°C. If you compare collecting serum and plasma samples to cell samples, the first is rather time efficient, whereas collecting cells in the laboratory from venous blood samples is rather time consuming. However, there are some drawbacks with serum and plasma samples; one is that it is relatively hard to detect cytokines in this kinds of samples since that type of biomolecules are produced at a lower concentration compared to, for example chemokines, and are acting more locally than the chemo attractive chemokines. Cells have receptors for both cytokines and chemokines on their surface [65].

The determination of circulating chemokine levels in epidemiological studies may be a tool for the identification of factors associated with the development of sensitization or allergic disease.

7.1.1. ELISA

One common method to measure biomolecules in fluids, actually all types of fluids, such as serum, plasma, blood, saliva, etc. is enzyme-linked immuno sorbent assay (ELISA). This method is based on two antibodies with two different epitopes that bind the same biomolecule, in a "sandwich"model. The first thing to do when performing an ELISA is to bind the antibodies to a surface, preferentially one in a well, in a 96-well plate used for the purpose. The binding is enhanced by adding a buffer. Thereafter, one must block the other surface to prevent unspecific binding to the plastic of the wells. This is often performed with bovine serum albumin or milk. The sample is added, and after incubation the capture antibody is added. ELISA has several ways of detection; one is to add streptavidin-conjugated horseradish peroxidase (HRP). The streptavidin will form a strong binding to the biotin-conjugated capture antibody. Then the addition of a substrate for the enzyme that is conjugated to the capture antibody; if HRP is used, TMB is a good substrate (although toxic) and HRP turns TMB to a yellow product and the reaction is incubated for about 15–30 min. The addition of a H_2SO_4 will stop the reaction and turn the liquid blue. The color of the product is relative to the concentration of the biomolecules in the sample and easily detected using an ELISA reader that measures optical density (OD). To further enhance the capability of your ELISA, you can add a standard curve with known concentration that you may relate your samples to.

7.1.2. Multiplex bead assay

Another good method to measure biomolecules in fluids is multiplex bead arrays. These bead arrays are based on the same principles as ELISA, but you couple the capture antibody to a bead instead of the well bottom. That antibody binds an epitope on the biomolecule of interest and a second detection antibody often conjugated with biotin is common; the biotin-conjugated antibody then reacts with streptavidin with a bound fluorescent molecule, often pycoerythrin (PE). The main advantage of the multiplex technology is that it enables several simultaneous analysis, that is, you are able to detect several biomolecules from the same sample at the same time by mixing beads with distinct fluorescent spectra (a mixture of two or more dyes trapped inside the beads) in the same well upon analysis. The detection method is also a bit different from ELISA, which is based on optical density, and the multiplex bead array is a flow cytometry-based system which aligns all beads in a single row to enable single-bead analysis. The single bead is excited with a laser to determine the bead emission, that is, the biomolecule you measure and the concentration of the biomolecule trapped on the bead. If you include samples with known concentration, you can create a standard curve and relate all the measured samples to that to determine the unknown concentration. Since this method can be labor and cost effective, it is possible to determine, for example, the immune status in quite large cohorts by collecting serum and plasma samples and measure biomolecules such as cytokines and chemokines.

8. What are the mechanisms behind probiotics in allergy prevention trials?

The mechanisms behind probiotic supplementation have not been totally mapped yet; various effects on the immune system have been reported after probiotic treatment in allergy prevention trials. There is no consensus among studies, possibly due to different study designs, when probiotics have been introduced prenatally, pre- and postnatally, or only postnatally. The probiotic strain is also of great importance. Evidence of increased CRP, total IgE, and IL-10 levels, which are characteristic of a low-grade inflammation has been presented [66]. Another study decreased that after supplementation during pregnancy with *L. rhamnosus* and *B. lactis*, IFN-γ in cord blood increased [67]. Anti-CD3/CD28-induced IL-2 mRNA expression at 13 months of age was showed after probiotic supplementation at weaning [68]. Although no allergy preventive effect was observed in some cohorts, an immune modulatory effect was detected [69]. Reduced TNF and IL-10 responses to house dust mite were found [70]. Boyle et al. demonstrated that prenatal *Lactobacillus GG* supplementation during the last month of pregnancy reduced heat-killed LGG-induced CD4+T cell proliferation [71], although no allergy preventive effects were observed [72]. Taken together, the studies indicate that several strains of *Lactobacillus* may modulate immunity in infants.

8.1. *Lactobacillus reuteri* and chemokines

The analysis of circulating chemokines is a useable tool to investigate the T helper (Th)1/Th2 imbalance in allergic disease and other diseases in vivo. Circulating levels of Th1-associated

CXC-chemokine ligand (CXCL)9, CXCL10, and CXCL11 and Th2-associated CC-hemokine ligand (CCL)17 and CCL22 have been related to allergic disease, sensitization, and probiotic supplementation [73]. Infants are born with a Th2 deviation of the immune system, which is also reflected in chemokine concentration early in life. The Th2-associated chemokines CCL17 and CCL22 have been shown to be the highest at birth and then decreased, whereas CCL18 and the Th1-associated chemokines increased with age. Allergic children have been observed to have high Th2-associated chemokine concentration, as expected. Interestingly, different allergic symptoms may be related to different chemokines. Furthermore, an imbalance in circulating Th1- and Th2-associated chemokines may precede the onset of sensitization, eczema, and recurrent wheeze from birth [73, 74]. Supplementation with specific probiotic strains [75] may be detected by the presence of strain in stool samples. The presence of *L. reuteri* in stool in the first week of life was associated with low CCL17 and CCL22 and high CXCL11 levels at 6 months of age. However, no other differences were observed between the probiotic and placebo groups. Low Th2-associated chemokine levels and high Th1-associated levels may be of benefit to counteract a Th2 deviation and could possibly imply a decreased tendency to develop allergic diseases. High Th1-associated chemokine levels were associated with day care. As discussed previously, day care is associated with reduced incidence of allergic diseases, possibly by inducing a Th1-associated immunity. Also, to keep in mind when investigating these chemokines is that Th1 and Th2 cytokines are likely important upstream mediators of these effects, as they induce the production of the respective chemokines. The names of the chemokines also indicate how they are regulated.

8.2. *Lactobacillus reuteri* and allergen responsiveness

Probiotic treatment with *Lactobacillus reuteri* [75] has been shown to be associated with lower secretion of allergen induced Th2- and Th1-related cytokines during infancy, as well as with low IL-10 and Th2-associated CCL22 responses [76]. In our study, the differences were more marked for responses to the perennial and ubiquitously present [9] cat allergen than the food allergen OVA and the seasonal birch allergen. Allergens may have different route and duration of exposure, which may imply different regulation. Also, in Sweden, it is uncommon to be allergic to house dust mite but however quite common to be allergic to birch and grass. Moreover, low mitogen induced Th2-like responses were also associated with *L. reuteri* supplementation. The lower cytokine and chemokine levels in the probiotic group could indicate an increased immune regulatory capacity, possibly implying a reduced atopic propensity, consistent with our previous findings in this cohort [75]. We also investigated if probiotic supplementation affected the pattern of cytokine release after stimulation in this study; however, the allergen- and mitogen-induced cytokine responses seemed to be independently associated with probiotic treatment and allergy development, since logistic regression indicated separate effects of treatment and allergy on immune responses. Possibly another mechanism than we were able to investigate is responsible for this effect. However, this could be due to the fact that only few allergic infants were included. In agreement with previous studies [77], allergic infants did show high Th2 responses after birch and food allergen stimulation, whereas probiotic supplementation showed less clear effects.

In this study, treatment reduced the incidence of clinical manifestations as well as sensitization, possibly reflected by the lower responses to allergen stimulation in probiotic-treated infants [75]. It is believed that some strains of probiotics can induce a Th1 immunity to counteract a deviated Th2 immunity in infants and allergic diseases. To investigate this hypothesis, Th1-associated factors were investigated in this cohort. The mRNA expression of the transcription factors T-bet and GATA-3, driving Th1 and Th2 differentiation, respectively, was not influenced by probiotic treatment, although T-bet expression correlated to the secretion of IFN-γ and the Th1-associated chemokine CXCL10. Neither Foxp3 nor Ebi3 mRNA expressions were affected by probiotic treatment, while Ebi3 and Foxp3 expressions were correlated to each other and associated with IL-10 secretion, supporting an immune regulatory role of Ebi3 [78].

The lower allergen responsiveness in the infants receiving probiotics, as compared to placebo, is similar to our previously reported observations of lower allergen-induced cytokine secretion during infancy in a country with a low incidence of allergies (Estonia) [27]. Thus, allergen-induced IL-5, -13, -10, and IFN-γ responses were lower in Estonian than in Swedish children. Living conditions are different, and besides that, lactobacilli were more often detected in fecal samples from Estonian than Swedish children [79]. A low lactobacilli colonization has been associated with allergic disease development [80].

8.3. *Lactobacillus reuteri* and Toll-like receptors

Can pre- and postnatal supplementation with *Lactobacillus reuteri* affect the innate cytokine and chemokine responses to bacterial products and the expression of associated receptors, i.e., TLR2, 4 and 9 In this study, TLR2 stimulation leads to lower IL-1β, IL-6, IL-10, CCL4, and CXCL8 responses in the probiotic treated infants [81]. These differences were not dependent on the differences in TLR2 mRNA expression in the probiotic and placebo groups. Probiotic supplementation may thus be associated with an increased immune regulatory capacity during infancy, in line with our previous findings showing lower allergen responsiveness in the probiotic-treated children [81].

Low responsiveness to stimulation with lipoteichoic acid after previous supplementation with the Gram positive bacteria *Lactobacillus reuteri* could be related to a phenomenon referred to in the literature as lipopolysaccharide tolerance [82]. Our results could suggest that such a downregulation occurs in vivo as a consequence of long-term exposure to TLR2 ligands, that is, supplementation with the Gram positive *Lactobacillus reuteri*. The expression of TLR receptors has been shown not to be involved in this phenomenon, but studies suggest that this is dependent on a downstream effect involving IRAK [83]. This would also explain why the TLR2 mRNA expression was not affected by probiotic supplementation, whereas studies of children growing up on a farm have shown that microbial exposure upregulate these receptors [14, 25, 26]. Our data, however, indicate that the TLR2 mRNA expression and LTA-induced cytokine and chemokine responses are not correlated. The lower responses to TLR2 stimulation could be dependent on an induction of regulatory macrophages responding to stimuli with lower secretion of proinflammatory cytokines and chemokines [84]. Whether this downregulation of TLR2 responses is also related to the decreased incidence of IgE-associated disease in probiotic-treated children is not known. The logistic regression analyses suggested, however, that the effects on TLR2 responsiveness were related to probiotic supplementation but not allergy development in this study. This could also be due to the fact that there were few allergic children included in these analyses, although we did detect higher levels of TLR2 mRNA expression in non-allergic than allergic infants at 12 months of age. Other studies suggest differences in TLR responsiveness between children who do or do not develop allergy [85–87].

That probiotic supplementation may be associated with an increased immune regulatory capacity during infancy is also in line with studies suggesting that immune regulatory mechanisms are established at a later age in Sweden compared to Estonia [27], a country with higher microbial exposure and a lower allergy prevalence than Sweden [9]. Comparatively, after allergen stimulation, Estonian infants responded with lower levels of cytokines, both Th1 and Th2, than Swedish infants [27]. Estonian infants also secrete lower levels of proinflammatory cytokines after LPS stimulation compared to Swedish infants (unpublished). Another study comparing countries with higher microbial exposure and less allergies with countries with less microbial exposure and more allergic diseases demonstrate that neonatal antigen presenting cells (APCs) are more quiescent in children born under traditional, i.e., Papua New Guinea, compared to modern environmental conditions, i.e. Australia [88]. This was reflected by less responsiveness to stimulation in vitro in APCs from newborns born in Papua New Guinea, while they exhibited higher baseline levels of activation and inhibitory markers in the resting state compared to APC from Australian neonates [88]. This quiescent function could potentially be a protective mechanism learned in utero. Thus, lower TLR-induced levels of proinflammatory cytokines and chemokines may be due to an enhanced immune regulatory capacity among infants living in conditions with a higher microbial burden.

Of course, there has been an effort in elucidating the passage ways that the bacteria colonize the body and affect the immune system. Until recently, the infant intestines were supposed to originate from perineal, vaginal, and fecal microbiota and before delivery thought to be sterile. However, the microbial colonization might already start before birth by microbial transfer through the placental barrier. DNA from a wide variety of microbial taxa in the human placenta, umbilical cord blood, amniotic fluid, and meconium have been found and sequenced. The bacteria may gain access through ascent from the vagina and/or through the blood stream for bacteria from intestinal or oral origin. So one might say that the sterile womb theory is history [89]. These findings suggest that normal colonization may already start before birth, colonization that is of benefit for the infant and not detrimental and leading to disease. Labeled *Enterococcus faecium* in an experimental animal study showed that beyond transplacental passage, bacteria can be transferred via the gastrointestinal canal [90]. As reviewed in [89], bacteria may travel via the bloodstream from the mouth, of course without causing sepsis, via the breast, external through the sebaceous skin to the breast milk. Internally, via the entero-mammary pathway that brings gut bacteria to the mammary gland via lymph and blood circulation.

Other possible effector mechanisms of probiotic supplementation could be dependent on epigenetic changes, although this needs further investigation. Thus, epigenetic regulation has been suggested as one of the underlying effector mechanisms for the allergy preventive effect of microbial exposure during pregnancy [91].

8.4. *Lactobacillus reuteri* and the composition of breast milk

Breast milk not only provides the necessary nutrients for growth and development, it also contains many important immunological components to provide the immunological immature infant for the surrounding environment and the challenges outside the womb. Such components include immune cells, antibodies (especially IgA antibodies), pro- and anti-inflammatory cytokines such as TNF, IL-10, and TGF-b, and factors that may modify immune responses to bacteria, e.g., soluble CD14 (sCD14).

How can probiotic supplementation change the composition of breast milk? Well, nutritional, metabolic, and immunological processes in the gut are reflected in the mammary gland and the milk through the entero-mammary link [89]. In addition, the immunological composition of breast milk differs between mothers, and the reasons for these differences and the consequences for the breastfed infants are not fully elucidated yet. When *Lactobacillus reuteri* was supplemented to pregnant mothers from gestational week 32 during pregnancy, supplementation was associated with low levels of TGF-b2 and slight and increased levels of IL-10 in colostrum. The slightly higher levels of IL-10 could be due to the reason that *L. reuteri* previously had been reported to induce IL-10-producing regulatory T cells in vitro [36].

9. Probiotics and epigenetic mechanisms?

Epigenetic modifications can alter the DNA sequence without heritable changes [92] and have been shown to be important in prenatal immune programming. Epigenetic modifications can alter the DNA compaction and open/close for gene transcription [92]. The most important mechanisms are posttranslational histone modifications and methylation of DNA CpG dinucleotide [92]. The methylation pattern is thus preserved with high fidelity through cell divisions, assuring preservation of cellular inheritance [93]. The epigenetic pattern varies between tissue and cell type, and also between individuals and over time, representing immune maturation, ageing and disease states. There are many examples that epigenetic are not permanent but changes over time. Some are implemented during only a short time to open or close chromatin state and access transcription of certain genes. In addition, the epigenetic state is reversible and with the appropriate enzymatic machinery, the whole epigenome can be modified [94]. Once these islands are methylated, gene transcription might not occur. Once removed, the promoter allows interaction with various transcription factors and allows gene activation. In T-cells, epigenetics are important for differentiation [95]. Of course, there are several ways of keeping/removing the epigenome. The major regulatory enzymes of DNA methylation are DNA methyltransferases (DNMTs). There are different DNMTs that play unique roles in the DNA methylation process [94]. DNA methylation patterns may be responsible for the Th2 skewing in neonates. Possibly, hypermethylation of the IFNG promoter may restrict expression of the IFNG gene. A permissive epigenetic state at the IL13 locus has been described for human naive neonatal CD4 cells as consistent with the Th2 skewing of the immune system early in life [96, 97]. Prenatal environmental exposures may also alter gene expression via epigenetic mechanisms, aiming to induce physiological adaptations to the anticipated postnatal environment, but potentially also increasing disease susceptibility in the offspring [98]. The maternal microbial environment could possibly influence infant immune maturation [13, 14, 20] and T effector and T regulatory immunity [17, 28]. Th1, Th2, and Th17 differentiation is controlled epigentically [95, 99, 100], and human T regulatory cell differentiation needs demethylation of the FOXP3 promoter [101]. Also, the immunological interaction between the mother infants is close during pregnancy [102, 103]. Children growing up in a traditional farming environment had a lower risk of respiratory allergic disease later in life, as discussed previously. There is increasing evidence that at least some of the protective effects are mediated through epigenetic modifications [16, 94].

10. Conclusion and future directions

Recently, the World Allergy Organisation wrote guidelines for probiotic use in prevention of allergic disease: World Allergy Organization-McMaster University Guidelines for Allergic Disease Prevention (GLAD-P): Probiotics [104]. After much research effort different strains of probiotics as supplementation during pregnancy and/or postnatal were used to prevent the development of allergic diseases in infants. There are some common guidelines to try to sum up the advances and bring them into practical guidelines in this field. Allergic diseases have a strong hereditary factor, the prevalence in infants without parents or siblings with allergic symptoms is 10% but reaches 20-30% if the first-degree has been made in trying to identify factors critical for allergy development. Of essential importance seems to be the gut microbiota. Colonization patterns differ between allergic and non-allergic infants, depending on delivery mode, and geographical factors influence this pattern. The gut microbiota and microbial environment have been reported to modulate immunity and may be one way to try to stop the escalating rate of allergic disease prevalence. WAO recommendations about probiotic supplementation for the prevention of allergy are intended to support parents, clinicians and other health care professionals in their decisions whether to use probiotics in pregnancy and during breastfeeding, and whether to give them to infants. "The WAO guideline panel determined that there is a likely net benefit from using probiotics resulting primarily from the prevention of eczema. The WAO guideline panel suggests: a) using probiotics in pregnant women at high risk of having an allergic child; b) using probiotics in women who breastfeed infants at high risk of developing allergy; and c) using probiotics in infants at high risk of developing allergy" [104].

Of course, there are many questions to answer and discuss. Several strains have been used in allergy prevention probiotic trials. There is a consensus that the strain is of importance, since different strains have different properties and also, as evident in allergy prevention trials, different outcome after use. Also, exactly when are the best "window of opportunity" and which population is the most susceptible for intervention methods?

Author details

Anna Forsberg

Address all correspondence to: anna.forsberg@liu.se

Unit for Autoimmunity and Immune Regulation (AIR), Department of Clinical and Experimental Medicine (IKE), Faculty of Health Sciences, Linköping University, Linköping, Sweden

References

[1] Schaub B, Lauener R, von Mutius E, The many faces of the hygiene hypothesis. J Allergy Clin Immunol 2006; 117: 969–77.

[2] Haahtela T, Holgate S, Pawankar R, Akdis CA, Benjaponpitak S, Caraballo L, Demain J, Portnoy J, von Hertzen L, The biodiversity hypothesis and allergic disease: world allergy organization position statement. World Allergy Organ J 2013; 6: 3.

[3] Ebert CS, Jr., Pillsbury HC, 3rd, Epidemiology of allergy. Otolaryngol Clin North Am 2011; 44: 537–48, vii.

[4] Chen W, Mempel M, Schober W, Behrendt H, Ring J, Gender difference, sex hormones, and immediate type hypersensitivity reactions. Allergy 2008; 63: 1418–27.

[5] Casimir GJ, Mulier S, Hanssens L, Zylberberg K, Duchateau J, Gender differences in inflammatory markers in children. Shock 2010; 33: 258–62.

[6] Pennell LM, Galligan CL, Fish EN, Sex affects immunity. J Autoimmun 2012; 38: J282–91.

[7] Postma DS, Gender differences in asthma development and progression. Gend Med 2007; 4 Suppl B: S133–46.

[8] Strachan DP, Hay fever, hygiene, and household size. BMJ 1989; 299: 1259–60.

[9] Böttcher MF, Björkstén B, Gustafson S, Voor T, Jenmalm MC, Endotoxin levels in Estonian and Swedish house dust and atopy in infancy. Clin Exp Allergy 2003; 33: 295–300.

[10] Bashir ME, Louie S, Shi HN, Nagler-Anderson C, Toll-like receptor 4 signaling by intestinal microbes influences susceptibility to food allergy. J Immunol 2004; 172: 6978–87.

[11] Foliaki S, Pearce N, Bjorksten B, Mallol J, Montefort S, von Mutius E, Antibiotic use in infancy and symptoms of asthma, rhinoconjunctivitis, and eczema in children 6 and 7

years old: International Study of Asthma and Allergies in Childhood Phase III. J Allergy Clin Immunol 2009; 124: 982–9.

[12] Kwon HK, Lee CG, So JS, Chae CS, Hwang JS, Sahoo A, Nam JH, Rhee JH, Hwang KC, Im SH, Generation of regulatory dendritic cells and CD4+Foxp3+ T cells by probiotics administration suppresses immune disorders. Proc Natl Acad Sci U S A 2010; 107: 2159–64.

[13] Hawrylowicz C, Ryanna K, Asthma and allergy: the early beginnings. Nat Med 2010; 16: 274–5.

[14] Ege MJ, Bieli C, Frei R, van Strien RT, Riedler J, Ublagger E, Schram-Bijkerk D, Brunekreef B, van Hage M, Scheynius A, Pershagen G, Benz MR, Lauener R, von Mutius E, Braun-Fahrlander C, Prenatal farm exposure is related to the expression of receptors of the innate immunity and to atopic sensitization in school-age children. J Allergy Clin Immunol 2006; 117: 817–23.

[15] Douwes J, Cheng S, Travier N, Cohet C, Niesink A, McKenzie J, Cunningham C, Le Gros G, von Mutius E, Pearce N, Farm exposure in utero may protect against asthma, hay fever and eczema. Eur Respir J 2008; 32: 603–11.

[16] von Mutius E, Vercelli D, Farm living: effects on childhood asthma and allergy. Nat Rev Immunol 2010; 10: 861–8.

[17] Schaub B, Liu J, Hoppler S, Schleich I, Huehn J, Olek S, Wieczorek G, Illi S, von Mutius E, Maternal farm exposure modulates neonatal immune mechanisms through regulatory T cells. J Allergy Clin Immunol 2009; 123: 774–82 e5.

[18] Fall T, Lundholm C, Ortqvist AK, Fall K, Fang F, Hedhammar A, Kampe O, Ingelsson E, Almqvist C, Early exposure to dogs and farm animals and the risk of childhood asthma. JAMA Pediatr 2015; 169: e153219.

[19] Björkstén B, Diverse microbial exposure – consequences for vaccine development. Vaccine 2012; 30: 4336–40.

[20] Conrad ML, Ferstl R, Teich R, Brand S, Blumer N, Yildirim AO, Patrascan CC, Hanuszkiewicz A, Akira S, Wagner H, Holst O, von Mutius E, Pfefferle PI, Kirschning CJ, Garn H, Renz H, Maternal TLR signaling is required for prenatal asthma protection by the nonpathogenic microbe *Acinetobacter lwoffii* F78. J Exp Med 2009; 206: 2869–77.

[21] Cao L, Wang J, Zhu Y, Tseu I, Post M, Maternal endotoxin exposure attenuates allergic airway disease in infant rats. Am J Physiol Lung Cell Mol Physiol 2010; 298: L670–7.

[22] Blümer N, Herz U, Wegmann M, Renz H, Prenatal lipopolysaccharide-exposure prevents allergic sensitization and airway inflammation, but not airway responsiveness in a murine model of experimental asthma. Clin Exp Allergy 2005; 35: 397–402.

[23] Gerhold K, Avagyan A, Seib C, Frei R, Steinle J, Ahrens B, Dittrich AM, Blumchen K, Lauener R, Hamelmann E, Prenatal initiation of endotoxin airway exposure prevents

subsequent allergen-induced sensitization and airway inflammation in mice. J Allergy Clin Immunol 2006; 118: 666–73.

[24] Cao L, Wang J, Zhu Y, Tseu I, Post M, Maternal endotoxin exposure attenuate allergic airway disease in infant rats. Am J Physiol Lung Cell Mol Physiol 2010; 298: L670–7.

[25] Roduit C, Wohlgensinger J, Frei R, Bitter S, Bieli C, Loeliger S, Buchele G, Riedler J, Dalphin JC, Remes S, Roponen M, Pekkanen J, Kabesch M, Schaub B, von Mutius E, Braun-Fahrlander C, Lauener R, Prenatal animal contact and gene expression of innate immunity receptors at birth are associated with atopic dermatitis. J Allergy Clin Immunol 2011; 127: 179–85 e1.

[26] Loss G, Bitter S, Wohlgensinger J, Frei R, Roduit C, Genuneit J, Pekkanen J, Roponen M, Hirvonen MR, Dalphin JC, Dalphin ML, Riedler J, von Mutius E, Weber J, Kabesch M, Michel S, Braun-Fahrlander C, Lauener R, Prenatal and early-life exposures alter expression of innate immunity genes: the PASTURE cohort study. J Allergy Clin Immunol 2012; 130: 523–30 e9.

[27] Böttcher MF, Jenmalm MC, Voor T, Julge K, Holt PG, Björkstén B, Cytokine responses to allergens during the first 2 years of life in Estonian and Swedish children. Clin Exp Allergy 2006; 36: 619–28.

[28] Vuillermin PJ, Ponsonby AL, Saffery R, Tang ML, Ellis JA, Sly P, Holt P, Microbial exposure, interferon gamma gene demethylation in naive T-cells, and the risk of allergic disease. Allergy 2009; 64: 348–53.

[29] Christensen HR, Frokiaer H, Pestka JJ, *Lactobacilli* differentially modulate expression of cytokines and maturation surface markers in murine dendritic cells. J Immunol 2002; 168: 171–8.

[30] McGovern N, Chan JK, Ginhoux F, Dendritic cells in humans – from fetus to adult. Int Immunol 2015; 27: 65–72.

[31] FAO/WHO, Health and nutritional properties of probiotics in food including powder milk with live lactic acid bacteria. Report of a joint FAO/WHO expert consultation on evaluation of health and nutritional properties in food including powder milk with live lactic acid bacteria, 2001.

[32] Björkstén B, Sepp E, Julge K, Voor T, Mikelsaar M, Allergy development and the intestinal microflora during the first year of life. J Allergy Clin Immunol 2001; 108: 516–20.

[33] Björkstén B, Naaber P, Sepp E, Mikelsaar M, The intestinal microflora in allergic Estonian and Swedish 2-year-old children. Clin Exp Allergy 1999; 29: 342–6.

[34] Karimi K, Inman MD, Bienenstock J, Forsythe P, *Lactobacillus reuteri*-induced regulatory T cells protect against an allergic airway response in mice. Am J Respir Crit Care Med 2009; 179: 186–93.

[35] O'Mahony C, Scully P, O'Mahony D, Murphy S, O'Brien F, Lyons A, Sherlock G, MacSharry J, Kiely B, Shanahan F, O'Mahony L, Commensal-induced regulatory T cells mediate protection against pathogen-stimulated NF-kappaB activation. PLoS Pathog 2008; 4: e1000112.

[36] Smits HH, Engering A, van der Kleij D, de Jong EC, Schipper K, van Capel TM, Zaat BA, Yazdanbakhsh M, Wierenga EA, van Kooyk Y, Kapsenberg ML, Selective probiotic bacteria induce IL-10-producing regulatory T cells in vitro by modulating dendritic cell function through dendritic cell-specific intercellular adhesion molecule 3-grabbing nonintegrin. J Allergy Clin Immunol 2005; 115: 1260–7.

[37] Renz H, Brandtzaeg P, Hornef M, The impact of perinatal immune development on mucosal homeostasis and chronic inflammation. Nat Rev Immunol 2012; 12: 9–23.

[38] Jenmalm MC, Childhood immune maturation and allergy development: regulation by maternal immunity and microbial exposure. Am J Reprod Immunol 2011; 66(Suppl. 1): 75–80.

[39] Sakaguchi S, Miyara M, Costantino CM, Hafler DA, FOXP3+ regulatory T cells in the human immune system. Nat Rev Immunol 2010; 10: 490–500.

[40] Miyara M, Yoshioka Y, Kitoh A, Shima T, Wing K, Niwa A, Parizot C, Taflin C, Heike T, Valeyre D, Mathian A, Nakahata T, Yamaguchi T, Nomura T, Ono M, Amoura Z, Gorochov G, Sakaguchi S, Functional delineation and differentiation dynamics of human CD4+ T cells expressing the FoxP3 transcription factor. Immunity 2009; 30: 899–911.

[41] Vignali DA, Collison LW, Workman CJ, How regulatory T cells work. Nat Rev Immunol 2008; 8: 523–32.

[42] Stiles ME, Holzapfel WH, Lactic acid bacteria of foods and their current taxonomy. Int J Food Microbiol 1997; 36: 1–29.

[43] Reuter G, The Lactobacillus and bifidobacterium microflora of the human intestine: composition and succession. Curr Issues Intest Microbiol 2001; 2: 43–53.

[44] Haarman M, Knol J, Quantitative real-time PCR analysis of fecal Lactobacillus species in infants receiving a prebiotic infant formula. Appl Environ Microbiol 2006; 72: 2359–65.

[45] Chung TC, Axelsson L, Lindgren SE, Dobrogosz WJ, In vitro studies on reuterin synthesis by *Lactobacillus reuteri*. Microbial Ecol Health Dis 1989; 2:137–44.

[46] Degnan FH, The US Food and Drug Administration and probiotics: regulatory categorization. Clin Infect Dis 2008; 46(Suppl. 2): S133–6; discussion S44–51.

[47] Kalliomäki M, Salminen S, Arvilommi H, Kero P, Koskinen P, Isolauri E, Probiotics in primary prevention of atopic disease: a randomised placebo-controlled trial. Lancet 2001; 357: 1076–79.

[48] Kukkonen K, Savilahti E, Haahtela T, Juntunen-Backman K, Korpela R, Poussa T, Tuure T, Kuitunen M, Probiotics and prebiotic galacto-oligosaccharides in the prevention of allergic diseases: a randomized, double-blind, placebo-controlled trial. J Allergy Clin Immunol 2007; 119: 192–8.

[49] Wickens K, Black PN, Stanley TV, Mitchell E, Fitzharris P, Tannock GW, Purdie G, Crane J, A differential effect of 2 probiotics in the prevention of eczema and atopy: a double-blind, randomized, placebo-controlled trial. J Allergy Clin Immunol 2008; 122: 788–94.

[50] West CE, Hammarström ML, Hernell O, Probiotics during weaning reduce the incidence of eczema. Pediatr Allergy Immunol 2009; 20: 430–7.

[51] Kim JY, Kwon JH, Ahn SH, Lee SI, Han YS, Choi YO, Lee SY, Ahn KM, Ji GE, Effect of probiotic mix (*Bifidobacterium bifidum, Bifidobacterium lactis, Lactobacillus acidophilus*) in the primary prevention of eczema: a double-blind, randomized, placebo-controlled trial. Pediatr Allergy Immunol 2010; 21: e386–93.

[52] Dotterud CK, Storro O, Johnsen R, Oien T, Probiotics in pregnant women to prevent allergic disease: a randomized, double-blind trial. Br J Dermatol 2010; 163: 616–23.

[53] Kalliomäki M, Kirjavainen P, Eerola E, Kero P, Salminen S, Isolauri E, Distinct patterns of neonatal gut microflora in infants in whom atopy was and was not developing. J Allergy Clin Immunol 2001; 107: 129–34.

[54] Cuello-Garcia CA, Brozek JL, Fiocchi A, Pawankar R, Yepes-Nunez JJ, Terracciano L, Gandhi S, Agarwal A, Zhang Y, Schunemann HJ, Probiotics for the prevention of allergy: a systematic review and meta-analysis of randomized controlled trials. J Allergy Clin Immunol 2015; 136: 952–61.

[55] Lee J, Seto D, Bielory L, Meta-analysis of clinical trials of probiotics for prevention and treatment of pediatric atopic dermatitis. J Allergy Clin Immunol 2008; 121: 116–21 e11.

[56] Kalliomäki M, Salminen S, Arvilommi H, Kero P, Koskinen P, Isolauri E, Probiotics in primary prevention of atopic disease: a randomised placebo-controlled trial. Lancet 2001; 357: 1076–9.

[57] Kalliomäki M, Salminen S, Poussa T, Arvilommi H, Isolauri E, Probiotics and prevention of atopic disease: 4-year follow-up of a randomised placebo-controlled trial. Lancet 2003; 361: 1869–71.

[58] Abrahamsson TR, Jakobsson T, Böttcher MF, Fredrikson M, Jenmalm MC, Björkstén B, Oldaeus G, Probiotics in prevention of IgE-associated eczema: a double-blind, randomized, placebo-controlled trial. J Allergy Clin Immunol 2007; 119: 1174–80.

[59] Kim JY, Kwon JH, Ahn SH, Lee SI, Han YS, Choi YO, Lee SY, Ahn KM, Ji GE, Effect of probiotic mix (*Bifidobacterium bifidum, Bifidobacterium lactis, Lactobacillus acidophilus*) in the primary prevention of eczema: a double-blind, randomized, placebo-controlled trial. Pediatr Allergy Immunol 2010;21: e386–93.

[60] Taylor AL, Dunstan JA, Prescott SL, Probiotic supplementation for the first 6 months of life fails to reduce the risk of atopic dermatitis and increases the risk of allergen sensitization in high-risk children: a randomized controlled trial. J Allergy Clin Immunol 2007; 119: 184–91.

[61] Soh SE, Aw M, Gerez I, Chong YS, Rauff M, Ng YP, Wong HB, Pai N, Lee BW, Shek LP, Probiotic supplementation in the first 6 months of life in at risk Asian infants – effects on eczema and atopic sensitization at the age of 1 year. Clin Exp Allergy 2009; 39: 571–8.

[62] Abrahamsson TR, Jakobsson T, Bjorksten B, Oldaeus G, Jenmalm MC, No effect of probiotics on respiratory allergies: a seven-year follow-up of a randomized controlled trial in infancy. Pediatr Allergy Immunol 2013; 24: 556–61.

[63] Papiernik M, Correlation of lymphocyte transformation and morphology in the human fetal thymus. Blood 1970; 36: 470–9.

[64] Abrahamsson TR, Not all probiotic strains prevent necrotising enterocolitis in premature infants. Lancet 2016; 387: 624–5.

[65] Peases JE, Williams TJ, Chemokines and their receptors in allergic disease. J Allergy Clin Immunol 2006; 118: 305–17.

[66] Marschan E, Kuitunen M, Kukkonen K, Poussa T, Sarnesto A, Haahtela T, Korpela R, Savilahti E, Vaarala O, Probiotics in infancy induce protective immune profiles that are characteristic for chronic low-grade inflammation. Clin Exp Allergy 2008; 38: 611–18.

[67] Prescott SL, Wickens K, Westcott L, Jung W, Currie H, Black PN, Stanley TV, Mitchell EA, Fitzharris P, Siebers R, Wu L, Crane J, Supplementation with *Lactobacillus rhamnosus* or *Bifidobacterium lactis* probiotics in pregnancy increases cord blood interferon-gamma and breast milk transforming growth factor-beta and immunoglobin A detection. Clin Exp Allergy 2008; 38: 1606–14.

[68] West CE, Hernell O, Andersson Y, Sjöstedt M, Hammarström ML, Probiotic effects on T-cell maturation in infants during weaning. Clin Exp Allergy 2012; 42: 540–9.

[69] Prescott SL, Wiltschut J, Taylor A, Westcott L, Jung W, Currie H, Dunstan JA, Early markers of allergic disease in a primary prevention study using probiotics: 2.5-year follow-up phase. Allergy 2008; 63: 1481–90.

[70] Taylor AL, Hale J, Wiltschut J, Lehmann H, Dunstan JA, Prescott SL, Effects of probiotic supplementation for the first 6 months of life on allergen- and vaccine-specific immune responses. Clin Exp Allergy 2006; 36: 1227–35.

[71] Boyle RJ, Mah LJ, Chen A, Kivivuori S, Robins-Browne RM, Tang ML, Effects of *Lactobacillus GG* treatment during pregnancy on the development of fetal antigen-specific immune responses. Clin Exp Allergy 2008; 38: 1882–90.

[72] Boyle RJ, Ismail IH, Kivivuori S, Licciardi PV, Robins-Browne RM, Mah LJ, Axelrad C, Moore S, Donath S, Carlin JB, Lahtinen SJ, Tang ML, *Lactobacillus GG* treatment during

pregnancy for the prevention of eczema: a randomized controlled trial. Allergy 2011; 66: 509–16.

[73] Abrahamsson TR, Sandberg Abelius M, Forsberg A, Björkstén B, Jenmalm MC, A Th1/Th2-associated chemokine imbalance during infancy in children developing eczema, wheeze and sensitization. Clin Exp Allergy 2011; 41: 1729–39.

[74] Abelius MS, Ernerudh J, Berg G, Matthiesen L, Nilsson LJ, Jenmalm MC, High cord blood levels of the T-helper 2-associated chemokines CCL17 and CCL22 precede allergy development during the first 6 years of life. Pediatr Res 2011; 70: 495–500.

[75] Abrahamsson TR, Jakobsson T, Böttcher MF, Fredrikson M, Jenmalm MC, Björkstén B, Oldeaus G, Probiotics in prevention of IgE-associated eczema: a double blind, randomized, placebo-controlled trial. J Allergy Clin Immunol 2007; 119: 1174–80.

[76] Forsberg A, Abrahamsson TR, Björkstén B, Jenmalm MC, Pre- and post-natal *Lactobacillus reuteri* supplementation decreases allergen responsiveness in infancy. Clin Exp Allergy 2013; 43: 434–42.

[77] Böttcher MF, Jenmalm MC, Björkstén B, Immune responses to birch in young children during their first 7 years of life. Clin Exp Allergy 2002; 32: 1690–8.

[78] Collison LW, Chaturvedi V, Henderson AL, Giacomin PR, Guy C, Bankoti J, Finkelstein D, Forbes K, Workman CJ, Brown SA, Rehg JE, Jones ML, Ni HT, Artis D, Turk MJ, Vignali DA, IL-35-mediated induction of a potent regulatory T cell population. Nat Immunol 2010; 11: 1093–101.

[79] Sepp E, Julge K, Vasar M, Naaber P, Björkstén B, Mikelsaar M, Intestinal microflora of Estonian and Swedish infants. Acta Paediatr 1997; 86: 956–61.

[80] Sjögren YM, Jenmalm MC, Böttcher MF, Björkstén B, Sverremark-Ekström E, Altered early infant gut microbiota in children developing allergy up to 5 years of age. Clin Exp Allergy 2009; 39: 518–26.

[81] Forsberg A, Abrahamsson TR, Bjorksten B, Jenmalm MC, Pre- and postnatal administration of *Lactobacillus reuteri* decreases TLR2 responses in infants. Clin Transl Allergy 2014; 4: 21.

[82] Biswas SK, Lopez-Collazo E, Endotoxin tolerance: new mechanisms, molecules and clinical significance. Trends Immunol 2009; 30: 475–87.

[83] Fan H, Cook JA, Molecular mechanisms of endotoxin tolerance. J Endotoxin Res 2004; 10: 71–84.

[84] Svensson J, Jenmalm MC, Matussek A, Geffers R, Berg G, Ernerudh J, Macrophages at the fetal-maternal interface express markers of alternative activation and are induced by M-CSF and IL-10. J Immunol 2011; 187: 3671–82.

[85] Prescott SL, Noakes P, Chow BW, Breckler L, Thornton CA, Hollams EM, Ali M, van den Biggelaar AH, Tulic MK, Presymptomatic differences in Toll-like receptor function in infants who have allergy. J Allergy Clin Immunol 2008; 122: 391–9, 99 e1–5.

[86] Tulic MK, Hodder M, Forsberg A, McCarthy S, Richman T, D'Vaz N, van den Biggelaar AH, Thornton CA, Prescott SL, Differences in innate immune function between allergic and nonallergic children: new insights into immune ontogeny. J Allergy Clin Immunol 2011; 127: 470–78 e1.

[87] Amoudruz P, Holmlund U, Saghafian-Hedengren S, Nilsson C, Sverremark-Ekstrom E, Impaired Toll-like receptor 2 signalling in monocytes from 5-year-old allergic children. Clin Exp Immunol 2009; 155: 387–94.

[88] Lisciandro JG, Prescott SL, Nadal-Sims MG, Devitt CJ, Richmond PC, Pomat W, Siba PM, Holt PG, Strickland DH, van den Biggelaar AH, Neonatal antigen-presenting cells are functionally more quiescent in children born under traditional compared with modern environmental conditions. J Allergy Clin Immunol 2012; 130: 1167–74 e10.

[89] Funkhouser LJ, Bordenstein SR, Mom knows best: the universality of maternal microbial transmission. PLoS Biol 2013; 11: e1001631.

[90] Jimenez E, Fernandez L, Marin ML, Martin R, Odriozola JM, Nueno-Palop C, Narbad A, Olivares M, Xaus J, Rodriguez JM, Isolation of commensal bacteria from umbilical cord blood of healthy neonates born by cesarean section. Curr Microbiol 2005; 51: 270–4.

[91] Brand S, Teich R, Dicke T, Harb H, Yildirim AO, Tost J, Schneider-Stock R, Waterland RA, Bauer UM, von Mutius E, Garn H, Pfefferle PI, Renz H, Epigenetic regulation in murine offspring as a novel mechanism for transmaternal asthma protection induced by microbes. J Allergy Clin Immunol 2011; 128: 618–25, e1–7.

[92] Jaenisch R, Bird A, Epigenetic regulation of gene expression: how the genome integrates intrinsic and environmental signals. Nat Genet 2003; 33(Suppl): 245–54.

[93] Kim JK, Samaranayake M, Pradhan S, Epigenetic mechanisms in mammals. Cell Mol Life Sci 2009; 66: 596–612.

[94] Harb H, Renz H, Update on epigenetics in allergic disease. J Allergy Clin Immunol 2015; 135: 15–24.

[95] Janson PC, Linton LB, Bergman EA, Marits P, Eberhardson M, Piehl F, Malmstrom V, Winqvist O, Profiling of CD4+ T cells with epigenetic immune lineage analysis. J Immunol 2011; 186: 92–102.

[96] Webster RB, Rodriguez Y, Klimecki WT, Vercelli D, The human IL-13 locus in neonatal CD4+ T cells is refractory to the acquisition of a repressive chromatin architecture. J Biol Chem 2007; 282: 700–9.

[97] Martino D, Maksimovic J, Joo JH, Prescott SL, Saffery R, Genome-scale profiling reveals a subset of genes regulated by DNA methylation that program somatic T-cell phenotypes in humans. Genes Immun 2012; 13: 388–98.

[98] Wadhwa PD, Buss C, Entringer S, Swanson JM, Developmental origins of health and disease: brief history of the approach and current focus on epigenetic mechanisms. Semin Reprod Med 2009; 27: 358–68.

[99] Wilson CB, Rowell E, Sekimata M, Epigenetic control of T-helper-cell differentiation. Nat Rev Immunol 2009; 9: 91–105.

[100] Janson PC, Winerdal ME, Winqvist O, At the crossroads of T helper lineage commitment - Epigenetics points the way. Biochim Biophys Acta 2009; 1790: 906–19.

[101] Janson PC, Winerdal ME, Marits P, Thorn M, Ohlsson R, Winqvist O, FOXP3 promoter demethylation reveals the committed Treg population in humans. PloS ONE 2008; 3: e1612.

[102] Jenmalm MC, Björkstén B, Cord blood levels of immunoglobulin G subclass antibodies to food and inhalant allergens in relation to maternal atopy and the development of atopic disease during the first 8 years of life. Clin Exp Allergy 2000; 30: 34–40.

[103] Sandberg M, Frykman A, Ernerudh J, Berg G, Matthiesen L, Ekerfelt C, Nilsson LJ, Jenmalm MC, Cord blood cytokines and chemokines and development of allergic disease. Pediatr Allergy Immunol 2009; 20: 519–27.

[104] Fiocchi A, Pawankar R, Cuello-Garcia C, Ahn K, Al-Hammadi S, Agarwal A, Beyer K, Burks W, Canonica GW, Ebisawa M, Gandhi S, Kamenwa R, Lee BW, Li H, Prescott S, Riva JJ, Rosenwasser L, Sampson H, Spigler M, Terracciano L, Vereda-Ortiz A, Waserman S, Yepes-Nunez JJ, Brozek JL, Schunemann HJ, World Allergy Organization-McMaster University Guidelines for Allergic Disease Prevention (GLAD-P): Probiotics. World Allergy Organ J 2015; 8: 4.

Chapter 5

The Synergistic Contribution of *Lactobacillus* and Dietary Phytophenols in Host Health

Danielle N. Kling, Guillermo E. Marcial,
Dana N. Roberson, Graciela L. Lorca and
Claudio F. Gonzalez

Additional information is available at the end of the chapter

http://dx.doi.org/10.5772/63787

Abstract

Phytophenols are found ubiquitously among all plants. They are important in diets rich in fruits and vegetables because these compounds provide health benefits to the host, ultimately decreasing the incidence of chronic diseases. These compounds act as natural antioxidants and provide anti-inflammatory, antiviral, antibiotic, and antineoplastic properties. Reactive oxygen species (ROS) are produced under normal physiological functions, and low/moderate levels are required for cellular turnover and signaling. However, when ROS levels become too high, oxidative stress can occur. Phytophenols quench ROS and ultimately avoid the damaging effects ROS elicit on the cell. The highest source of bioavailable phytophenols comes from our diet as a component usually esterified in plant fiber. For phytophenols to be absorbed by the body, they must be released by esterases, or other related enzymes. The highest amount of esterase activity comes from the gastrointestinal (GI) microbiota; therefore, the host requires the activity of mutualistic bacteria in the GI tract to release absorbable phytophenols. For this reason, mutualistic bacteria have been investigated for beneficial properties in the host. Our laboratory has begun studying the interaction of *Lactobacillus johnsonii* N6.2 with the host since it was found to be negatively correlated with type 1 diabetes (T1D). Analyses of this strain have revealed two important characteristics: (1) It has the ability to release phytophenols from dietary fiber through the secretion of two strong cinnamoyl esterases and (2) *L. johnsonii* also has the ability to generate significant amounts of H_2O_2, controlling the activity of indoleamine 2,3-dioxygenase (IDO), an immunomodulatory enzyme.

Keywords: *Lactobacillus*, *Lactobacillus johnsonii* N6.2, Indolamine 2,3-dioxygenase, 5-hydroxytryptamine, reactive oxygen species, esterase

1. Phytophenols

Phytophenols, also called polyphenols or simply phenols, are a unique group of monocyclic and polycyclic phytochemicals found within fruits, vegetables, and other plants as a component of plant fiber. Phytophenols are ubiquitously found as secondary metabolites in plants and are therefore consumed in relatively high quantities. They are a very diverse and multifunctional group of active plant compounds with substantial health potential in many areas, and numerous scientific studies demonstrate that increasing the intake of plant foods rich in fiber can minimize the incidence of modern diseases [1–3].

Consumption of foods and beverages containing phytophenols may impact nutrient levels in the body by preventing their oxidation. Their activity is based on functional groups' capacity to accept a free radical's negative charge [4, 5]. In order to be absorbed by intestinal epithelial cells, phytophenols attached to fiber can only be released by the enzymatic activities of the gastrointestinal (GI) microbiota [6–9] because the phenolic esterase enzymes necessary to release antioxidant phytophenols from plant fiber are not produced by the host GI system. It has been shown *in vitro* that after hydrolysis with purified enzymes, more biologically active compounds can be released, including hydroxytyrosol and elenolic acid from oleuropein [10, 11] and dihydroxyphenyllactic acid from rosmarinic and salvianolic acids [12, 13]. Nevertheless, very little is known about the modifications that these natural compounds undergo after ingestion.

All phytophenols arise from a common intermediate, phenylalanine, or a close precursor, shikimic acid [14]. Often they are present in conjugated forms, with sugar residues linked to hydroxyl groups, although in some cases, direct links of the sugar to an aromatic carbon do exist. In addition, associations with other compounds are also common, including linkages with carboxylic and organic acids, amines, and lipids, as well as associations with other phenols [15].

Plants produce an impressive array of phenolic compounds, and it is thought that these plant-based constituents have a stronger biological antioxidant effect when compared to synthetic antioxidants. This is mainly because phytophenols are part of the normal function of living plants and therefore are thought to have better compatibility with the body [4, 16, 17]. Although there are more than 8000 identified polyphenolic compounds, they can be sorted into four main classes: phenolic acids, flavonoids, stilbenes, and lignans [18]. **Figure 1** illustrates the different groups, which are divided by the number of rings they contain as well as the structural elements that bind these rings together.

Phenolic acids are derivatives of either benzoic acid or cinnamic acid and can thus be divided into two classes. They make up about a third of the polyphenolic compounds found in human diets. These phenolic compounds can be found in all plant-based material, although they are most commonly found in acidic fruits [19]. Flavonoids are the most abundant polyphenolic compounds found in our diet and are also the most well-studied group. More than 4000 varieties have been accounted for, often contributing to the color of flowers, fruits, and leaves [20]. Six subclasses exist, as shown in **Figure 2**, based upon variations in structure: flavonols, flavones, flavanones, flavanols, anthocyanins, and isoflavones.

http://dx.doi.org/10.5772/63787

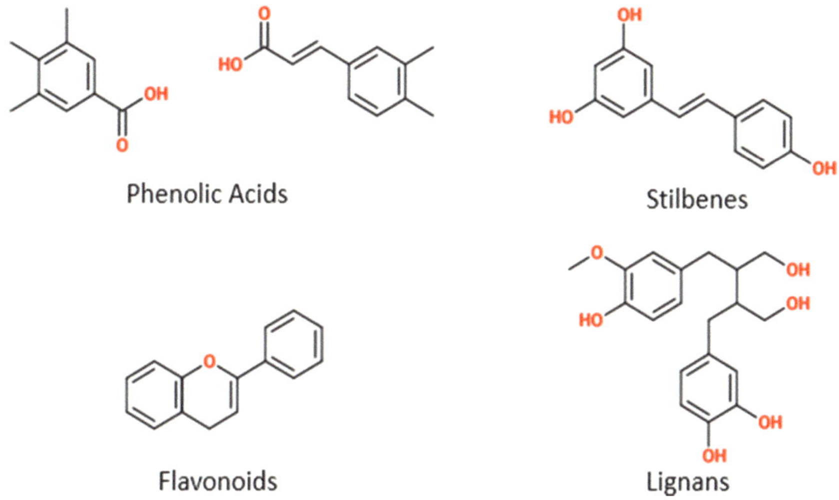

Figure 1. Chemical structures of the different classes of polyphenols, broadly divided into four classes [14].

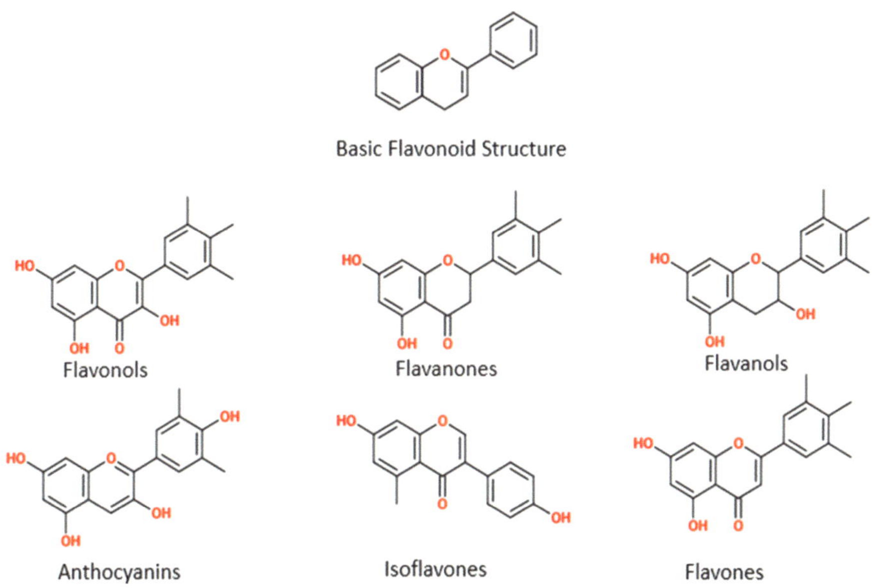

Figure 2. Chemical structures of subclasses of flavonoids [14].

Stilbenes contain two phenyl moieties connected by a two-carbon methylene bridge. Their synthesis is typically initiated as a result of injury or infection in plants, and as a consequence, their occurrence in our diet is much lower than either phenolic acids or flavonoids. The best studied stilbene is resveratrol, found mainly in grapes and as a result also in red wine. Lignans are diphenolic compounds formed by the dimerization of two cinnamic acid residues, as seen in **Figure 1**.

Estimating the total polyphenol content is most accurately done through analysis of every individual phytophenolic compound. Due to the large diversity in phytophenolics, the only way to complete this task is through a compilation of the literature data. Fortunately, the USDA database contains a nearly complete source of food composition data [21–23]. This database combined with other literature sources for the remaining phytophenolic compounds was used to develop the Phenol-Explorer database. This recently developed database is the most complete source on the content of polyphenols in foods, including glycosides, esters, and aglycones of flavonoids, phenolic acids, lignans, stilbenes, and other polyphenols [24].

The occurrence of dietary phenolics in plants is not uniform, even at the cellular level. Insoluble phytophenols are often found in cells walls, while soluble phytophenols are found within the vacuoles of plant cells [25]. In many instances, plant-based foods contain a variable mixture of polyphenols. Some polyphenols, such as flavanones and isoflavones, are found only in specific foods, whereas others such as quercetin are found in nearly all plant products. Conventionally, the outer tissues of a plant contain higher levels of phenolics than the inner tissues [26].

Various other factors can affect the concentration of dietary phytophenols, including ripeness of the plant when harvested, environmental factors, storage, and processing of plant materials [14]. Before harvesting, abiotic factors such as soil type, exposure to sunlight, and amount of rainfall can alter phenolic compounds in plants. In addition, the degree of ripeness when harvested can be positively or negatively correlated with the concentration of polyphenols, depending upon which compound is under observation [27]. Storage of plant-based foods also affects polyphenol levels, and the oxidation of polyphenols over time can be beneficial (as in the case of black tea) or harmful (as in the case of browning of fruit) to polyphenolic compound concentrations [27]. Cooking also has a major effect on phytophenolic compounds, and depending on how the material is processed, cooking may account for a 30–80% loss of phenolic content [28].

Bioavailability is described as the proportion of the nutrient that follows natural pathways to be digested, absorbed, and metabolized in the body. For phytophenols, there is no relationship between the quantity of phenolic compounds found in food and their bioavailability, and every one of the numerous known polyphenols differs in its bioavailability. Furthermore, the most ubiquitous phytophenols found in plant-based foods are not necessarily the same as those that show the highest concentration of metabolites in tissues. Often, polyphenols are present in a form that cannot directly be absorbed by the body, including esters, glycosides, or polymers [29]. Due to the microbial modification of phytophenols during absorption in the intestinal cells and later in the liver, the compounds reaching the bloodstream and bodily tissues are drastically different from those originally ingested. As a consequence, identifying all the metabolites and subsequently evaluating their activity is a difficult task. It is the chemical structure of the phytophenolic compound that determines absorption rate and extent rather than the concentration of the compound found in the diet [30]. Evidence does indirectly suggest that phenols are absorbed to some extent through the gut barrier due to an increase in antioxidant capacity of plasma after ingestion of phytophenol-rich foods [31, 32].

The potential pharmacological properties of these natural plant compounds have been demonstrated *in vitro* and include anti-inflammatory [9], antioxidant [33–35], antineoplastic

http://dx.doi.org/10.5772/63787

[10, 36], antiviral [37], and antibiotic [38] properties. Although several mechanisms of action combine to provide the widespread health benefits offered by phytophenols, their role as antioxidants is the mostly frequently studied mechanism. The intestinal inflammatory process is primarily a consequence of the overproduction of inflammatory mediators, triggered by an excess of reactive oxygen species (ROS) [39–41].

ROS are the by-products of cellular redox processes in the body. These free radical compounds contain one or more unpaired electrons in their outer orbit, creating instability that leads to significant reactivity. ROS species include superoxide ($O^{2\bullet-}$), hydroxyl ($^{\bullet}OH$), peroxyl ($ROO^{\bullet}$), lipid peroxyl ($LOO^{\bullet}$), and alkoxyl ($RO^{\bullet}$) radicals. Oxygen free radicals can also be converted to other non-radical reactive species, which are dangerous for health due to their tendency to lead to free radical reactions in living organisms. These species include hydrogen peroxide (H_2O_2), ozone (O_3), singlet oxygen ($1/2O_2$), and hypochlorous acid (HOCl). ROS are capable of modifying structural proteins or inactivating enzymes, and as a consequence disrupting normal physiologic functions in the body [42–44]. Production of free radicals is a normal part of our physiology and occurs continually to keep the body functioning properly. Processes that generate ROS include activities of the immune system, metabolism, and inflammation responses, along with stress, pollution, radiation, diet, toxins, exhaust fumes, and smoking. [4, 16, 42, 45].

Excessive production of ROS can easily overwhelm both the enzymatic and non-enzymatic antioxidant defense systems, leading to oxidative stress and inflammation. It has been widely discussed in scientific literature that increasing the intake of natural antioxidants minimizes the deleterious effects of ROS [34, 46–48]. Evidence collected from feeding assays using diets rich in antioxidant plant phenolics supports this claim [2, 7, 49]. The intake of phytophenols has been shown to minimize the production of ROS and mitigate their harmful impact on the GI system [3, 33, 50].

Oxidative stress leads to disease through four destructive pathways: membrane lipid peroxidation, protein oxidation, DNA damage, and disturbance of reducing equivalents in the cell [4]. These steps often lead to altered signaling pathways and cell destruction. Oxidative stress has been connected to various diseases such as cancer, cardiovascular diseases, neurological disorders, diabetes, and aging. Each molecule in the body is at risk of damage by ROS, and damaged molecules can impair cellular functioning and lead to cell death, which ultimately results in diseased states [43, 44, 51]. Due to the antioxidant properties of phytophenolic compounds, they are associated with the prevention of a large array of diseases, including cardiovascular disease, cancer, diabetes, rheumatoid arthritis, neurodegenerative diseases, GI diseases, renal disorders, pulmonary disorders, eye disorders, infertility, and pregnancy complications, as well as slowing the progression of aging [4].

Although reduction of ROS has been shown to decrease risk of a huge array of diseases, the classical model of ROS generation and resulting oxidative stress contrasts with some emerging scientific evidence. Benefits of ROS can in fact occur when these species are present in low/moderate concentrations, as part of normal physiological functions [43]. The majority of cells produce superoxide and hydrogen peroxide constitutively, while other cells possess inducible ROS release systems. Beneficial effects can include defense against infectious agents by phagocytosis, killing of cancer cells by macrophages and cytotoxic lymphocytes, detoxification of xenobiotics by Cytochrome P450, generation of ATP in mitochondria (energy production), cell growth, and the induction of mitogenic responses at low concentrations. ROS also plays a role in cellular signaling, including activation of several cytokines and growth factors, non-receptor tyrosine kinase activation, protein tyrosine phosphatase activation, release of calcium from intracellular stores, and activation of nuclear transcription factors. ROS can also initiate vital actions such as gene transcription and regulation of soluble guanylate cyclase activity in cells [44, 50].

Reactive oxygen species (ROS) are known to play a dual role in biological systems; they are well documented for playing a role as both deleterious and beneficial species [43, 44, 52]. We hypothesize that redox homeostasis in the GI tract is dependent on the dynamic interplay between the generation of ROS and the ROS quencher ability of antioxidant phytophenols released by intestinal microbes. Although there are possible benefits to maintain low levels of ROS in the proper functioning of the body, the diet and lifestyle of the majority results in increased levels of ROS in the body are known to be harmful and can lead to the progression of disease. In this way, it is critical to maintain the proper balance of ROS in the body, and phenolic compounds have been shown to reestablish a healthy level of ROS. Next, we turn to the vital interaction of phytophenols and microflora of the gut system that can lead to creation of redox balance critical to health.

2. Lactic acid bacteria

The group known as lactobacilli is composed of several genera of bacteria (*Leuconostoc, Pediococcus, Lactococcus,* and *Streptococcus*), *Lactobacillus* being the largest order in the phylum Firmicutes and the class Bacilli [53]. These free living lactic acid bacteria flourish in different biological niches such as soil, plants (fruits, beverage, and silage) and fermented foods (cheese, fermented milk, yogurt, meat products, alcoholic beverages, and pickled products). They are also associated with mammals as members of the microbial community characteristic of the oral cavity, GI system, urinary tract, skin, etc. [54–57]. The genus *Lactobacillus* is composed of nutritionally fastidious gram-positive, non-spore-forming rods or coccobacilli, catalase-negative, aerotolerant or anaerobic bacteria. The main characteristic of their homo- or hetero-fermentative metabolism is the production of lactic acid as the primary end fermentation product. The genus *Lactobacillus* is represented by over 212 species described to date, including several industrially relevant microorganisms such as *L. acidophilus, L. bulgaricus, L. casei, L. lactis, L. paracasei, L. plantarum, L. reuteri, L. fermentum, L. salivarius, L. rhamnosus, L. delbrueckii,* and *L. johnsonii.*

The *Lactobacillus* genus is widely studied because of the bacterias' capacity to produce lactic acid. Thus, most studies regarding their physiology were centered on acidifying bacteria such as *L. delbrueckii subsp. bulgaricus,* which in combination with *Streptococcus thermophilus* acidify milk in a few hours. This process is critical to optimize the production of fermented dairy products such as cheese and yogurt, or other non-dairy products such as pickles, sauerkraut, and sourdough bread.

The extensive use of these bacteria in food and beverage industries drove the scientific attention toward the evaluation of their impact on health, mainly on the GI system's integrity and responsiveness. Regardless, lactic acid bacteria were safely used for centuries to modify food flavor and texture, modern genomics bring back to light the scientific discussion toward their impact on human health [54, 58].

Studies of the human microbiome revealed that lactobacilli could occupy different microhabitats in the human body, such as the buccal cavity and nasal fossa, but they mainly thrive in the gut and the urogenital tract [59]. In women, it was observed that variations of estrogen and glycogen stimulates the growth of lactic acid bacteria. Depletion of vaginal lactobacilli could give rise to adverse microbial flora colonization inducing urogenital infection [60]. Gustafsson *et al.* evaluated the population of lactobacilli in healthy fertile and postmenopausal women in correlation with hormone levels [57]. They demonstrated that *L. crispatus* is the most abundant bacteria and, together with *L. vaginalis, L. jensenii* and *L. gasseri* are responsible in protecting the urogenital tract against vaginal infection. This effect was associated with the capacity of these *Lactobacillus* species to produce H_2O_2, which negatively affects the viability of pathogenic bacteria [61, 62]. The GI system is home to many different kinds of microorganisms, which globally is referred as the gut microbiota. Among these microbes, one of the most abundant groups, in this complex microbial population, is *Lactobacillus*. Although it is not the most abundant genus in the microflora, it is considered one of the most important genus due to potential beneficial effects associated with them. Scientific studies revealed that the *Lactobacillus* abundance in the gut microbiota changes according to the portion of the GI tract. The highest presence of *Lactobacillus* sequences was found in the jejunum and ileum lumen, 16% respect to the total microbiota. Their abundance in the colon/rectal lumen decreased to 9.9%. Surprisingly, *Lactobacillus* sequences were lower than 0.5% in the fecal samples studied [63–66]. The main *Lactobacillus* strains found in feces are *L. acidophilus, L. crispatus, L. gasseri, L. reuteri, L. brevis, L. sakei, L. curvatus, L. casei, L. paracasei, L. rhamnosus, L. delbrueckii, L. brevis, L. johnsonii, L. plantarum,* and *L. fermentum* [67]. In the GI context, these bacteria interact with other intestinal microbes, with food components and with the GI mucosa. The consequences of these interactions are endless; in addition, it is extremely difficult to isolate the effects and study them separately. Probably one of the most complex and interesting systems effected is the host immune system. Commensals can help in educating and maturing the host immune response and prompt the immunological defensive arsenal. All members of the *Lactobacillus* group are classified as GRAS (generally recognized as safe) organisms; consequently, they are considered innocuous or beneficial for health. The specific mechanisms by which these bacteria are considered beneficial are still the subject of important discrepancies and the center of scientific debates.

Lactobacilli are excellent organic acid producers, converting sugars into lactic acid and other by-products such as acetate, ethanol, CO_2, butyrate, and succinate. They produce small molecules, as well, such as H_2O_2, or compounds such as diacetyl, or acetaldehyde [67]. Several of these metabolites are bioactive, with beneficial effects for the human GI. At the same time, they are essential for the dairy industry because they provide flavoring and display natural preservative properties [68]. They help to maintain the integrity of GI layers, favoring the renewal of the epithelium. A continuous renewal of the GI layers is critical to maintain an adequate barrier function to minimize several significant human diseases, including autoimmunity and cancer. According to recently published studies, the production of low amounts of H_2O_2 at the GI level is beneficial to the host. Besides its well-characterized antimicrobial activity, this molecule could directly down-regulate the early stages of the host inflammatory response and improve epithelial cell restitution and healing via the oxidation of cysteine residues in the host tyrosine phosphatases [62, 69].

Other important metabolites synthesized by *Lactobacillus* species are larger molecules such as polysaccharides (viscosifying agents) [70] and enzymes (proteases, bacteriocins, esterases, and lipases) [6, 71, 72], which improve dairy product quality (flavor development, texture modification) and provide beneficial effects to boost human health [73]. *L. helveticus* is considered one of the most efficient species associated with proteolysis in cheese ripening. *L. helveticus* also produces bioactive peptides with antihypertensive and antimicrobial activity [74]. Indeed, *Lactobacillus* antimicrobial activity is directly related to its ability to secrete bacteriocins. A subset of *Lactobacillus* strains produce these kind of antimicrobial peptides such as *L. sakei* (bavaricin, sakacin) [75], *L. curvatus* (curvaticin), *L. plantarum* (pediocin), *L. salivairus* (bacteriocins) [76], and *L. acidophilus* (acidocin) [77]. These antimicrobials may play an essential role in regulating the composition of the microbial communities within the GI system, influencing the host's health; however, not all of them showed promising effects on human [71].

Maintenance of the GI redox homeostasis is essential in minimizing human diseases. The production of enzymes, which could increase the amount of free and active antioxidant agents in the GI lumen, is another important characteristic associated with several *Lactobacillus* strains. These enzymes, such as esterases and/or lipases, are synthesized by the intestinal microbiota and can release redox quenchers like the above-described phytophenols that are ingested with the host diet. Thus, the ingestion of probiotic bacteria able to produce these enzymes is a healthy and natural alternative to modulate the redox status in the GI tract. Lactobacilli are excellent producers of lipases and esterases, and several of the best producing strains were selected by the dairy industry due to their contribution in cheese ripening. The esterases are active toward a wide range of ester substrates from free fatty acids to tri-, di-, and monoacylglyceride substrates. Cinnamoyl esterases (CE) are one of the most important enzymes involved in releasing antioxidant molecules from dietary fibers. These enzymes break down the ester linkages between hydroxycinnamates and sugars, commonly found in the fiber of dietary plants, releasing phenolics such as hydroxycinnamic, ferulic, coumaric, and caffeic acids with high ROS scavenging activity. Genes encoding various esterases have been described in *L. fermentum* and *L. reuteri*, *L. leichmanni*, and *L. farciminis*, and the first two species are frequently found in animal and human feces. These enzymes have also demonstrated to be active toward soluble polyphenols such as chlorogenic acid to release caffeic and quinic acids [78]. The accumulation of the enzymatic products released (monophenols) in *Lactobacillus* cultures suggests that these microorganisms do not (or do so extremely slowly) metabolize the phenolic acids released. The enzymatic action correlates directly with increased amounts of phenolics (i.e., caffeic acid) detected in the bloodstream of model animals fed with fibers in combination with probiotics formulated with those strains [78]. Guglielmetti *et al.* studied the activity of CE produced by *L. helveticus* MIMLh5 on soluble phenolics, such as chlorogenic acid, to enrich food with free caffeic acid [79]. *L. helveticus* enzymes are mainly intracellular, but some of them could be surface-associated as observed in *L. fermentum* [80]. *L. plantarum*, frequently found in plant-derived food products where hydroxycinnamoyl esters are abundant, produces the enzyme Lp_0796 (esterase), which hydrolyzes the four model substrates for feruloyl esterases (methyl ferulate, methyl caffeate, methyl *p*-coumarate, and methyl sinapinate). This esterase is generally present among several *L. plantarum* strains and provides new insights into the metabolism of hydroxycinnamic compounds in this bacterial species [81]. Further studies on *L. plantarum* showed another esterase encoded by the *est_1092* gene is able to hydrolyze hydroxycinnamic esters, such as methyl ferulate or methyl caffeate, and is active on a broad range of phenolic esters [82]. *L. acidophilus* produces a novel CE with high similarity (70%) with the main CE characterized in *L. johnsonii* LJ1228 [72]. Other *L. acidophilus* and *L. johnsonii* strains displayed, as well, high CE activity [79]. One strain of *L. johnsonii* showed high ferulic acid esterase activity, stimulates insulin production, and alleviates symptoms caused by diabetes [83]. However, there is no direct evidence to associate the ability to release phenolics with the capacity to stimulate insulin production. The strain *L. johnsonii* N6.2 presented two different proteins with ferulic acid esterase activity. These enzymes showed high affinities and catalytic efficiencies toward aromatic compounds such as ethyl ferulate and chlorogenic acid [6]. *L. johnsonii* NCC533 also hydrolyzes rosmarinic acid, the main components of rosemary extracts, and it is ascribed to many health benefits.

The released monophenols (caffeic acid or other cinnamic acids) may exert its biological activities on the host, either at the level of the colonic mucosa itself, or in other tissues and organs, possibly after further modification by mammalian enzymes in the liver [80]. The release and solubilization of these phenolics, from fiber, also favor its absorption and further modification by other GI commensals. *In vitro* fermentation assays demonstrate that the fecal microbiota can efficiently metabolize caffeic, chlorogenic, and caftaric acids. With the use of highly sensitive analytical techniques, it was possible to identify two major metabolites: 3-hydroxyphenylpropionic (3-HPP) and benzoic acids (BA) once the original compounds were fully metabolized. Similar metabolic patterns were observed for other polyphenolic acids, suggesting a large and important metabolic flexibility of the gut microbiota [84]. Evidence for a metabolic pathway leading to the formation of BA from 3-HPP is supported by the established quality of intestinal microorganisms to carry out biological dehydroxylation of 3-HPP to 3-phenylpropionic acid, which can itself be further β-oxidized into BA by the colonic microbiota [85]. Alternatively, the absorbed cinnamic and phenylpropionic acids undergo β-oxidation in the liver to produce BA, which is subsequently conjugated to glycine to form hippuric acid in the liver [86].

The capacity of lactic acid bacteria to transform phenolic compounds into smaller novel molecules able to be absorbed in the GI system reoriented modern research to use combinations of probiotics and prebiotic products together. A large variety of dietary fibers were used for this purpose. Yet, the microbial metabolism of the released compounds by different bioconversion pathways, such as glycosylation, deglycosylation, ring cleavage, methylation, glucuronidation, and sulfate conjugation, depends on the microbial strains and substrates used. The results of such combinations are a large array of new metabolites, many of them recognized as bioactive molecules. This strategy demonstrates to have the potential to produce extracts with a high-added value from plant-based matrices (soybean, apple, cereals, among others).

Studies of apple juice fermentation to manage hyperglycemia, hypertension, and modulation of microbiota composition were also carried out. Apple juice, fermented by *L. acidophilus*, showed outstanding effects enhancing the free radical-scavenging activity in blood samples. *Lactobacillus* fermented samples inhibited *H. pylori in vitro*. However, the fermented extracts did not exert inhibitory effects on the beneficial intestinal species such as *Bifidobacterium longum*. Thus, these data provided biochemical rationale for the development of new fermented food to reduce hyperglycemia (diabetes) and other chronic diseases [87]. The development of probiotics with therapeutic and preventative effects for various diseases and metabolic disorders is the trend of new healthy nutrition. The main limitation for oral probiotics is the harsh conditions of the GI system. For that, the beneficial bacteria have to reach the intestines alive, colonize, and locally release enzymes or bioactive metabolites.

The benefits of *Lactobacillus* intake is not only linked to the capacity to hydrolyze phytophenols inside the lower GI system but also to prehydrolyze those present in plant extract (juice, fruits, etc.) and increased the phenolic content in food and beverages. Predigestion will enhance their absorption once they reach the small intestine to exert their healing properties. For example, the use of three *Lactobacillus* strains (*L. johnsonii* LA1, *L. reuteri* SD2112, and *L. acidophilus* LA-5) improved the bioavailability of the dietary phenolics present in barley and oat flour by 20-fold [88]. The free ferulic acid in the pretreated cereals increased from 1 μg/g dried weight up to 39–56 μg/g dried weight. Comparing the three strains used, *L. johnsonii* demonstrate to be more active in releasing phenolic acids than the other strains. These data showed that cereal fermentation with specific probiotic strains can significantly increase the quantity of free phenolic acids, improving their bioavailability [89]. *L. johnsonii* NCC 533 synthesizes esterases and a hydroxycinnamate decarboxylase responsible for the biotransformation of chlorogenic and caffeic acids. The complete hydrolysis of 5-caffeoylquinic acid *in vitro* occurred during the first 16 h of incubation. After 48 h, caffeic acid was completely transformed to 4-vinylcatechol (4-VC). In this case, the bacteria increased the presence of caffeic acid and simultaneously generated flavor compounds from plant phytophenols [90]. These data provide solid evidence that the same microorganism is able to hydrolyze caffeoyl quinic acids into 4-VC, combining chlorogenate esterase and a hydroxycinnamate decarboxylase activity [6, 91]. Similar results have been reported in the case of some *L. brevis* strains [92].

The ability of lactic acid bacteria to metabolize dietary phytophenols prompts the use of new component combinations in fermented products. Several of these new blends were formulated with plant extracts rich in aromatic compounds. Example of this is the addition of green tea in bioyogurts fermented with selected lactic acid bacteria. Species such as *St. thermophilus, L. acidophilus* LA-5, *B. animalis* subsp. *lactis* BB-12, or acidophilus enhanced the antioxidant capacity of these preparations in dose-dependent manner. Similar studies were carried out with different tea extracts, green, white, and black tea (*Camellia sinensis*) in yogurt combined with *L. acidophilus* LA-5, *Bifidobacterium* Bb-12, *L. casei* LC-01, *S. thermophilus* Th-4, and *L. delbrueckii* ssp. *bulgaricus*. In general, the three types of tea extracts did not significantly affect the viability of the bacteria used during storage [93]. The tea extracts could be successfully used as a functional additives in fermented food, adding extra value to the known health benefits of probiotics. Others extracts prepared from olive, garlic, onion, and citrus were also evaluated using similar formulations [94].

3. A model case study, *Lactobacillus johnsonii* N6.2

The intestinal epithelium is one of the most immunologically active surfaces of the body due to the high abundance of microbes and food antigens that are constantly exposed to the GI system. The mucosal surface of the intestinal epithelium is the first line of defense from invading pathogens in the GI tract. Breaching this barrier and subsequently activating aberrant immune signaling have been involved in many diseases, both locally and systematically related. In this context, it has been proposed that there is a complex interplay between gut resident microbiota [95, 96], gut permeability [97], and altered immune function in the development of type 1 diabetes [98].

Currently, our scientific efforts are directed on characterizing a strain of *Lactobacillus* (*L. johnsonii* N6.2). This lactobacilli is abundant in GI microbiome in a line of animals used as a T1D model, in contrast to the scarcity observed in the counterpart diabetes prone animals. Type 1 diabetes (T1D), also referred to as diabetes mellitus type 1, is an autoimmune disease in which pancreatic β-cells produce little to no insulin due to their destruction. Its more commonly known and more prevalent counterpart, type 2 diabetes, occurs when the body becomes resistant to insulin. Both of these conditions result in increased blood glucose levels, called hyperglycemia. Insulin is the hormone responsible for absorbing sugar, in the form of glucose, from circulating blood to be stored in skeletal muscles and fat cells. Although type 1 diabetes has a genetic component and primarily occurs in adolescents and children, it is possible for adults to develop the disease too. Five to 10 percent of diabetes cases in adults are the result of T1D, and an estimated 80 people per day are newly diagnosed with T1D [99, 100]. Unfortunately, recently epidemiological studies have suggested that the incidence of T1D is increasing up to 3–4% globally every year, most notably among youths [101, 102].

L. johnsonii N6.2 was discovered when it was negatively correlated with diabetes development when analyzing the stool samples from BioBreeding diabetes-prone (BB-DP) and BioBreeding diabetes-resistant (BB-DR) rats. Stool embodies a representative microbiome of an individual and is a useful sample for understanding the microbial diversity of the GI tract. Currently, it is estimated that more than 1000 microbial species encompassing more than 100 trillion microorganisms colonize the GI system, collectively outnumbering human genes by 150-fold [103]. These microorganisms grow more in number and diversity progressing through the GI tract. The BioBreeding rat is popular model when studying type 1 diabetes, as it spontaneously develops this disease through its genetic predisposition. After using culture-independent methods, it was found that two genera, *Bifidobacterium* and *Lactobacillus*, showed a higher abundance in BB-DR rats [104]. Quantitative PCR of 16S rRNA revealed a higher abundance of *Bifidobacterium* and *Lactobacillus* in BB-DR samples [104]. However, it was unknown whether the higher abundance of these bacteria was just the common microflora of a "healthy" gut or if they played a part in preventing the onset of T1D. Further analyses of the *Lactobacillus* strains in the BB-DR rat model revealed that those with CE activity, such as *L. johnsonii* N6.2 and *L. reuteri* TD1, were negatively correlated with T1D development [6].

As it was described before, the release of antioxidant compounds by probiotic bacteria is relevant since an enhanced oxidative stress response triggered by the excessive production of reactive oxygen species is observed in T1D and other diseases [105–107]. This characteristic was relevant in the study because a low dosage of ferulic acid stimulates the release of insulin and alleviates symptoms common to T1D in rodents [83, 108, 109]. Therefore, it would seem plausible that orally administering lactic acid bacteria containing CE qualities would help reduce blood glucose levels and ultimately prevent the onset of diabetes. To confirm this, a feeding experiment of *L. johnsonii* N6.2 and *L. reuteri* TD1 on BioBreeding rats was conducted to determine whether these strains were responsible for the lack of T1D development. While *L. johnsonii* N6.2-fed rats were associated with reduced diabetes onset, *L. reuteri* T1D showed similar diabetes development characteristics as vehicle-fed control groups [110]. A feruloyl esterase screening assay of bacterial stool sample isolates from BB-DR rats on MRS media supplemented with feruloyl esters demonstrates that *L. johnsonii* N6.2 contained the highest feruloyl esterase activity [6]. Enzymatic screening of two purified *L. johnsonii* proteins, Lj0536 and Lj1228, showed high preference and good enzymatic activity using aromatic esters as substrates (**Figure 3**). Lj1228 displayed the best hydrolytic activity with ethyl ferulate, chlorogenic acid, and rosmarinic acid, while Lj0536 showed a preference to ethyl ferulate. Sequence analyses of these proteins revealed a 42% similarity and the classical serine nucleophilic motif characteristic for some feruloyl esterases [111, 112]. Biochemical analyses of these enzymes suggested that they maintain excellent activity in the presence of emulsifiers. Their activity was tested in the presence of conjugated and deconjugated bile salts of which none of the compounds assayed decreased their activity. Interestingly, with increasing concentrations of

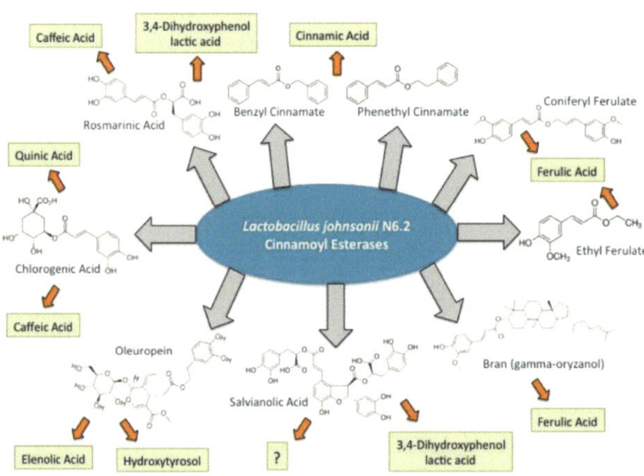

Figure 3. *L. johnsonii* LJ0536 hydrolyze a wide range of substrates. The product(s) of hydrolysis for each substrate are boxed.

sodium glycocholate, Lj0536 showed increased activity. In this condition, both enzymes were active against a wide variety of substrates, showing the highest affinity toward aromatic esters.

L. johnsonii post-weaning feedings has demonstrated a decreased incidence of diabetes in BB-DP rats compared to vehicle-fed controls and *L. reuteri* TD1-fed rats [110]. With this in mind, it was then determined what type of altered environment *L. johnsonii* created compared to healthy controls and diabetic animals (including those animals from *L. johnsonii* feedings and controls that developed T1D). The first thing that was noticed was the modification of the intestinal microbiota as determined by real-time quantification. While all animals showed an abundance of *Lactobacillus* in stool samples, differences in species seem to differ among feeding groups (*L. johnsonii, L. reuteri,* and vehicle control). Vehicle control animals displayed a predominance of *L. murinus* (65%), while 88% and 92% of *L. johnsonii* and *L. reuteri*, respectively, corresponded to the fed bacteria in each group. Analyses of ileal mucosa unveiled a significant increase of the *Lactobacillus* population in all rats that did not develop diabetes, and a significant increase of enterobacteria was found in all diabetic animals. Since no differences in the microbiota were obtained in stool samples, but were statistically significant in ileal mucosa, the positive effect of *L. johnsonii* N6.2 could be exhibited primarily in the intestinal mucosa [110].

As it was observed that an altered intestinal microbiota was associated with diabetes onset, as previously suggested [95, 96], gut permeability and barrier function were investigated next between *L. johnsonii*-fed, healthy controls, and diabetic animals. It was previously reported that changes in intestinal morphology and permeability, partly due to decreased levels of claudin-1, were observed before the onset of T1D [97]. Claudin-1 is an intercellular tight junction protein responsible for cell-to-cell adhesion in epithelial cell layers. This protein is important in strengthening the physical barrier that keeps the contents of gut lumen from passing into the lamina propria. It has been suggested that unregulated passage of environmental antigens through the intercellular space of the intestinal epithelial could trigger the autoimmune response that contributes to T1D. Expression analysis of the claudin-1 gene in *L. johnsonii*-fed animals exposed its higher abundance when compared to healthy controls or diabetic animals [110]. Furthermore, a significant increase in goblet cells was unveiled in healthy controls and *L. johnsonii*-fed animals compared to those that developed diabetes. Goblet cells produce mucin, the main constituent of the mucosal lining of the GI tract. This feature is important when considering the harsh environment of the GI tract and the constant exposure to potential invading pathogens and inflammatory antigens. The mucosal layer serves as one's first line of defense against these threats by acting as a physical, viscous, and continuously moving layer that rests above epithelial cells. Most harmful substances get trapped in the mucous and before even making it to the epithelial layer, get swept down the intestines. The increase in claudin-1 and goblet cell levels in *L. johnsonii*-fed animals strengthens and physically protects the epithelial cell layer and undoubtedly intensifies intestinal barrier function contributing to the decrease in diabetes onset.

Among the destructive properties of reactive oxygen species (ROS) generated during early disease development is its ability to disrupt the function of epithelial tight junction proteins [113]. To determine the extent of the oxidative stress environment, ileal mucosal hexanoyllysine levels were quantified by ELISA and a significant increase of levels was observed in diabetic animals when compared to healthy controls and *L. johnsonii*-fed animals [110]. Due to the difference in the oxidative environment between diabetic and non-diabetic animals, the expression of genes involved in ROS detoxification pathways were also quantified. It was evident that *L. johnsonii* helps the host to cope with intestinal oxidative stress response as levels of superoxide dismutase 2, catalase, glutathione reductase, and glutathione peroxide were induced in diabetic animals. Meanwhile, superoxide dismutase and glutathione peroxidase were induced in healthy controls compared to *L. johnsonii*-fed groups. Taken collectively, catalase and glutathione reductase were negatively correlated with a healthy status, while superoxide dismutase 2 and glutathione peroxidase were negatively correlated with *L. johnsonii* feeding. Also among the stress response genes assayed was inducible nitric oxide synthase (iNOS), which produces nitric oxide in the presence of ROS. The mRNA levels of iNOS were significantly reduced in *L. johnsonii*-fed rats compared to healthy controls and those that developed diabetes. When further examining the iNOS protein levels via Western blot, *L. johnsonii*-fed rats and healthy controls showed similar levels of detection, suggesting that expression of iNOS is associated with healthy status. Amid the inducers of iNOS expression is INFγ, a pro-inflammatory cytokine [114, 115]. It was hypothesized that a negative correlation existed between pro-inflammatory cytokines, specifically INFγ, and the reduced stress response due to *L. johnsonii* feeding. This hypothesis was proven as diabetic animals showed a significant increase in INFγ gene expression compared to healthy animals; meanwhile, healthy controls and *L. johnsonii*-fed animals did not show any statistical differences.

Since it has been determined that *L. johnsonii* N6.2 feedings can promote a healthy gut microbiota and strengthen epithelial barrier function, it was next examined whether *L. johnsonii* could influence immune function. At the intestinal mucosal layer, resident microbiota and host cells reside in constant homeostasis, epithelial cells tightly controlled by the recognition and tolerance of local bacteria. Host cells recognize the resident microbiota or their associated components through pattern recognition receptors (Toll-like receptor, TLR) and/or by cytoplasmic nucleotide-binding oligomerization domain (NOD)-like receptors, which can subsequently initiate an immune response. Of the first things noticed with *L. johnsonii* administration was the overexpression of pro-inflammatory chemokine mRNA levels, particularly CCL20 (MIP3A), CXCL8 (IL-8), and CXCL10 (IP-10), suggesting that *L. johnsonii* may prime the innate immune system to become more resistant to a subsequent strong inflammatory response [116]. Investigation of the ability of *L. johnsonii* to activate TLR and NOD-like receptor revealed that exposure to *L. johnsonii* created a 4.2- and 10-fold increased expression of TLR7 and TLR9, respectively. Because both of these receptors are involved in nucleic acid recognition, cell free extracts and purified *L. johnsonii* nucleic acid extracts were tested on their ability to induce expression of these TLRs. In both cases, cell-free extracts and purified *L. johnsonii* nucleic acid were able to increase the mRNA levels of TLR7 and TL9, suggesting that the ability for epithelial cells to sense foreign nucleic acids may be involved in the observed increased of some chemokine levels. This also suggests that *L. johnsonii* predominantly exerts its signaling capability through RNA/DNA recognition, as opposed to other cell components, such as peptidoglycan that is sensed by TLR2 and NOD2. Lastly, consequences of TLR9 induction by *L. johnonii* were determined by exploring the expression of Frizzled 5 receptor (fzd5), which is responsible for Paneth cell maturation, and INF-α, which is secreted by TLR9 activity and induces the chemokine CXCL10 [117–119]. Paneth cells are located at the base of intestinal glands throughout the small intestines and secrete antimicrobial peptides. *L. johnsonii* administration showed higher levels of Paneth cells in agreement with the higher levels of fzd5, and a higher level of INF-α, in agreement with the observed increased levels of CXCL10 [116]. As discovered in this study, *L. johnsonii* may be able to prime the immune system by activating an innate immune response early on and therefore protecting the host from more prominent stimuli later on.

As more is studied about *L. johnsonii* N6.2, it has been found that its protective functions are very diverse, supporting its probiotic qualities. In addition to the activation of innate immune response, adaptive immune response stimulation was discovered when diabetes-resistant *L. johnsonii*-fed rats were correlated with a T helper 17 (Th17) cell bias [120]. Th17 cells protect the host from extracellular pathogens by recruiting neutrophils and macrophages to the site of infection. This activity could aid in defending the host from aberrant microflora that could ultimately trigger the autoimmune response leading to T1D. While experimenting with other host-effected pathways, our recent focus has been on the ability of *L. johnsonii* to modulate the tryptophan catabolism pathway. This pathway involves the rate-limiting enzyme indoleamine 2,3-dioxygenase (IDO), which is the first enzyme along the pathway that breaks down tryptophan into kynurenine. Kynurenine is a potent aryl hydrocarbon receptor (AhR) ligand; however, the largest source of AhR ligands is found in the diet among which are vegetable and fruit phytophenols [121–123]. Interestingly, IDO induction has also been linked to AhR [124–126]. AhR is a ligand-activated, basic helix-loop-helix transcriptional activator that is associated with many diseases, including autoimmunity [127–129]. Since it was previously found that *L. johnsonii* associates with the ileal mucosa and its colonization correlated with decreased expression of pro-inflammatory cytokine INFγ, the ileal tissue seemed to suggest the best site for observing *L. johnsonii* effects on host cells [110, 130]. More importantly, INFγ has been noted as a primary inducer of IDO in many cell types. Indeed, while surveying different tissues via quantification of the IDO gene expression, the ileum appeared to have a decreased appearance of IDO transcripts in *L. johnsonii*-fed animals compared to control animals [130]. Healthy control rats expressed a 4.7-fold higher level of IDO transcripts, while diabetic animals expressed 11.8-fold increase in mRNA levels compared to *L. johnsonii*-fed animals [130]. This correlated with an observed decrease in blood serum kynurenine levels through HPLC in *L. johnsonii*-fed animals compared to healthy controls and diabetic animals [130]. However, since this study was performed at 120 days, after diabetes onset, it could not reveal early developmental or physiological effects of the bacterial feeding in the host. To address this, a study was completed to evaluate the effects of *L. johnsonii* feedings in a prediabetic host. As a reliable indicator of IDO activity, systemic kynurenine: tryptophan ratios were quantified via HPLC in 30- and 60-day-old prediabetic BBDP rats. At both ages, serum kynurenine levels decreased significantly from the controls while only at 30 days of age did serum tryptophan levels show a significant increase [130]. To verify that IDO activity was responsible for the reduced systemic kynurenine: tryptophan ratios between bacterial-fed groups and controls, the activity of a related enzyme more commonly found in the liver, tryptophan 2,3-dioxygenase (TDO), was examined. TDO, unlike IDO, was previously reported to be unresponsive to inflammatory stimuli and is important in homeostatic control of tryptophan levels under normal conditions. However, recently TDO expression has been correlated to neurological diseases, such as Alzheimer's, and various cancers, such as ovarian carcinoma, breast, and gliomas [121, 131]. After examining activity levels from tissue lysates, there was not a significant difference between the TDO activities in *L. johnsonii*-fed rats and vehicle-fed controls. IDO is widely distributed throughout the human host, and therefore, significant levels can be found throughout the GI tract. Since this enzyme, and its downstream catabolite kynurenine, is activated during inflammatory conditions, it could be involved in the inflammatory response associated with diabetes. Interestingly, we have reported that *L. johnsonii* feedings can reduce the expression of INFγ, a pro-inflammatory cytokine, in the ileum of rats after diabetes onset [110]. Upon performing Western blots of lysates of the colon, cecum, duodenum, jejunum, ileum, liver, and pancreas, it was found that the colon and ileum had variable, but overall decreased, levels of IDO in *L. johnsonii*-fed animals compared to control animals [130]. This correlates well with reduced ileal INFγ expression and overall decreased inflammation in *L. johnsonii*-fed hosts. At this point, it appeared that *L. johnsonii* effected IDO activity and subsequent systemic kynurenine concentrations.

L. johnsonii produces an inhibitor of IDO affecting the enzymatic activity and the products synthesized downstream the pathway. Diluted cell-free supernatant (CFS) of *L. johnsonii* was incubated with purified recombinant IDO, and the resulting kynurenine concentrations were quantified. Increasing concentrations of *L. johnsonii* CFS caused an increased inhibition of IDO activity. Furthermore, CFS from *L. johnsonii* N6.2 most potently inhibited IDO when compared to other enteric *Lactobacillus* species CFS effect on IDO activity [130]. This observation stimulated the characterization of *L. johnsonii* N6.2 supernatant in order to locate the IDO inhibitor. It was found that increased concentrations of hydrogen peroxide (H_2O_2) correlated with increased *L. johnsonii* culture incubation time before centrifugation and collection of the CFS [130]. Upon increasing concentrations of catalase, which decreases the pool of H_2O_2, IDO activity increased, supporting the role of H_2O_2 in CFS as an inhibitor of IDO. Likewise, upon increasing concentrations of H_2O_2, IDO activity decreased in a dose-dependent manner. This strongly supported H_2O_2 as an inhibitor of IDO enzyme activity. This enzyme contains heme in the catalytic center to carry out its dioxygenase activity. When the active ferrous centers are oxidized to its inactive ferric form, the dioxygenase activity of IDO is restricted [132]. This causes an accumulation of tryptophan and a decrease in kynurenine levels that can be detected throughout the host. Hydrogen peroxide has the ability to oxidize the reactive heme ferrous centers of IDO, rendering the enzyme inactive. In this current study, the biological relevance of H_2O_2 was tested by measuring the levels of H_2O_2 in the GI tract of *L. johnsonii*-fed animals. Since ileal IDO levels were reduced, the hypothesis was that an increase of hydrogen peroxide would be found in these tissues compared to other sites of the body. This could potentially explain the difference in IDO expression of the ileum compared to other sites of the GI tract. Indeed, when measuring H_2O_2 levels from GI contents, the ileum contained higher levels compared to other sections of the digestive tract [130]. Since *L. johnsonii* most strongly associates with the host mucosa at this site, it further supports the hypothesis of the ability of *L. johnsonii* to produce an inhibitor of IDO [110]. Upon RNA-seq analysis of *L. johnsonii* grown under different aeration conditions, a gene (T285_08005) regulating H_2O_2 production was identified. The encoding protein contained a Per-Arnst-Sim (PAS) domain and regulated the H_2O_2 production from heterodimeric FMN reductases, FRedA and FRedB (WP_004898036.1 and WP_011162530.1, respectively) [62].

After experiencing reduced kynurenine production and IDO inhibition in response to *L. johnsonii*, it was hypothesized that other tryptophan metabolite concentrations could be effected. Tryptophan is a precursor to the neurotransmitter 5-hydroxytryptamine (5-HT, serotonin), which is predominantly produced in enterochromaffin cells along the GI epithelium. IDO also has the enzymatic activity to catalyze 5-HT to 5-hydroxykynuramine, aiding in increased 5-HT turnover [133, 134]. Using ELISA, 5-HT levels in ileum tissue lysates and blood serum collected from 60-day-old BBDP rats were quantified. Serotonin levels were significantly elevated, both locally and peripherally, in *L. johnsonii*-fed animals [130].

Figure 4 most accurately summarizes the work our group has done in characterizing *Lactobacillus johnsonii* N6.2, starting with its discovery in 2008 and most recently revealing its regulating effects on IDO. This bacterial genera was correlated with a reduced diabetes onset when comparing BioBreeding diabetes-prone and diabetes-resistant rats [104]. It was identified that *Lactobacillus* strains that contain CE activity were more correlated with diabetes resistance, and through subsequent feeding assays of these potential bacterial targets, *L. johnsonii* N6.2 was identified as being negatively associated with T1D [6, 110]. Since this discovery, *L. johnsonii* N6.2 has been characterized in regard to its diabetes resistance. *L. johnsonii* strengthens gut permeability through a higher abundance of the tight junction claudin-1 levels and goblet cells, and it reduces GI stress by reducing the expression of oxidative stress genes and inflammatory INF-γ levels [110]. Among the most recent and most interesting findings of the qualities of *L. johnsonii* is its ability to modulate IDO activity through its production of H_2O_2 [130]. However, this bacterium's esterase activity has the ability to quench its own H_2O_2 production through the release of phytophenols. These antioxidants have the potential to eliminate part of the pool of produced H_2O_2, along with other even more dangerous ROS that precede chronic diseases. In the case of *L. johnsonii* N6.2, sufficient H_2O_2 production is observed in the ileum, where *L. johnsonii* is localized [110, 130]. Conversely, reduced levels of oxidative stress genes are observed in the ileum of *L. johnsonii*-fed rats [6, 110]. Thus, one of the main probiotic properties of *L. johnsonii* could be its ability to maintain redox homeostasis in the GI tract. This balance is dependent on the dynamic interplay between the generation of H_2O_2 and the ROS quenching ability of antioxidant phytophenols released by this bacterium. The H_2O_2 released by this bacterium in the intestinal lumen would stimulate oxidative stress defense mechanisms in host cells, while controlling the activity of IDO [130, 132]. Meanwhile, enzymes unique to *L. johnsonii* will increase the pool of free, bioavailable antioxidant phytophenols in the intestinal lumen. The phenolic released will differentially quench the most reactive ROS.

Although *L. johnsonii* N6.2 was found and characterized in regards to its correlation with reduced T1D onset, it has the potential to expand its beneficial functions into the realm of other chronic diseases. IDO is an immunoregulatory enzyme whose altered activity has been

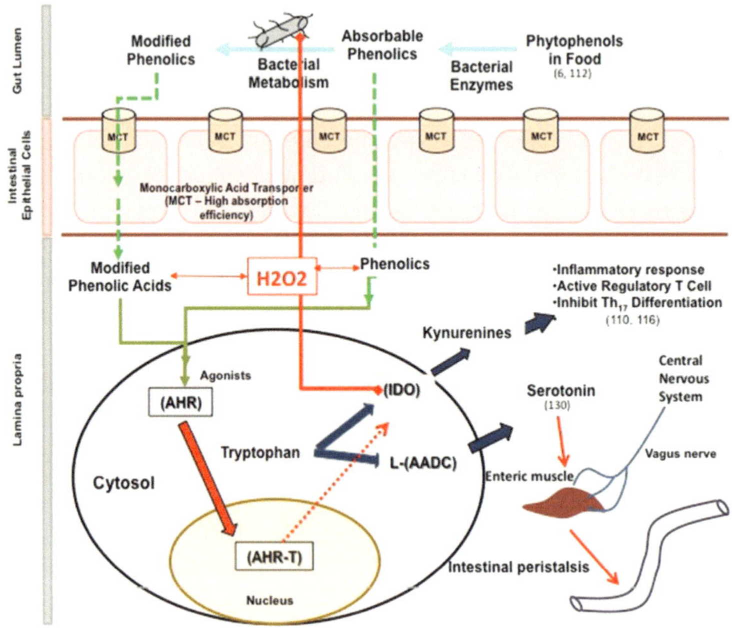

Figure 4. Gastrointestinal (GI) epithelium with proposed mechanisms of phytophenol and H_2O_2 action. This figure summarizes the results published by the group between 2009 and 2014.

observed in a multitude of diseases, including autoimmunity and cancer [135–137]. *L. johnsonii* N6.2 has the ability to regulate IDO activity by inactivating its redox-sensitive heme centers through H_2O_2 production [130]. The effect of this inactivation has the potential to expand over into other chronic disease and reduce their occurrence. This makes regulators of IDO an important immunotherapy target in preventing some of today's most serious diseases. Resident microbiota provide many protective functions for the host, such as outcompeting pathogenic threats, releasing necessary resources from digested foods, and maintaining GI homeostasis. It is to no surprise that disturbances to microfloral composition could dictate disease onset. There are numerous probiotics in the market, encompassing many different genera. These probiotics exert beneficial properties through their unique enzymes, their released metabolites, or a combination of both as in the case of *L. johnsonii* N6.2. Therefore, probiotic administration serves as an important defense in preventing some of the most common and chronic diseases.

Acknowledgements

This material is based upon work that is supported by the National Institute of Food and Agriculture, US Department of Agriculture, under award number 2015-67017-23182, and Juvenile Diabetes Research Foundation under award number 1-INO-2014-176-A-V.

http://dx.doi.org/10.5772/63787

Author details

Danielle N. Kling[1], Guillermo E. Marcial[1,3], Dana N. Roberson[1], Graciela L. Lorca[1,2] and Claudio F. Gonzalez[1,2*]

*Address all correspondence to: cfgonzalez@ufl.edu

1 Department of Microbiology and Cell Science, IFAS, University of Florida, Gainesville, USA

2 Genetics Institute, University of Florida, Gainesville, USA

3 CERELA-Conicet, Tucuman, Argentina

References

[1] Zamora-ros R, Cherubini A, Urp M, Bandinelli S, Ferrucci L, Andres-lacueva C. High concentrations of a urinary biomarker of polyphenol intake are associated with decreased mortality in older adults. J Nutr. 2013;143:1445–50.

[2] Sansbury LB, Wanke K, Albert PS, Kahle L, Schatzkin A, Lanza E. The effect of strict adherence to a high-fiber, high-fruit and -vegetable, and low- fat eating pattern on adenoma recurrence. Am J Epidemiol. 2009;170(5):576–84.

[3] Davis CD, Milner JA. Gastrointestinal microflora, food components and colon cancer prevention. J Nutr Biochem. 2009;20(10):743–52.

[4] Sen S, Chakraborty R. The role of antioxidants in human health. Oxidative Stress: Diagnostics, Prevention, and Therapy; 2011. p. 1–37.

[5] Watson R, Preedy V, Zibadi S. Polyphenols in Human Health and Disease. 1st ed. London: Academic Press; 2013. 1488p.

[6] Kin KL, Lorca GL, Gonzalez CF. Biochemical properties of two cinnamoyl esterases purified from a Lactobacillus johnsonii strain isolated from stool samples of diabetes-resistant rats. Appl Environ Microbiol. 2009;75(15):5018–24.

[7] Topakas E, Vafiadi C, Christakopoulos P. Microbial production, characterization and applications of feruloyl esterases. Process Biochem. 2007;42(4):497–509.

[8] Aura A-M. Microbial metabolism of dietary phenolic compounds in the colon. Phytochem Rev. 2008;7(3):407–29.

[9] Russell W, Scobbie L, Chesson A, Richardson A, Stewart C, Duncan S, et al. Anti-inflammatory implications of the microbial transformation of dietary phenolic compounds. Nutr Cancer. 2008;60(5):636–42.

[10] Sirianni R, Chimento A, De Luca A, Casaburi I, Rizza P, Onofrio A, et al. Oleuropein and hyrdroxytyrosol inhibit MCF-7 breast cancer cell proliferation interfering with ERK1/2 activation. Mol Nutr Food Res. 2010;54(6):833–40.

[11] Ciafardini G, Marsilio V, Lanza B, Pozzi N. Hydrolysis of oleuropein by Lactobacillus plantarum strains associated with olive fermentation. Appl Environ Microbiol. 1994;60(11):4142–7.

[12] Hlid RABEL, Respy VAC, Age NIP, Aab THR, Ansen CARLRIKH. Hydrolysis of rosmarinic acid from rosemary extract with esterases and Lactobacillus johnsonii in vitro and in a gastrointestinal model. J Agric Food Chem. 2009;57(17):7700–5.

[13] Yang J, Zhang G, Tian J, Li C, Jiang W, Xing Y, et al. Cardioprotective effect of SMND-309, a novel derivate of salvianolic acid B on acute myocardial infarction in rats. Basic Clin Pharmacol Toxicol. 2009;317–23.

[14] Pandey KB, Rizvi SI. Plant polyphenols as dietary antioxidants in human health and disease. Oxid Med Cell Longev. 2009;2(5):270–8.

[15] Kondratyuk T, Pezzuto J. Natural product polyphenols of relevance to human health. Pharm Biol. 2004;42:46–63.

[16] Sen S, Chakraborty R, Sridhar C, Reddy YSR, De B. Free radicals, antioxidants, diseases and phytomedicines: current and future prospect. Int J Pharm Sci. 2010;3(1):91–100.

[17] Krishnaiah D, Sarbatly R, Bono A. Phytochemical antioxidants for health and medicine —a move towards nature. Biotechnol Mol Biol Rev. 2007;1(September):97–104.

[18] Spencer JPE, Abd MM, Mohsen E, Minihane A, Mathers JC. Biomarkers of the intake of dietary polyphenols: strengths, limitations and application in nutrition research. Br J Nutr. 2008;44:12–22.

[19] Shahidi F, Naczk M. Food Phenolics: Sources, Chemistry, Effects, Applications. Lancaster, PA: Technomic Publishing Co Inc; 1995.

[20] Groot H De, Rauen U. Tissue injury by reactive oxygen species and the protective effects of flavonoids. Fundam Clin Pharmacol. 1998;12:249–55.

[21] Human B, Rock L, Cranberries OS. USDA Database for the Proanthocyanidin Content of Selected Foods; 2004.

[22] Bhagwat S, Haytowitz DB, Holden JM. USDA Database for the Flavonoid Content of Selected Foods; 2011.

[23] Bhagwat S, Haytowitz DB, Holden JM. USDA Database for the Isoflavone Content of Selected Foods; 2008.

[24] Neveu V, Perez-Jimenez J, Vos F, Crespy V, Du Chaffaut L, Mennen L. Phenol-Explorer: an online comprehensive database on polyphenol contents in foods. Databases. 2010.

[25] Wink M. Campartmentation of secondary metabolites and xenobiotics in plant vacuoles. Adv Bot Res. 1997;25:141–69.

[26] Gbmez-cordovi C, Estrella I, Fermentaciones I De, Csic I, Cierva CJ De, Madrid E-. Importance of phenolic compounds for the characterization of fruit juices. J Agric Food Chem. 1992;40:1531–5.

[27] Manach C, Scalbert A, Morand C, Rémésy C, Jime L. Polyphenols: food sources and bioavailability. Am J Clin Nutr. 2004;79:727–47.

[28] Crozier A, Lean MEJ, Mcdonald MS, Black C. Quantitative analysis of the flavonoid content of commercial tomatoes, onions, lettuce, and celery. J Agric Food Chem. 1997;45:590–5.

[29] Archivio MD, Filesi C, Benedetto R Di, Gargiulo R, Giovannini C, Masella R. Polyphenols, dietary sources and bioavailability. Ann 1st Super Sanita. 2007;43:348–61.

[30] Setchell K, Faughnan MS, Avades T, Zimmer-nechemias L, Brown NM, Wolfe BE. Comparing the pharmacokinetics of daidzein and genistein with the use of 13 C-labeled tracers in premenopausal women. Am J Clin Nutr. 2003;77:411–9.

[31] Duthie G, Pederson M, Gardner P, Morrice P, Jenkinson A, McPhail D, et al. The effect of whisky and wine consumption on total phenolic content and antioxidant capacity of plasma from health volunteers. Eur J Clin Nutr. 1998;52:733–6.

[32] Young JF, Nielsen SE, Haraldsdóttir J, Daneshvar B, Lauridsen ST, Knuthsen P, et al. Effect of fruit juice intake on urinary quercetin excretion and biomarkers of antioxidative` status. Am J Clin Nutr. 1999;69:87–94.

[33] Edward WCÆ, Birch J. Radical scavenging activity of lipophilized products from transesterification of flaxseed oil with cinnamic acid or ferulic acid. Lipids. 2009;44(9): 807–15.

[34] Nanjundaiah SM, Nayaka H, Annaiah M, Dharmesh SM. Gastroprotective effect of ginger rhizome (Zingiber officinale) extract: role of gallic acid and cinnamic acid in H +, K+, -ATPase/H. pylori inhibition and anti-oxidative mechanism. Evid Based Complement Altern Med. 2009;

[35] Moon D, Kim M, Lee J, Hyun Y, Kim G. Rosmarinic acid sensitizes cell death through suppression of TNF-a-induced NF-kB activation and ROS generation in human leukemia U937 cells. Cancer Lett. 2010;288(2):183–91 [Elsevier Ireland Ltd].

[36] Ding M, Yuan Y. Study on the mechanisms of an extract of Salvia miltiorrhiza on the regulation of permeability of endothelial cells exposed to tumour necrosis factor-a. J Pharm Pharmacol. 2007;59(7):1027–33.

[37] Lee-huang S, Huang PL, Zhang D, Lee JW, Bao J, Sun Y, et al. Discovery of small-molecule HIV-1 fusion and integrase inhibitors oleuropein and hydroxytyrosol: part II. Integrase inhibition. Biochem Biophys Res Commun. 2009;354(4):872–8.

[38] Bioactive berry compounds—novel tools against human pathogens. Appl Microbiol Biotechnol. 2005;67(1):8–18.

[39] Crosier A, Jaganath I, Clifford M. Dietary phenolics: chemistry, bioavailability and effects on health. Nat Prod Rep. 2009;26(8):1001–41.

[40] Omatsu T, Naito Y, Handa O. Involvement of reactive oxygen species in indomethacin-induced apoptosis of small intestinal epithelial cells. J Gastroenterol. 2009;44(19):30–4.

[41] Suschek CV, Gummersbach C, Hemmrich K, Kro K, Fehsel K, Pallua N. New aspects of adipogenesis: radicals and oxidative stress. Differentiation. 2009;77(2):115–20.

[42] Pham-huy LA, He H, Pham-huy C. Free radicals, antioxidants in disease and health. Int J Biochem. 2008;4(2):89–96.

[43] Valko M, Leibfritz D, Moncol J, Cronin MTD, Mazur M, Telser J. Free radicals and antioxidants in normal physiological functions and human disease. Int J Biochem. 2007;39:44–84.

[44] Fang Y, Yang S, Wu G. Free radicals, antioxidants, and nutrition. Nutrition. 2002;18:872–9.

[45] Sarma A, Mallick A, Ghosh A. Free radicals and their role in different clinical conditions: an overview. Int J Pharma Sci. 2010;1(3):185–92.

[46] Jaganathan SK, Mandal M. Antiproliferative Effects of honey and of its polyphenols. J Biomed Biotechnol. 2009;8306–16.

[47] Jemai H, El Feki A, Sayadi S. Antidiabetic and antioxidant effects of hydroxytyrosol and oleuropein from olive leaves in alloxan-diabetic rats. J Agric Food Chem. 2009;57(19):8798–804.

[48] Mueller M, Lukas B, Novak J, Simoncini T, Genazzani A, Jungbauer A. Oregano: a source for peroxisome proliferator-activated receptor gamma antagonists. J Agric Food Chem. 2008;56(24):1621–30.

[49] Tian J, Fu F, Li G, Wang Y, Gao Y, Liu Z, et al. SMND-309, a novel derivate of salvianolic acid B, ameliorates cerebral infarction in rats: characterization and role. Brain Res. 2009;1263:114–21.

[50] Lu Y, Foo LY. Salvianolic acid L, a potent phenolic antioxidant from Salvia officinalis. Tetrahedron Lett. 2001;42(46):8223–5.

[51] Devasagayam T, Tilak J, Boloor K, Sane K, Ghaskadbi S, Lele R. Free radicals and antioxidants in human health: current status and future prospects. Assoc Physicians India. 2004;52:794–804.

[52] Shi Y, Yao S, Zhongjian J, Nianyun L, Rongliang Z. Dietary polyphenols act as scavengers of reducing radicals. Food Chem. 2011;124:1322–7.

[53] Hammes WP, Hertel C. The genera lactobacillus and carnobacterium. In: The Prokaryotes [Internet]. New York, NY: Springer US; 2006. p. 320–403. Available from: http://link.springer.com/10.1007/0-387-30744-3_10.

[54] Canchaya C, Claesson MJ, Fitzgerald GF, van Sinderen D, O'Toole PW. Diversity of the genus Lactobacillus revealed by comparative genomics of five species. Microbiology [Internet]. 2006;152(Pt 11):3185–96. Available from: http://www.ncbi.nlm.nih.gov/pubmed/17074890.

[55] Claesson MJ, van Sinderen D, O'Toole PW. The genus Lactobacillus—genomic basis for understanding its diversity. FEMS Microbiol Lett [Internet]. 2007;269(1):22–8. Available from: http://www.ncbi.nlm.nih.gov/pubmed/17343688.

[56] Walter J. Ecological role of lactobacilli in the gastrointestinal tract: implications for fundamental and biomedical research. Appl Environ Microbiol [Internet]. 2008;74(16):4985–96. Available from: http://aem.asm.org/cgi/doi/10.1128/AEM.00753-08.

[57] Gustafsson RJ, Ahrné S, Jeppsson B, Benoni C, Olsson C, Stjernquist M, et al. The Lactobacillus flora in vagina and rectum of fertile and postmenopausal healthy Swedish women. BMC Womens Health [Internet]. 2011;11(1):17. Available from: http://www.biomedcentral.com/1472-6874/11/17.

[58] Pot B, Felis GE, Bruyne K De, Tsakalidou E, Papadimitriou K, Leisner J, et al. The genus Lactobacillus. In: Holzapfel WH, Wood BJB, editors. Lactic Acid Bacteria [Internet]. Chichester, UK: John Wiley & Sons, Ltd; 2014. p. 249–353. Available from: http://doi.wiley.com/10.1002/9781118655252.

[59] Huttenhower C, Gevers D, Knight R, Abubucker S, Badger JH, Chinwalla AT, et al. Structure, function and diversity of the healthy human microbiome. Nature [Internet]. 2012;486(7402):207–14. Available from: http://www.nature.com/doifinder/10.1038/nature11234.

[60] Forsum U, Holst E, Larsson PG, Vasquez A, Jakobsson T, Mattsby-Baltzer I. Bacterial vaginosis – a microbiological and immunological enigma. APMIS [Internet]. 2005;113(2):81–90. Available from: http://www.ncbi.nlm.nih.gov/pubmed/15723682.

[61] Petrova MI, Lievens E, Malik S, Imholz N, Lebeer S. Lactobacillus species as biomarkers and agents that can promote various aspects of vaginal health. Front Physiol [Internet]. 2015;6:81. Available from: http://www.ncbi.nlm.nih.gov/pubmed/25859220.

[62] Valladares RB, Graves C, Wright K, Gardner CL, Lorca GL, Gonzalez CF. H2O2 production rate in Lactobacillus johnsonii is modulated via the interplay of a heterodimeric flavin oxidoreductase with a soluble 28 Kd PAS domain containing protein. Front Microbiol [Internet]. 2015;6(July):1–14. Available from: http://journal.frontiersin.org/Article/10.3389/fmicb.2015.00716/abstract.

[63] Hayashi H, Sakamoto M, Benno Y. Phylogenetic analysis of the human gut microbiota using 16S rDNA clone libraries and strictly anaerobic culture-based methods. Microbiol

Immunol [Internet]. 2002;46(8):535–48. Available from: http://www.ncbi.nlm.nih.gov/pubmed/12363017.

[64] Hayashi H, Takahashi R, Nishi T, Sakamoto M, Benno Y. Molecular analysis of jejunal, ileal, caecal and recto-sigmoidal human colonic microbiota using 16S rRNA gene libraries and terminal restriction fragment length polymorphism. J Med Microbiol [Internet]. 2005;54(Pt 11):1093–101. Available from: http://www.ncbi.nlm.nih.gov/pubmed/16192442.

[65] Wang M, Ahrné S, Jeppsson B, Molin G. Comparison of bacterial diversity along the human intestinal tract by direct cloning and sequencing of 16S rRNA genes. FEMS Microbiol Ecol [Internet]. 2005;54(2):219–31. Available from: http://www.ncbi.nlm.nih.gov/pubmed/16332321.

[66] Ley RE, Turnbaugh PJ, Klein S, Gordon JI. Microbial ecology: human gut microbes associated with obesity. Nature [Internet]. 2006;444(7122):1022–3. Available from: http://www.nature.com/doifinder/10.1038/4441022a.

[67] Moon S-K, Wee Y-J, Choi G-W. A novel lactic acid bacterium for the production of high purity L-lactic acid, Lactobacillus paracasei subsp. paracasei CHB2121. J Biosci Bioeng [Internet]. 2012;114(2):155–9. Available from: http://www.ncbi.nlm.nih.gov/pubmed/22578598.

[68] Steele J, Broadbent J, Kok J. Perspectives on the contribution of lactic acid bacteria to cheese flavor development. Curr Opin Biotechnol [Internet]. 2013;24(2):135–41. Available from: http://www.ncbi.nlm.nih.gov/pubmed/23279928.

[69] Hertzberger R, Arents J, Dekker HL, Pridmore RD, Gysler C, Kleerebezem M, et al. H2O2 production in species of the Lactobacillus acidophilus group: a central role for a novel NADH-dependent flavin reductase. Appl Environ Microbiol [Internet]. 2014;80(7):2229–39. Available from: http://www.ncbi.nlm.nih.gov/pubmed/24487531.

[70] Yang T, Wu K, Wang F, Liang X, Liu Q, Li G, et al. Effect of exopolysaccharides from lactic acid bacteria on the texture and microstructure of buffalo yoghurt. Int Dairy J [Internet]. 2014;34(2):252–6. Available from: http://linkinghub.elsevier.com/retrieve/pii/S0958694613002239.

[71] Dobson A, Cotter PD, Ross RP, Hill C. Bacteriocin production: a probiotic trait? Appl Environ Microbiol [Internet]. 2012;78(1):1–6. Available from: http://aem.asm.org/cgi/doi/10.1128/AEM.05576-11.

[72] Baick S-C, Kim C-H. Assessment of characteristics and functional properties of lactobacillus species isolated from kimchi for dairy use. Korean J food Sci Anim Resour [Internet]. 2015;35(3):339–49. Available from: http://www.ncbi.nlm.nih.gov/pubmed/26761848.

[73] Sharma R, Sanodiya BS, Bagrodia D, Pandey M, Sharma A, Bisen PS. Efficacy and potential of lactic acid bacteria modulating human health. Int J Pharma Bio Sci. 2012;3(4):935–48.

[74] Beganović J, Kos B, Leboš Pavunc A, Uroić K, Džidara P, Šušković J. Proteolytic activity of probiotic strain Lactobacillus helveticus M92. Anaerobe [Internet]. 2013;20:58–64. Available from: http://www.ncbi.nlm.nih.gov/pubmed/23454496.

[75] Todorov SD, Rachman C, Fourrier A, Dicks LMT, van Reenen CA, Prévost H, et al. Characterization of a bacteriocin produced by Lactobacillus sakei R1333 isolated from smoked salmon. Anaerobe [Internet]. 2011;17(1):23–31. Available from: http://www.ncbi.nlm.nih.gov/pubmed/20152920.

[76] Svetoch EA, Eruslanov BV, Levchuk VP, Perelygin VV, Mitsevich EV, Mitsevich IP, et al. Isolation of Lactobacillus salivarius 1077 (NRRL B-50053) and characterization of its bacteriocin, including the antimicrobial activity spectrum. Appl Environ Microbiol [Internet]. 2011;77(8):2749–54. Available from: http://www.ncbi.nlm.nih.gov/pubmed/21378051.

[77] Kanatani K, Oshimura M, Sano K. Isolation and characterization of acidocin A and cloning of the bacteriocin gene from Lactobacillus acidophilus. Appl Environ Microbiol [Internet]. 1995;61(3):1061–7. Available from: http://www.ncbi.nlm.nih.gov/pubmed/7793908.

[78] Donaghy J, Kelly PF, McKay AM. Detection of ferulic acid esterase production by Bacillus spp. and lactobacilli. Appl Microbiol Biotechnol [Internet]. 1998;50(2):257–60. Available from: http://www.ncbi.nlm.nih.gov/pubmed/9763694.

[79] Guglielmetti S, De Noni I, Caracciolo F, Molinari F, Parini C, Mora D. Bacterial cinnamoyl esterase activity screening for the production of a novel functional food product. Appl Environ Microbiol [Internet]. 2008;74(4):1284–8. Available from: http://www.ncbi.nlm.nih.gov/pubmed/18165367.

[80] Couteau D, McCartney AL, Gibson GR, Williamson G, Faulds CB. Isolation and characterization of human colonic bacteria able to hydrolyse chlorogenic acid. J Appl Microbiol [Internet]. 2001;90(6):873–81. Available from: http://www.ncbi.nlm.nih.gov/pubmed/11412317.

[81] Esteban-Torres M, Reverón I, Mancheño JM, de Las Rivas B, Muñoz R. Characterization of a feruloyl esterase from Lactobacillus plantarum. Appl Environ Microbiol [Internet]. 2013;79(17):5130–6. Available from: http://www.ncbi.nlm.nih.gov/pubmed/23793626.

[82] Esteban-Torres M, Landete JM, Reverón I, Santamaría L, de las Rivas B, Muñoz R. A Lactobacillus plantarum esterase active on a broad range of phenolic esters. Appl Environ Microbiol [Internet]. 2015;81(9):3235–42. Available from: http://www.ncbi.nlm.nih.gov/pubmed/25746986.

[83] Balasubashini MS, Rukkumani R, Viswanathan P, Menon VP. Ferulic acid alleviates lipid peroxidation in diabetic rats. Phytother Res [Internet]. 2004;18(4):310–4. Available from: http://www.ncbi.nlm.nih.gov/pubmed/15162367.

[84] Gonthier M-P, Remesy C, Scalbert A, Cheynier V, Souquet J-M, Poutanen K, et al. Microbial metabolism of caffeic acid and its esters chlorogenic and caftaric acids by human faecal microbiota in vitro. Biomed Pharmacother = Biomédecine pharmacothérapie [Internet]. 2006;60(9):536–40. Available from: http://www.ncbi.nlm.nih.gov/pubmed/16978827.

[85] Pagella JH, Chen XB, MacLeod NA, Orskov ER, Dewey PJ. Excretion of benzoic acid derivatives in urine of sheep given intraruminal infusions of 3-phenylpropionic and cyclohexanecarboxylic acids. Br J Nutr [Internet]. 1997;77(4):577–92. Available from: http://www.ncbi.nlm.nih.gov/pubmed/9155507.

[86] Chesson A, Provan GJ, Russell WR, Scobbie L, Richardson AJ, Stewart C. Hydroxycinnamic acids in the digestive tract of livestock and humans. J Sci Food Agric [Internet]. 1999;79(3):373–8. Available from: http://doi.wiley.com/10.1002/%28SICI%291097-0010%2819990301%2979%3A3%3C373%3A%3AAID-JSFA257%3E3.0.CO%3B2-6.

[87] Ankolekar C, Johnson K, Pinto M, Johnson D, Labbe RG, Greene D, et al. Fermentation of whole apple juice using lactobacillus acidophilus for potential dietary management of hyperglycemia, hypertension, and modulation of beneficial bacterial responses. J Food Biochem [Internet]. 2012;36(6):718–38. Available from: http://doi.wiley.com/10.1111/j.1745-4514.2011.00596.x.

[88] Huynh N, Van Camp J, Smagghe G, Raes K. Improved release and metabolism of flavonoids by steered fermentation processes: a review. Int J Mol Sci [Internet]. 2014;15(11):19369–88. Available from: http://www.mdpi.com/1422-0067/15/11/19369/.

[89] Hole AS, Rud I, Grimmer S, Sigl S, Narvhus J, Sahlstrøm S. Improved bioavailability of dietary phenolic acids in whole grain barley and oat groat following fermentation with probiotic Lactobacillus acidophilus, Lactobacillus johnsonii, and Lactobacillus reuteri. J Agric Food Chem [Internet]. 2012;60(25):6369–75. Available from: http://www.ncbi.nlm.nih.gov/pubmed/22676388.

[90] Bel-Rhlid R, Thapa D, Kraehenbuehl K, Hansen CE, Fischer L. Biotransformation of caffeoyl quinic acids from green coffee extracts by Lactobacillus johnsonii NCC 533. AMB Express [Internet]. 2013;3:28. Available from: http://www.ncbi.nlm.nih.gov/pubmed/23692950.

[91] Bel-Rhlid R, Crespy V, Pagé-Zoerkler N, Nagy K, Raab T, Hansen C-E. Hydrolysis of rosmarinic acid from rosemary extract with esterases and Lactobacillus johnsonii in vitro and in a gastrointestinal model. J Agric Food Chem [Internet]. 2009;57(17):7700–5. Available from: http://www.ncbi.nlm.nih.gov/pubmed/19658402.

[92] Curiel JA, Rodríguez H, Landete JM, de las Rivas B, Muñoz R. Ability of Lactobacillus brevis strains to degrade food phenolic acids. Food Chem [Internet]. 2010;120(1):225–9. Available from: http://linkinghub.elsevier.com/retrieve/pii/S030881460901190X.

[93] Muniandy P, Shori AB, Baba AS. Comparison of the effect of green, white and black tea on Streptococcus thermophilus and Lactobacillus spp. in yogurt during refrigerated storage. J Assoc Arab Univ Basic Appl Sci [Internet]. 2015; Available from: http://linkinghub.elsevier.com/retrieve/pii/S1815385215000334.

[94] Michael M, Phebus RK, Schmidt KA. Plant extract enhances the viability of Lactobacillus delbrueckii subsp. bulgaricus and Lactobacillus acidophilus in probiotic nonfat yogurt. Food Sci Nutr [Internet]. 2015;3(1):48–55. Available from: http://doi.wiley.com/10.1002/fsn3.189.

[95] Brugman S, Klatter FA, Visser JTJ, Wildeboer-Veloo ACM, Harmsen HJM, Rozing J, et al. Antibiotic treatment partially protects against type 1 diabetes in the Bio-Breeding diabetes-prone rat. Is the gut flora involved in the development of type 1 diabetes? Diabetologia [Internet]. 2006;49(9):2105–8. Available from: http://www.ncbi.nlm.nih.gov/pubmed/16816951.

[96] Schwartz RF, Neu J, Schatz D, Atkinson MA, Wasserfall C. Comment on: Brugman S et al. (2006) Antibiotic treatment partially protects against type 1 diabetes in the Bio-Breeding diabetes-prone rat. Is the gut flora involved in the development of type 1 diabetes? Diabetologia 49:2105–2108. Diabetologia [Internet]. 2007;50(1):220–1. Available from: http://www.ncbi.nlm.nih.gov/pubmed/17119915.

[97] Neu J, Reverte CM, Mackey AD, Liboni K, Tuhacek-Tenace LM, Hatch M, et al. Changes in intestinal morphology and permeability in the biobreeding rat before the onset of type 1 diabetes. J Pediatr Gastroenterol Nutr [Internet]. 2005;40(5):589–95. Available from: http://www.ncbi.nlm.nih.gov/pubmed/15861021.

[98] Caicedo RA, Li N, Des Robert C, Scumpia PO, Hubsher CP, Wasserfall CH, et al. Neonatal formula feeding leads to immunological alterations in an animal model of type 1 diabetes. Pediatr Res [Internet]. 2008;63(3):303–7. Available from: http://www.ncbi.nlm.nih.gov/pubmed/18091354.

[99] National Diabates Statistics Report, 2014 [Internet]. Centers of Disease Control and Prevention. 2014 [cited 2015 Jan 1]. Available from: http://www.cdc.gov/diabetes/pubs/statsreport14/national-diabetes-report-web.pdf.

[100] Prime Group for JDRF [Internet]. 2011 [cited 2015 Jan 1]. Available from: http://www2.jdrf.org/site/DocServer/KW-T1D_Factsheet.pdf?docID=1024.

[101] Patterson CC, Gyürüs E, Rosenbauer J, Cinek O, Neu A, Schober E, et al. Trends in childhood type 1 diabetes incidence in Europe during 1989–2008: evidence of non-uniformity over time in rates of increase. Diabetologia [Internet]. 2012;55(8):2142–7. Available from: http://www.ncbi.nlm.nih.gov/pubmed/22638547.

[102] Bell RA, Mayer-Davis EJ, Beyer JW, D'Agostino RB, Lawrence JM, Linder B, et al. Diabetes in non-Hispanic white youth: prevalence, incidence, and clinical characteristics: the SEARCH for Diabetes in Youth Study. Diabetes Care [Internet]. 2009;32(Suppl 2):S102–11. Available from: http://www.ncbi.nlm.nih.gov/pubmed/19246575.

[103] Qin J, Li R, Raes J, Arumugam M, Burgdorf KS, Manichanh C, et al. A human gut microbial gene catalogue established by metagenomic sequencing. Nature [Internet]. 2010;464(7285):59–65. Available from: http://www.ncbi.nlm.nih.gov/pubmed/20203603.

[104] Roesch LFW, Lorca GL, Casella G, Giongo A, Naranjo A, Pionzio AM, et al. the Onset Diabet Rat Model. 2010;3(5):536–48.

[105] Malaguti C, La Guardia PG, Leite ACR, Oliveira DN, de Lima Zollner RL, Catharino RR, et al. Oxidative stress and susceptibility to mitochondrial permeability transition precedes the onset of diabetes in autoimmune non-obese diabetic mice. Free Radic Res [Internet]. 2014;48(12):1494–504. Available from: http://www.ncbi.nlm.nih.gov/pubmed/25236567.

[106] Babu PVA, Liu D, Gilbert ER. Recent advances in understanding the anti-diabetic actions of dietary flavonoids. J Nutr Biochem [Internet]. 2013;24(11):1777–89. Available from: http://www.ncbi.nlm.nih.gov/pubmed/24029069.

[107] Lightfoot YL, Chen J, Mathews CE. Oxidative stress and beta cell dysfunction. Methods Mol Biol [Internet]. 2012;900:347–62. Available from: http://www.ncbi.nlm.nih.gov/pubmed/22933078.

[108] Balasubashini MS, Rukkumani R, Menon VP. Protective effects of ferulic acid on hyperlipidemic diabetic rats. Acta Diabetol. 2003;40:118–22.

[109] Adisakwattana S, Moonsan P, Yibchok-Anun S. Insulin-releasing properties of a series of cinnamic acid derivatives in vitro and in vivo. J Agric Food Chem [Internet]. 2008;56(17):7838–44. Available from: http://www.ncbi.nlm.nih.gov/pubmed/18651742.

[110] Valladares R, Sankar D, Li N, Williams E, Lai K-K, Abdelgeliel AS, et al. Lactobacillus johnsonii N6.2 mitigates the development of type 1 diabetes in BB-DP rats. PLoS One [Internet]. 2010;5(5):e10507. Available from:/pmc/articles/PMC2865539/?report=abstract.

[111] Crepin VF, Faulds CB, Connerton IF. Production and characterization of the Talaromyces stipitatus feruloyl esterase FAEC in Pichia pastoris: identification of the nucleophilic serine. Protein Expr Purif [Internet]. 2003;29(2):176–84. Available from: http://linkinghub.elsevier.com/retrieve/pii/S1046592803000500.

[112] Lai K-K, Stogios PJ, Vu C, Xu X, Cui H, Molloy S, et al. An inserted α/β subdomain shapes the catalytic pocket of Lactobacillus johnsonii cinnamoyl esterase. PLoS One [Internet]. 2011;6(8):e23269. Available from: http://www.ncbi.nlm.nih.gov/pubmed/21876742.

[113] Elamin E, Masclee A, Juuti-Uusitalo K, van Ijzendoorn S, Troost F, Pieters H-J, et al. Fatty acid ethyl esters induce intestinal epithelial barrier dysfunction via a reactive oxygen species-dependent mechanism in a three-dimensional cell culture model. PLoS One [Internet]. 2013;8(3):e58561. Available from: http://www.ncbi.nlm.nih.gov/pubmed/23526996.

[114] Tate DJ, Patterson JR, Velasco-Gonzalez C, Carroll EN, Trinh J, Edwards D, et al. Interferon-gamma-induced nitric oxide inhibits the proliferation of murine renal cell carcinoma cells. Int J Biol Sci [Internet]. 2012;8(8):1109–20. Available from: http://www.ncbi.nlm.nih.gov/pubmed/22991499.

[115] Riquelme P, Tomiuk S, Kammler A, Fändrich F, Schlitt HJ, Geissler EK, et al. IFN-γ-induced iNOS expression in mouse regulatory macrophages prolongs allograft survival in fully immunocompetent recipients. Mol Ther [Internet]. 2013;21(2):409–22. Available from: http://www.ncbi.nlm.nih.gov/pubmed/22929659.

[116] Kingma SDK, Li N, Sun F, Valladares RB, Neu J, Lorca GL. Lactobacillus johnsonii N6.2 Stimulates the innate immune response through Toll-Like receptor 9 in Caco-2 cells and increases intestinal crypt Paneth cell number in biobreeding diabetes-prone rats. J Nutr. 2011;1–3:4–9.

[117] van Es JH, Jay P, Gregorieff A, van Gijn ME, Jonkheer S, Hatzis P, et al. Wnt signalling induces maturation of Paneth cells in intestinal crypts. Nat Cell Biol [Internet]. 2005;7(4):381–6. Available from: http://www.ncbi.nlm.nih.gov/pubmed/15778706.

[118] Veckman V, Miettinen M, Pirhonen J, Sirén J, Matikainen S, Julkunen I. Streptococcus pyogenes and Lactobacillus rhamnosus differentially induce maturation and production of Th1-type cytokines and chemokines in human monocyte-derived dendritic cells. J Leukoc Biol [Internet]. 2004;75(5):764–71. Available from: http://www.ncbi.nlm.nih.gov/pubmed/14966192.

[119] Hilbert T, Bongartz J, Weisheit C, Knüfermann P, Baumgarten G, Hoeft A, et al. Beta2-adrenoceptor stimulation suppresses TLR9-dependent IFNA1 secretion in human peripheral blood mononuclear cells. PLoS One [Internet]. 2013;8(5):e65024. Available from: http://www.ncbi.nlm.nih.gov/pubmed/23724117.

[120] Lau K, Benitez P, Ardissone A, Wilson TD, Collins EL, Lorca G, et al. Inhibition of type 1 diabetes correlated to a Lactobacillus johnsonii N6.2-mediated Th17 bias. J Immunol [Internet]. 2011;186(6):3538–46. Available from: http://www.ncbi.nlm.nih.gov/pubmed/21317395.

[121] Opitz CA, Litzenburger UM, Sahm F, Ott M, Tritschler I, Trump S, et al. An endogenous tumour-promoting ligand of the human aryl hydrocarbon receptor. Nature [Internet]. 2011;478(7368):197–203. Available from: http://www.ncbi.nlm.nih.gov/pubmed/21976023.

[122] Bessede A, Gargaro M, Pallotta MT, Matino D, Servillo G, Brunacci C, et al. Aryl hydrocarbon receptor control of a disease tolerance defence pathway. Nature [Inter-

net]. 2014;511(7508):184–90. Available from: http://www.ncbi.nlm.nih.gov/pubmed/24930766.

[123] Denison MS, Nagy SR. Activation of the aryl hydrocarbon receptor by structurally diverse exogenous and endogenous chemicals. Annu Rev Pharmacol Toxicol [Internet]. 2003;43(1):309–34. Available from: http://www.annualreviews.org/doi/abs/10.1146/annurev.pharmtox.43.100901.135828.

[124] Vogel CFA, Goth SR, Dong B, Pessah IN, Matsumura F. Aryl hydrocarbon receptor signaling mediates expression of indoleamine 2,3-dioxygenase. Biochem Biophys Res Commun [Internet]. 2008;375(3):331–5. Available from: http://www.ncbi.nlm.nih.gov/pubmed/18694728.

[125] Jux B, Kadow S, Esser C. Langerhans cell maturation and contact hypersensitivity are impaired in aryl hydrocarbon receptor-null mice. J Immunol [Internet]. 2009;182(11):6709–17. Available from: http://www.ncbi.nlm.nih.gov/pubmed/19454665.

[126] Nguyen NT, Kimura A, Nakahama T, Chinen I, Masuda K, Nohara K, et al. Aryl hydrocarbon receptor negatively regulates dendritic cell immunogenicity via a kynurenine-dependent mechanism. Proc Natl Acad Sci U S A [Internet]. 2010;107(46):19961–6. Available from: http://www.ncbi.nlm.nih.gov/pubmed/21041655.

[127] Monteleone I, Rizzo A, Sarra M, Sica G, Sileri P, Biancone L, et al. Aryl hydrocarbon receptor-induced signals up-regulate IL-22 production and inhibit inflammation in the gastrointestinal tract. Gastroenterology [Internet]. 2011;141(1):237–48, 248.e1. Available from: http://www.ncbi.nlm.nih.gov/pubmed/21600206.

[128] Veldhoen M, Hirota K, Westendorf AM, Buer J, Dumoutier L, Renauld J-C, et al. The aryl hydrocarbon receptor links TH17-cell-mediated autoimmunity to environmental toxins. Nature [Internet]. 2008;453(7191):106–9. Available from: http://www.ncbi.nlm.nih.gov/pubmed/18362914.

[129] Nakahama T, Kimura A, Nguyen NT, Chinen I, Hanieh H, Nohara K, et al. Aryl hydrocarbon receptor deficiency in T cells suppresses the development of collagen-induced arthritis. Proc Natl Acad Sci U S A [Internet]. 2011;108(34):14222–7. Available from: http://www.ncbi.nlm.nih.gov/pubmed/21825138.

[130] Valladares R, Bojilova L, Potts AH, Cameron E, Gardner C, Lorca G, et al. Lactobacillus johnsonii inhibits indoleamine 2,3-dioxygenase and alters tryptophan metabolite levels in BioBreeding rats. FASEB J [Internet]. 2013;27(4):1711–20. Available from: http://www.ncbi.nlm.nih.gov/pubmed/23303207.

[131] Pilotte L, Larrieu P, Stroobant V, Colau D, Dolusic E, Frédérick R, et al. Reversal of tumoral immune resistance by inhibition of tryptophan 2,3-dioxygenase. Proc Natl Acad Sci U S A [Internet]. 2012;109(7):2497–502. Available from: http://www.ncbi.nlm.nih.gov/pubmed/22308364.

[132] Freewan M, Rees MD, Plaza TSS, Glaros E, Lim YJ, Wang XS, et al. Human indoleamine 2,3-dioxygenase is a catalyst of physiological heme peroxidase reactions: implications

for the inhibition of dioxygenase activity by hydrogen peroxide. J Biol Chem [Internet]. 2013;288(3):1548–67. Available from: http://www.ncbi.nlm.nih.gov/pubmed/23209301.

[133] Godbout JP, Moreau M, Lestage J, Chen J, Sparkman NL, O'Connor J, et al. Aging exacerbates depressive-like behavior in mice in response to activation of the peripheral innate immune system. Neuropsychopharmacology [Internet]. 2008;33(10):2341–51. Available from: http://www.ncbi.nlm.nih.gov/pubmed/18075491.

[134] Corona AW, Norden DM, Skendelas JP, Huang Y, O'Connor JC, Lawson M, et al. Indoleamine 2,3-dioxygenase inhibition attenuates lipopolysaccharide induced persistent microglial activation and depressive-like complications in fractalkine receptor (CX(3)CR1)-deficient mice. Brain Behav Immun [Internet]. 2013;31:134–42. Available from: http://www.ncbi.nlm.nih.gov/pubmed/22926082.

[135] Shibata Y, Hara T, Nagano J, Nakamura N, Ohno T, Ninomiya S, et al. The role of indoleamine 2,3-dioxygenase in diethylnitrosamine-induced liver carcinogenesis. PLoS One [Internet]. 2016;11(1):e0146279. Available from: http://www.ncbi.nlm.nih.gov/pubmed/26727596.

[136] Masaki A, Ishida T, Maeda Y, Suzuki S, Ito A, Takino H, et al. Prognostic significance of tryptophan catabolism in adult T-cell leukemia/lymphoma. [Rinshō ketsueki] Japanese J Clin Hematol [Internet]. 2015;56(11):2295–304. Available from: http://www.ncbi.nlm.nih.gov/pubmed/26666715.

[137] Ben-Haj-Ayed A, Moussa A, Ghedira R, Gabbouj S, Miled S, Bouzid N, et al. Prognostic value of indoleamine 2,3-dioxygenase activity and expression in nasopharyngeal carcinoma. Immunol Lett [Internet]. 2016;169:23–32. Available from: http://www.ncbi.nlm.nih.gov/pubmed/26608400.

Chapter 6

Pili in Probiotic Bacteria

Vengadesan Krishnan, Priyanka Chaurasia and Abhiruchi Kant

Additional information is available at the end of the chapter

http://dx.doi.org/10.5772/63087

Abstract

The ability to adhere to intestinal epithelial tissue and mucosal surfaces is a key criterion in selecting probiotics. Adhesion is considered to be a prerequisite for successful colonization and survival in the gastrointestinal tract to provide persistent beneficial effects to the host. Bacteria express a multitude of surface components that mediate adherence. Pili or fimbriae are surface adhesive components implicated in initiating bacterial adhesion and mediating interaction with the host. These nonflagellar proteinaceous fiber appendages were identified and explored over several decades in pathogenic bacteria, and many distinct types are known. However, the presence of pili in probiotics and/or commensalic bacteria has only recently been recognized. Thus knowledge about pili in probiotics is relatively limited, but structural and functional data have begun to emerge. Availability of these data in the future would enable us to understand the pili-mediated adhesion strategies of probiotics. This knowledge could be utilized to develop antiadhesion-based therapies against bacterial infections as well as probiotic designs for beneficial effects. This chapter will briefly summarize the current knowledge of pili in probiotics with emphasis on members of lactobacilli and bifidobacteria.

Keywords: Adhesion, Bifidobacteria, Lactobacilli, Pili, Probiotics

1. Introduction

Bacterial colonization of humans seems to commence at birth and evolves throughout life. It depends on several factors including mode of birth, age, geographical location, local environment, diet, stress, illness, medications, and antibiotic treatment. Bacteria colonize all parts of the human body that are exposed to external environment. Specifically, the gastrointestinal tract (GIT) harbors more than 1000 species, and this complex microbial community is referred to as the "gut microbiota" [1, 2]. The gut microbiota are well recognized because of their impact on health and disease. However, knowledge on the precise mechanism(s) by which the microbiota exerts its influence remains largely unknown. *Lactobacillus* and *Bifidobacterium* species constitute a major part of the microbiota and are believed to play an essential role in modulating immune system, resisting pathogen colonization, metabolism, and energy balance [3, 4]. Some members of these two genera are also popular as probiotics. Though the specific contribution of these members to the beneficial effects is subject to investigation and speculation, it is widely accepted that their presence in the GIT often confers health benefits. The molecular mechanisms that allow these members to colonize the GIT have not yet been elucidated in detail, though their persistence was shown to be essential for the beneficial effects.

Most pathogenic bacteria are known to express multitude of surface components for establishing contacts and mediating interactions with the host for bacterial colonization. Among these, long, hair-like filamentous structures known as pili or fimbriae have been often implicated in adhesion processes and shown to be required for bacterial colonization on host tissues (for reviews, see [5–11]). Typically, these structures are made up of building blocks called pilins or fimbrilins. Genes for these pilins along with other genes required for the pilus assembly are located in the same place in the genome called pilus gene cluster or Pathogenicity Island. Distinct pilus structures (e.g., chaperone-mediated, type IV, Curli, and CS1) are known in Gram-negative pathogens. Their structure, function, and biogenesis have been well explored to some extent. The details of pili have begun to emerge for Gram-positive pathogens a decade ago (for reviews, see [8, 10–15]). The sortase-mediated pili seem to be conserved across the Gram-positive pathogens. Some of the pilus types (e.g., type IV) exist both in the Gram-negative and Gram-positive pathogens. The pilus types have been majorly categorized based on secretion systems, biogenesis, architecture, and function. The sortase-mediated pili differ from other known types by being a covalent polymer in which pilin subunits are covalently tethered to each other by sortase-mediated isopeptide bonds. The pili and their components in the pathogens are recognized as virulence factors as they play a key role in pathogenesis. Also, they are considered as potential vaccine candidates because of their immunogenic properties.

Although the focus is traditionally on pili in pathogenic bacteria for last few decades, they have been recently identified in many gut commensalic bacteria and often shown to be essential for their colonization and persistence in the the GIT and for immune modulation. Although the pili in pathogenic bacteria are regularly reviewed, this chapter attempts to give a brief overview of pili in beneficial bacteria, which is relatively recent.

2. Sortase-mediated pili

As demonstrated first in pathogen *Corynebacterium diptheriae* [15, 16], the sortase-mediated pilus (SpaA-type) model consists of three different types of pilins (one major pilin and two ancillary pilins). Typically, the loci for the pilins and at least one sortase are located together in the genome as a pilus operon or gene cluster (**Figure 1A**). Similar to microbial surface component recognizing adhesive matrix molecules (MSCRAMMs), the pilin precursors contain signal sequence at the N-terminal and sorting signal at the C-terminal. The C-terminal sorting signal is composed of a conserved LPXTG (Leu-Pro-any-Thr-Gly) motif, a hydrophobic domain, and a positively charged tail (**Figure 1B**). Multiple copies of major pilin form the pilus backbone like beads on a string (**Figure 1C**). Hence, they are also referred to as backbone or shaft pilins. The major pilins often contain a conserved YPKN (Tyr-Pro-Lys-Asn)-like motif close to the N-terminal (**Figure 1B**). The pilin-specific sortase, whose gene is located in the pilus gene cluster, generates the covalently cross-linked pilus shaft as follows. Prior to polymerization into pilus fibers, the prepilins or pilin precursors are exported across the membrane through the Sec apparatus. These precursors are then embedded into the membrane by their C-terminal hydrophobic domain and positively charged tail. The membrane-bound pilin-specific sortase forms acyl-enzyme intermediate by cleaving the LPXTG motif of major pilin between threonine and glycine, and creates a thioester bond between its catalytic cysteine residue and the nascent C-terminal threonine. This intermediate receives nucleophilic attack from the lysine residue of pilin motif of another major pilin that results in an amide bond formation between the cleaved threonine and lysine side chain. The repeated reaction promotes the growth of pilus structure on the cell surface (**Figure 1**). The ancillary pilins are incorporated into the pilus structure, presumably by similar transpeptidation reaction. Ancillary pilin 1, which is larger in size, is generally located at the pilus tip. This pilin, also known as tip pilin, often plays a role in adhesion to host. Ancillary pilin 2 or basal pilin is often observed at the base of pilus and smaller in size. These basal pilins are shown to contain a pilin-like motif for their incorporation into the pilus base [21]. A different transpeptidase known as housekeeping sortase, which is not part of the pilus gene cluster, anchors the assembled pilus structure on the cell wall. Similar to pilin-specific sortase transpeptidase reaction, the housekeeping sortase forms acyl-enzyme intermediate with basal pilin. This intermediate receives nucleophilic attack from the peptidoglycan cross-bridge that results in the formation of covalent link between the carboxyl threonine in the basal pilin and the free amino group of the cell wall lipid II precursors.

The pilins are commonly made up of two building blocks, which are variants of immunoglobulin fold known as CnaA [17] and CnaB [18], often with intradomain isopeptide bond [19] (for reviews, see [20–22]) (**Figure 2**). In addition, the tip pilins also contain adhesin modules such as von Willebrand factor type A domain (vWFA) with two inserted arms [23, 24] and thioester containing domains [25–27] (**Figure 2**). The pilus model of *C. diptheriae* appears to be conserved across the Gram-positive pathogenic strains (e.g., *Streptococcus agalactiae, Streptococcus pyogenes, Streptococcus pneumoniae, Streptococcus parasanguinis, Streptococcus salivarius, Streptococcus sanguinis, Enterococcus faecalis, Enterococcus faecium, Bacillus cererus*, and *Actinomyces naeslundi*) with some variations in number of pilus gene clusters, number of pilins, number of pilin-specific sortases, and pilus architecture. They majorly participate in cellular adhesion and colonization processes. More than one sortase-mediated pilus gene cluster are often present in the same bacterial strains suggesting their different cellular targets and functions.

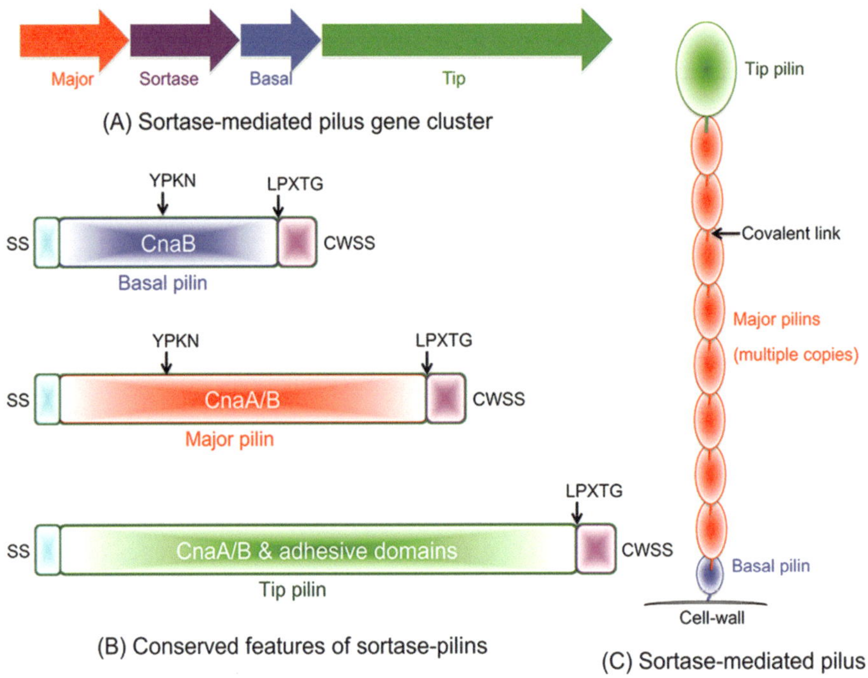

Figure 1. Schematic diagram of typical sortase-mediated pili. (A) Pilus gene cluster for sortase-mediated pilus assembly. It encodes genes for a major (red), basal (blue), tip (green) pilins, and a pilin-specific sortase (purple). More than one sortase (e.g., SpaD- and SpaH-pilus gene cluster in *C. diphtheriae*) and less than three pilins (e.g., type 1 and 2 pilus gene clusters in *A. oris*) have also been observed. In the pilus gene cluster, differences in the order of gene's arrangement and the presence of transposon elements in the vicinity are often observed. (B) Conserved features of sortase pilins. Signal sequence (SS) and LPXTG-containing cell wall sorting signal (CWSS) are at the N- and C-terminals of all the (basal, major, and tip) pilins. In addition, the basal and major pilins have pilin motif (YPKN) in the vicinity of N-terminals. A conserved element called E-box (LXET) has also been observed in the sortase pilins. The basal pilins consist of 1–3 CnaB domains (Figure 2A). The major pilins contain 2–4 CnaA/B domains. CnaB domains are often at the N- and C-terminals, and CnaA at the middle (Figure 2B). The tip plins have adhesive domains (vWFA/thioester containing domains) in addition to CnaA/B domains (Figure 2C). (C) Sortase-mediated pilus structure. The pilus is made up of three distinct types of pilins: basal (blue), major (red), and tip (green) pilin. In the pilus, the pilins are tethered to each other by sortase-mediated covalent links (see the text for details). Multiple copies of the major pilins form the pilus shaft in a head-to-tail fashion like beads on a string. The tip pilin is often located at tip projecting adhesive domain for favoring adhesion. The basal pilin is often located at the base of pilus shaft and helping for anchoring the polymerized pilus on the cell wall through the housekeeping sortase.

The sortase-mediated pili, which are being actively investigated in Gram-positive pathogens and considered as virulence factors, have been detected in several gut commensals as mentioned in the following sections. The pilus-like gene clusters were earlier noticed in probiotic *Lactobacillus johnsonii* NCC 533 [28], but first received attention through probiotic *Lactobacillus rhamnosus* GG in 2009 [29, 30]. Since then, it has been identified in several species and strains of probiotic and other commensal bacteria by genomic analysis and shown to be essential for their adherence and colonization in GIT. Their presence was further confirmed by imaging analysis in the *L. rhamnosus* GG [29, 31], genus of *Bifidobacterium* [32, 33], *Lacococcus lactis* IL1403 and TIL448 [34, 35], and recently in *Lactobacillus ruminis* ATCC 25644 [36]. Hence, the view of surface piliation has now been expanded to include its role also as a niche-adaptation factor.

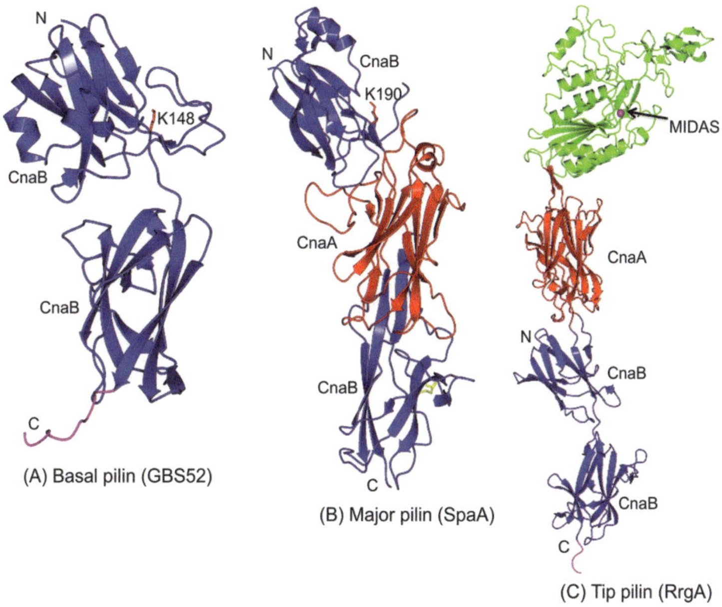

Figure 2. Three-dimensional structures of sortase-pilins from pathogenic bacteria. (A) Basal pilin, GBS52 (PDB id: 3PHS), from *S. agalactiae*. It consists of two CnaB domains, and the lysine from the pilin motif is shown as stick (in red). A proline-rich C-terminal tail is shown in magenta. (B) Major pilin, SpaA (PDB id: 3HR6), from *C. diphtheriae* consists of three domains. CnaB domains (in blue) are at N- and C-terminals, and CnaA (in red) at the middle. Pilin motif lysine is shown in stick (red). (C) Tip pilin, RrgA (PDB id: 2WW8), from *S. pneumoniae* contains four domains. CnaB domains (in blue) are at the terminals and CnaA (in red) at the middle. Metal (pink)-ion-dependent adhesion site (MIDAS) containing vWFA domain with two inserted arms are shown in green.

2.1. Pili in *L. rhamnosus* GG

L. rhamnosus GG is one the of well-documented and widely used probiotic strains [37]. The pilus-like protrusions in *L. rhamnosus* GG were initially seen in 2009 [30]. *L. rhamnosus* GG contains two pilus gene clusters *SpaCBA* and *SpaFED* as shown by comparative genomic analysis [29] (**Figure 3A**). The *SpaCBA* encodes a major pilin SpaA, two ancillary pilins SpaB and SpaC, and a pilin-specific sortase (SrtC1). As further confirmed by western blotting and immunogold electron microscopy [29, 31], the SpaCBA pilus of *L. rhamnosus* GG has similar morphology to the three-pilins architecture model of *C. diptheriae* [15, 16]. The repeating SpaA makes the pilus backbone. The cell wall anchoring SpaB and adhesive SpaC ancillary pilins are found at the base and tip of the pilus, respectively (**Figure 3C**). However, in contrast to the pili from most Gram-positive pathogens, the tip pilin (SpaC) and, to a lesser extent, basal pilin (SpaB) are found sporadically throughout the SpaCBA pilus backbone. Such a distribution is thought to enhance adherence to the intestinal mucosa and epithelial layer and thereby then extend the relative longevity and transient colonization of *L. rhamnosus* GG cells in the gut. The SpaCBA pilus was demonstrated to be pivotal for efficient adherence to mucus [29, 38, 39], collagen [40], and Caco-2 intestinal epithelial cell line and biofilm formation [41]. The immunomodulation of SpaCBA pili includes toll-like receptor 2 (TLR2)-dependent activation and dendritic cell cytokine production [42], dampening endogenous interleukin (IL)-8 mRNA levels [41], eliciting macrophage-mediated anti-inflammatory cytokine mRNA expression [43], inducing TLR-related gene expression in a human fetal intestine model [44], and stimulating cellular responses in intestinal epithelial cells [45]. Interestingly, the SpaC plays a role in most of the SpaCBA pili-triggered host cell immune responses. The surface piliation apparently provides a niche-specific fitness to *L. rhamnosus* GG cells for extending their transient colonization in the gut [46]. Presumably, this is an advantage over nonpiliated probiotic bacteria. For example, the non-SpaCBA piliated *L. rhamnosus* LC705, which is genetically similar to *L. rhamnosus* GG, shows decreased adherence to intestinal mucus in the comparative study [29]. More recently, the key role of *L. rhamnosus* GG pili in interaction with β-lactoglobulin has also been demonstrated [47].

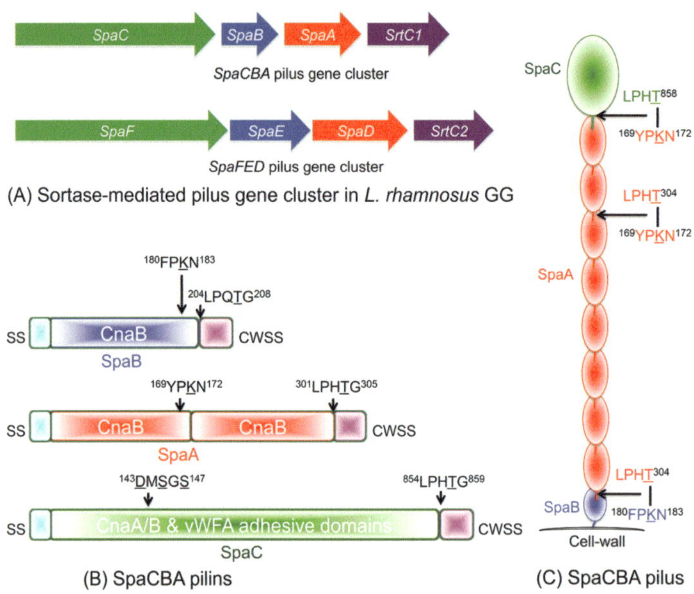

Figure 3. Schematic diagram of sortase-mediated pili in *L. rhamnosus* GG. (A) *SpaCBA* and *SpaFED* pilus gene clusters identified in *L. rhamnosus* GG. Each cluster encodes a tip pilin (SpaC/SpaF), major pilin (SpaA/SpaD), basal pilin (SpaB/SpaE), and pilin-specific sortase (SrtC1/SrtC2). (B) Predicted elements required for the pilus assembly in the SpaCBA pilins. The basal pilin SpaB contains a single CnaB domain with FPKN pilin motif and LPQTG-containing CWSS at C-terminal. Residue numbers and positions were labeled and marked by arrow. The major pilin SpaA contain two CnaB domains, and its pilin and sorting motif are marked. The tip pilin SpaC contains a vWFA domain and its MIDAS (DMSGS) motif is marked. (C) The SpaCBA pilus model consists of SpaA, SpaB, and SpaC. The possible sortase-mediated intercovalent link is marked by arrow with details of residues involved. A possible mode of association for SpaC and SpaB along the pilus shaft other than at the tip and base of the pilus needs to be further shown by a high-resolution imaging technique or structural studies.

Similar to *SpaCBA*, the *SpaFED* operon encodes the pilus backbone (SpaD), the pilus tip (SpaF) and the base (SpaE) pilins, as well as a putative sortase enzyme (SrtC2) required for pilus assembly (**Figure 3A**). Though the recombinant SpaF has been shown to bind intestinal mucus [39], the genes associated with the spaFED pilus gene cluster are not constitutively expressed in the tested laboratory conditions [31]. Thus, the native form of the SpaFED pilus remains hypothetical, not only in *L. rhamnosus* GG, but also in other strains carrying the spaFED operon (e.g., *L. rhamnosus* LC705) [31, 46]. However, *L. rhamnosus* GG SpaFED pili can be readily produced as an assembled structure in recombinant *L. lactis* [48].

Obtaining three-dimensional structural insights into pilus assembly and adhesion mechanisms through the structural biology techniques has been instrumental for Gram-negative pathogens in the past (for reviews, see [5, 8, 49, 50]), and it was begun much later for Gram-positive pathogens in 2007 ([19, 51], for reviews, see [11, 20–22]). The structures of individual major as well as ancillary pilins from several pathogenic strains have been determined (for recent review, see [21]) (**Figure 2**). A Cryo-EM study on *S. pneumoniae* pili has also supported the sortase-mediated three pilins architectural model [52]. According to current structural knowledge, the basal pilins consist of 1–3 CnaB domains often with intradomain isopeptide bonds (**Figure 2A**). Conserved proline-rich C-terminal tails in the known basal pilins suggest their likely role in pilus anchoring via housekeeping sortase. The presence of a pilin-like motif with a lysine in the basal pilin indicates that they could be incorporated into the pilus base by sortase (**Figure 2**). The major pilins are made of 2–4 CnaB/A domains (**Figure 2**). The CnaB domains are at the N- and C-terminals, whereas the CnaA domain is in the middle. The pilin motif is present at the C-terminal region of N-terminal CnaB domain (**Figure 2B**). The N-terminal domain in many pilins seems to be flexible with no or slow forming internal isopeptide bond. In some crystal structure studies, a fiber-like pilus arrangement in the crystal packing has been observed though the sortase-mediated intermolecular amide bond between the backbone pilins was absent. The tip pilins contain adhesive domains at the tip in addition to CnaA and CnaB domains that form a stalk and connect adhesive domains to the pilus shaft (**Figure 2C**). These adhesive domains are often a modified vWFA domain with two inserted arms [23, 24], and thioester containing domain [25]. The complicated domains arrangement and folding in tip pilins makes difficult to predict them from their sequence.

Detailed structural knowledge is yet to emerge for pili and related components for probiotic bacteria. However, preliminary crystallographic data are available for some of the pilins (SpaA [53], SpaD [54], and SpaC [55]) in *L. rhamnosus* GG. Our initial analysis of ongoing structural investigations on pilus constituents of *L. rhamnosus* GG and comparison with their counterparts in pathogens suggest that SpaA may consist of two CnaB domains (**Figure 3B**), and SpaD contains three domain with CnaB domains at the terminals and CnaA domain in the middle. Though it is yet to be validated, it is tempting us to describe Lys171 from the pilin motif SpaA as the possible linking lysine that could involve in the SpaA–SpaA and SpaA–SpaC pilins covalent association during SpaCBA pilus shaft polymerization by pilin-specific SrtC1 (**Figure 3B** and **C**). Similarly, Lys182 in SpaB seems a likely candidate for its incorporation into the pilus (**Figure 3B** and **C**). Such a linking lysine is yet to be predicted for SpaC for its incorporation other than at the pilus tip. In contrast to known pathogenic tip pilins (e.g., GBS104 [24] and RrgA [23]), but similar to eukaryotic proteins (e.g., integrins, complement C2a, and Fb), the vWFA domain predicted in SpaC [55] seems not to have the two inserted arms, suggesting both possible differences and similarities in binding mechanism via a metal-ion-containing vWFA adhesin domain. Certainly, knowledge generated from our ongoing structural investigations would provide new insights into pilus assembly and adhesion mechanisms in *L. rhamnosus* GG, and serves as a model for probiotics.

2.2. Pili in *L. ruminis*

L. ruminis, one of the dominating *Lactobacillus* species in the mammalian intestines, is routinely isolated from the feces of human, cattle, and pigs. It is one of the few motile members known in lactobacilli. It is also recognized as an autochthonous microbiota in the GIT. The pilus gene identified in the human-derived intestinal isolate *L. rumini* ATCC 25644 has been named as *lrpCBA* (*L.* rumini *p*ilus) [36] since they appear to be different from the known lactobacillar pilus types (SpaCBA and SpaFED) at the primary structural level. The *LrpCBA* pilus operon encodes tip (lrpC), basal (lrpB), and major (lrpA) pilins and a pilin-specific sortase (SrtC). Sequence of *L. ruminis* pilins displays the common pilin features such as LPXTG-like motifs, E-box motif, and pilin motifs (in major and basal pilins) [36] (**Figure 2**). The expression and surface localization of *lrpCBA* pilus gene product have further confirmed by immunoblot analysis and immune-electron microscopic visualization (for details, see [36]). Interestingly, the pilus genes have also been detected in *L. ruminis* ATCC 27782 from bovine gut origin [56], but the microarray analysis showed that the corresponding genes were upregulated in human strain compared with the bovine isolate. The ability of LrpCBA pilus to adhere to gut epithelial cells and extracellular matrix (ECM) proteins, and immune-modulation activities has been demonstrated using recombinant-piliated lactococci (for details, see [36]). Interestingly, the tip pilin LrpC supports *L. ruminis* binding to ECM-related substrates but not to the mucosal surfaces.

2.3. Pili in other *Lactobacillus* species

The presence of sortase-mediated pilus gene clusters has been reported in many strains of *Lactobacillus casei* [57–60] and *Lactobacillus paracasei* [61], which are members of the normal human gut microbiota and used extensively as probiotics and in the food industries. Although the pilus expression and function are yet to be studied in detail, the most analyzed strains in the *L. casei* and *L. paracasei* group show that they contain *SpaCBA* and *SpaFED* pilus gene clusters. In contrast, only few strains in *L. rhamnosus* group have *SpaCBA* cluster (e.g., *L. rhamnosus GG* and LMS2-1 strain). However, several *L. paracasei* strains including COM0101 are shown to have truncated SpaC gene [60]. The transposon genes, which are present in the vicinity of the *SpaCBA* cluster in *L. rhamnosus*, seem to be absent in the *L. casei* suggesting that L. *rhamnosus* GG and LMS2-1 could have acquired the *SpaCBA* pilus gene cluster through horizontal gene transfer (HGT) from *L. casei* [57, 62]. This is further evidenced by the presence of high nucleotide sequence identity in spaCBA cluster of *L. rhamnosus* and *L. casei* [57, 62].

2.4. Pili in *L. lactis*

L. lactis is another widely used species as starter in dairy fermentation and best characterized strain in lactic acid bacteria (LAB). They seem to present in nutrient-rich ecological niches (gut mucus, milk, and plants). A functional pilus operon (*pil*) has been shown to present in *L. lactis* IL1403 [34, 63]. It encodes tip (YhgD), major (YhgE), and basal (YhhB) pilins and a pilin-specific sortase (SrtC). The presence of pilus structures has been confirmed by immunogold electron microscopy and atomic force microscopy (AFM) analyses. The major YhgE and basal YhhB pilins display typical LPXTG motifs and pilin motifs. Additionally, the YhgE has an E-box. The pili were also shown to promote biofilm formation by confocal laser scanning microscopy (CLSM). The occurrence of pili in few other *L. lactis* isolates from clinical and vegetal environments was also visualized by by transmission electron microscopy (TEM) analysis [34]. Later, a proteomic analysis study has also detected pilus genes (YhgE2, YhhB2, ORF4, and SrtC2) in a vegetal isolate *L. lactis* subsp. *lactis* TIL448 [35]. The YhgE2 was shown to play a major role in intestinal epithelial Caco-2 cells adhesion. The pilus biogenesis and morphology were further analyzed by immunoblot, electron micrograph, transcriptional, and AFM experiments [35, 64].

2.5. Pili in bifidobacteria

Bifidobacteria are the common components of the gut microbiota of a broad range of hosts [65]. Several members of bifidobacteria are typical inhabitants of the infant intestine [66], which is thought to be sterile at birth. Identification of many bifidobacterial strains in the stools of healthy infants suggests that they could be the first colonizers in the GIT subsequent to birth. Genomic analysis has revealed pilus genes cluster in several bifidobacterial strains [67]. Interestingly, many pilus gene clusters are flanked by transposon elements indicating their acquisition by HGT. The presence of pilus structures was further examined by AFM and transcription analysis in *Bifidobacterium bifidum, Bifidobacterium dentium, Bifidobacterium longum* subsp. *longum, Bifidobacterium adolescentis*, and *Bifidobacterium animalis* subsp. *lactis* [67]. The pilus gene clusters often found to contain one major pilin (FimA or FimP) and one or two ancillary pilins (FimB or FimQ) with a pilin-specific sortase. Many of these pilus genes are similar to the (two-pilins) pilus gene clusters identified in Gram-positive pathogens such as *Actinomyces oris* [68, 69] and *Bacillus cereus* [70], which lack basal pilus genes differing from the three-pilins architectural model of *C. diphtheriae* [15, 16]. *A. oris* encodes two different fimbriae (types 1 and 2). Type 1 fimbria, which mediates the interaction of actinomyces to tooth enamel, consists of the major pilin (FimP) and tip pilin (FimQ). Whereas, the type 2 fimbria that mediate interaction with oral streptococci and host cell for causing dental plaque is made of major pilin (FimA) and tip pilin (FimB). Similarly, *B. cereus* pili is composed of major pilin BcpA and the tip pilin (BcpB). In the two-pilin sortase-mediated pili model, the last major pilin may function as the pilus base. The three-dimensional structures for major pilins for *A. oris* are available while they are yet to be elucidated for tip pilins. The major pilins of bifidobacteria have typical pilin motif and LPXTG motif required for pilus polymerization [67]. The role of pili in adherence, immunomodulation, and bacterial aggregations was further extensively explored in *B. bifidum* PRL2010, which contains three different pilus gene clusters (*pil1*, *pil2*, and *pil3*)

[71]. Apart from sortase-mediated pili, the presence of type IV pili has also been reported in bifidobacteria (e.g., *Bifidobacterium breve* UCC2003 [32]), which is described below.

3. Tad pili

The Tad (tight adherence) pili, which was first described in *Aggregatibacter (Actinobacillus) actinomycetemcomitans* [72], is a specialized subtype of type IV pili (for reviews, see [5, 7, 8, 73, 74]). Tad pili in this bacterium were shown to mediate adhesion to surfaces and essential for colonization and pathogenesis. Apart from adhesion, the type IV pili have been implicated in several functions such as aggregation, biofilm formation, twitching motility, DNA uptake, and electron transfer. Type IV pili are found to be present in Gram-negative (e.g., enteropathogenic *Escherichia coli, Salmonella enterica, Pseudomonas aeruginosa, Neisseria meningitides,* and *Vibrio cholerae*) as well as Gram-positive bacteria (*Clostridium perfringens, Mycobacterium tuberculosis,* and *Ruminococcus albus*). Type IV pili are typically 6–8 nm in diameter and several micrometers long. The type IV pilus is comprised of homopolymers of a single (major) pilin subunit (**Figure 4**). The major pilins in Tad pili are relatively smaller in size (~7 kDa) compared with other known pilus types in type IV. The flexible homopolymer filaments in type IV often have tendency to form characteristic helical bundles by lateral interactions. Some pili possess an adhesive or ancillary pilins at the pilus tip or can be decorated with pseudopilins along the pilus.

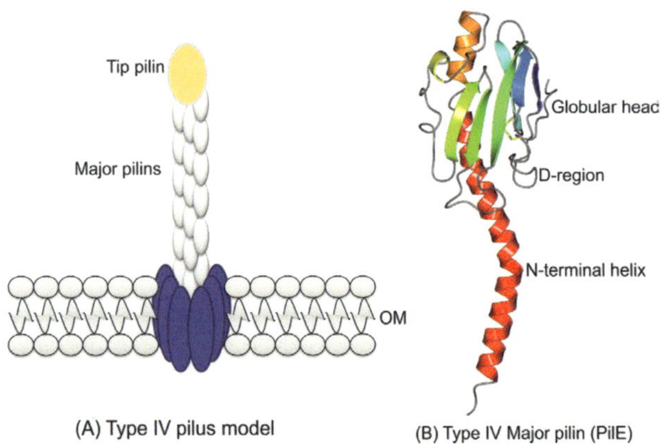

Figure 4. Schematic diagram of type IV pilus structure. (A) Type IV (gonococcal) pilus model. Major pilins form the filament majorly by hydrophobic interactions between their N-terminal helices in the filament core. The globular head of major pilins pack on the filament surface. (B) Type IV major pilin, PilE (PDB id: 1AY2), from *N. gonorrhoeae* showing N-terminal helix (in red) and globular head with D-region.

Type IV pilus assembly is a complex process, which requires protein products from multiple genes (~14) including minor pilins, prepilin peptidase, ATPase, inner membrane core proteins, and accessory proteins. Many of the core genes are conserved across different bacterial species. Tad pili seem to differ from other type IV pilus types by lacking four core homologous minor pilins. The type IV pilins are synthesized as precursors with a leader peptide and transported across the inner membrane into the periplasmic space, where they are retained in the inner membrane through their N-terminal hydrophobic segments. The globular domain is folded with stabilizing intramolecular disulfide bonds. A dedicated prepilin peptidase cleaves the positively charged leader sequence and methylates the N-terminal amine to generate the mature pilin. The methylated, positively charged N-terminal residue is thought to attract negatively charged glutamate (at fifth position) of adjacent major pilin in the growing pilus fiber. This results in vertical displacement between one pilin and the next. The assembly ATPase associated with the cytoplasmic part of the inner membrane protein undergoes conformational change during ATP hydrolysis and pushes the pilus filament out of the membrane, providing a gap for the next major pilin. Type IV pili is further complicated by divergence and divided into two classes (types IVa and IVb) based on the length of leader peptides and mature pilins. The pilins of type IVa are typically 150–160 residues long with a short leader peptide (<10 residues), whereas the pilins of type IVb are either long (180–200 residues) or short (40–50 residues) with longer leader peptides (~15–30 residues). The Tad pili are monophyletic subclass of type IVb pili [73]. The pilins of Tad pili are short with 40–50 residues long.

Though the sequence and structural diversity are associated with the pilins in type IV, they share a common lollipop-like architecture consisting of an extended N-terminal helical stick followed by a globular head containing a β-sheet with 4–7 strands [74] (**Figure 4B**). The N-terminal half of the helix is hydrophobic and multifunctional regulatory domain. It protrudes from the globular head and forms the central hydrophobic core of the growing filament during the pilus assembly. Prior to assembly, it acts as transmembrane segment to retain individual pilin in the cytoplasmic membrane. The C-terminal half of the helix is amphipathic and embedded in the globular head. For many pili, a hypervariable C-terminal loop known as D-region or disulfide-bonded loop (DSL) performs an essential role in surface adherence (**Figure 4B**). The conserved disulfide bridge in the D-region observed in several Gram-negative major pilins appears to be off in Gram-positive pilins (e.g., PilA1 in *Chlostrodium difficle* [75]). The Tad genes are also widespread in the genomes of Gram-positive species (*C. diphtheriae, Thermobifida fusca,* and *Streptomyces coelicolor*). Recently, they have been identified in probiotic *B. breve.*

3.1. Tad pili in *B. breve*

Apart from sortase-dependent pili, *B. breve* UCC2003 was recently shown to contain the type IVb or Tad pilus gene cluster named tad_{2003} [32]. The presence of pili was further confirmed by immunogold transmission electron microscopy and shown to be essential for efficient gut colonization in a murine model by mutational analysis [32]. Specifically, the Tad locus is highly conserved among all sequenced bifidobacterial strains supporting a ubiquitous pilus-mediated host colonization and persistence mechanism for intestinal bifidobacteria. The structural data are yet to come for pilins of Tad pilus from beneficial bacteria for shedding light on their structure and function.

4. Future perspectives

Adhesion of bacteria to host surfaces is a prerequisite and crucial step for bacterial colonization, which may result in pathogenic or commensal relationship. The pili have been often implicated in initiating adhesion and mediating interaction with host. Understanding pilus structure and function, and their mediated interactions with the host has been achieved to a certain extent in pathogenic strains. The pili and their components are recognized as virulence factors in pathogenic strains, and also considered as potential vaccine candidates in combating bacterial infection. Recent identification of such surface organelles in probiotic or commensal bacteria gives a new perspective as a niche-adaption factor as well. The sortase-mediated pili initially discovered in Gram-positive pathogens appear to be widespread among commensals. The Tad pili, which are known to present in both Gram-negative and Gram-positive pathogens, have also been detected in some commensal strains. It may not be a surprise if additional pilus type comes in the future from the fast-growing technology and genomes for gut microbiota. Available preliminary data suggest that the pili from pathogenic and beneficial bacteria share several sequence and structural features. The presence of transposable element in several pilus gene clusters indicates that the pathogenic and commensal bacteria may be acquired from each other during the evolution. The challenge is now to understand the differences between the (enemy) pathogenic and (friendly) beneficial bacteria in their pili-mediated adhesion strategies and interactions with the host. This knowledge is crucial in optimizing probiotics and targeting adhesion-based therapies for human health. The journey of pilus research in probiotics has begun with the prototype SpaCBA pili in *L. rhamnosus* GG. The ongoing and future research hopefully would shed light in this area.

Acknowledgments

This work was funded by the Regional Centre for Biotechnology (RCB) and the Department of Biotechnology (DBT) (Grant No. BT/PR5891/BRB/10/1098/2012), India.

Author details

Vengadesan Krishnan[1*], Priyanka Chaurasia[1,2] and Abhiruchi Kant[1,2]

*Address all correspondence to: kvengadesan@rcb.res.in

1 Regional Centre for Biotechnology, NCR Biotech Science Cluster, Faridabad, India

2 Department of Biotechnology, Manipal University, Manipal, Karnataka, India

References

[1] Gerritsen J, Smidt H, Rijkers GT, de Vos WM. Intestinal microbiota in human health and disease: the impact of probiotics. Genes & Nutrition. 2011;6:209–40. doi:10.1007/s12263-011-0229-7.

[2] Qin J, Li R, Raes J, Arumugam M, Burgdorf KS, Manichanh C, et al. A human gut microbial gene catalogue established by metagenomic sequencing. Nature. 2010;464:59–65. doi:10.1038/nature08821.

[3] Chow J, Lee SM, Shen Y, Khosravi A, Mazmanian SK. Host-bacterial symbiosis in health and disease. Advances in Immunology. 2010;107:243–74. doi:10.1016/B978-0-12-381300-8.00008-3.

[4] Ventura M, O'Flaherty S, Claesson MJ, Turroni F, Klaenhammer TR, van Sinderen D, et al. Genome-scale analyses of health-promoting bacteria: probiogenomics. Nature Reviews Microbiology. 2009;7:61–71. doi:10.1038/nrmicro2047.

[5] Craig L, Li J. Type IV pili: paradoxes in form and function. Current Opinion in Structural Biology. 2008;18:267–77. doi:10.1016/j.sbi.2007.12.009.

[6] Kline KA, Dodson KW, Caparon MG, Hultgren SJ. A tale of two pili: assembly and function of pili in bacteria. Trends in Microbiology. 2010;18:224–32. doi:10.1016/j.tim.2010.03.002.

[7] Pelicic V. Type IV pili: e pluribus unum? Molecular Microbiology. 2008;68:827–37. doi:10.1111/j.1365-2958.2008.06197.x.

[8] Proft T, Baker EN. Pili in Gram-negative and Gram-positive bacteria – structure, assembly and their role in disease. Cellular and Molecular Life Science. 2009;66:613–35. doi:10.1007/s00018-008-8477-4.

[9] Sauer FG, Mulvey MA, Schilling JD, Martinez JJ, Hultgren SJ. Bacterial pili: molecular mechanisms of pathogenesis. Current Opinion in Microbiology. 2000;3:65–72.

[10] Scott JR, Zahner D. Pili with strong attachments: Gram-positive bacteria do it differently. Molecular Microbiology. 2006;62:320–30. doi:10.1111/j.1365-2958.2006.05279.x.

[11] Hendrickx AP, Budzik JM, Oh SY, Schneewind O. Architects at the bacterial surface – sortases and the assembly of pili with isopeptide bonds. Nature Reviews Microbiology. 2011;9:166–76. doi:10.1038/nrmicro2520.

[12] Danne C, Dramsi S. Pili of Gram-positive bacteria: roles in host colonization. Research in Microbiology. 2012;163:645–58. doi:10.1016/j.resmic.2012.10.012.

[13] Mandlik A, Swierczynski A, Das A, Ton-That H. Pili in Gram-positive bacteria: assembly, involvement in colonization and biofilm development. Trends in Microbiology. 2008;16:33–40. doi:10.1016/j.tim.2007.10.010.

[14] Telford JL, Barocchi MA, Margarit I, Rappuoli R, Grandi G. Pili in Gram-positive pathogens. Nature Reviews Microbiology. 2006;4:509–19. doi:10.1038/nrmicro1443.

[15] Ton-That H, Schneewind O. Assembly of pili in Gram-positive bacteria. Trends in Microbiology. 2004;12:228–34. doi:10.1016/j.tim.2004.03.004.

[16] Ton-That H, Marraffini LA, Schneewind O. Sortases and pilin elements involved in pilus assembly of *Corynebacterium diphtheriae*. Molecular Microbiology. 2004;53:251–61.

[17] Symersky J, Patti JM, Carson M, House-Pompeo K, Teale M, Moore D, et al. Structure of the collagen-binding domain from a *Staphylococcus aureus* adhesin. Nature Structural Biology. 1997;4:833–8.

[18] Deivanayagam CC, Rich RL, Carson M, Owens RT, Danthuluri S, Bice T, et al. Novel fold and assembly of the repetitive B region of the *Staphylococcus aureus* collagen-binding surface protein. Structure. 2000;8:67–78.

[19] Kang HJ, Coulibaly F, Clow F, Proft T, Baker EN. Stabilizing isopeptide bonds revealed in Gram-positive bacterial pilus structure. Science. 2007;318:1625–8.

[20] Kang HJ, Baker EN. Structure and assembly of Gram-positive bacterial pili: unique covalent polymers. Current Opinion in Structural Biology. 2012;22:200–7.

[21] Krishnan V. Pilins in Gram-positive bacteria: a structural perspective. IUBMB Life. 2015;67:533–43. doi:10.1002/iub.1400.

[22] Vengadesan K, Narayana SV. Structural biology of Gram-positive bacterial adhesins. Protein Science 2011;20:759–72. doi:10.1002/pro.613.

[23] Izoré T, Contreras-Martel C, El Mortaji L, Manzano C, Terrasse R, Vernet T, et al. Structural basis of host cell recognition by the pilus adhesin from *Streptococcus pneumoniae*. Structure. 2010;18:106–15.

[24] Krishnan V, Dwivedi P, Kim BJ, Samal A, Macon K, Ma X, et al. Structure of *Streptococcus agalactiae* tip pilin GBS104: a model for GBS pili assembly and host interactions. Acta Crystallographica Section D, Biological Crystallography. 2013;69:1073–89. doi:10.1107/S0907444913004642.

[25] Linke-Winnebeck C, Paterson NG, Young PG, Middleditch MJ, Greenwood DR, Witte G, et al. Structural model for covalent adhesion of the *Streptococcus pyogenes* pilus through a thioester bond. The Journal of Biological Chemistry. 2014;289:177–89. doi:10.1074/jbc.M113.523761.

[26] Pointon JA, Smith WD, Saalbach G, Crow A, Kehoe MA, Banfield MJ. A highly unusual thioester bond in a pilus adhesin is required for efficient host cell interaction. The Journal of Biological Chemistry. 2010;285:33858–66. doi:10.1074/jbc.M110.149385.

[27] Walden M, Crow A, Nelson MD, Banfield MJ. Intramolecular isopeptide but not internal thioester bonds confer proteolytic and significant thermal stability to the *S. pyogenes* pilus adhesin Spy0125. Proteins. 2014;82:517–27. doi:10.1002/prot.24420.

[28] Pridmore RD, Berger B, Desiere F, Vilanova D, Barretto C, Pittet AC, et al. The genome sequence of the probiotic intestinal bacterium *Lactobacillus johnsonii* NCC 533. Proceedings of the National Academy of Sciences of the United States of America. 2004;101:2512–7.

[29] Kankainen M, Paulin L, Tynkkynen S, von Ossowski I, Reunanen J, Partanen P, et al. Comparative genomic analysis of *Lactobacillus rhamnosus* GG reveals pili containing a human-mucus binding protein. Proceedings of the National Academy of Sciences of the United States of America. 2009;106:17193–8. doi:10.1073/pnas.0908876106.

[30] Lebeer S, Verhoeven TL, Francius G, Schoofs G, Lambrichts I, Dufrene Y, et al. Identification of a gene cluster for the biosynthesis of a long, galactose-rich exopolysaccharide in *Lactobacillus rhamnosus* GG and functional analysis of the priming glycosyltransferase. Appled and Environmental Microbiology. 2009;75:3554–63. doi:10.1128/AEM.02919-08.

[31] Reunanen J, von Ossowski I, Hendrickx AP, Palva A, de Vos WM. Characterization of the SpaCBA pilus fibers in the probiotic *Lactobacillus rhamnosus* GG. Applied and Environmental Microbiology. 2012;78:2337–44.

[32] O'Connell Motherway M, Zomer A, Leahy SC, Reunanen J, Bottacini F, Claesson MJ, et al. Functional genome analysis of *Bifidobacterium breve* UCC2003 reveals type IVb tight adherence (Tad) pili as an essential and conserved host-colonization factor. Proceedings of the National Academy of Sciences of the United States of America. 2011;108:11217–22. doi:10.1073/pnas.1105380108.

[33] Turroni F, Foroni E, Serafini F, Viappiani A, Montanini B, Bottacini F, et al. Ability of *Bifidobacterium breve* to grow on different types of milk: exploring the metabolism of milk through genome analysis. Applied and Environmental Microbiology. 2011;77:7408–17. doi:10.1128/AEM.05336-11.

[34] Oxaran V, Ledue-Clier F, Dieye Y, Herry JM, Pechoux C, Meylheuc T, et al. Pilus biogenesis in *Lactococcus lactis*: molecular characterization and role in aggregation and biofilm formation. PLoS One. 2012;7:e50989. doi:10.1371/journal.pone.0050989.

[35] Meyrand M, Guillot A, Goin M, Furlan S, Armalyte J, Kulakauskas S, et al. Surface proteome analysis of a natural isolate of *Lactococcus lactis* reveals the presence of pili able to bind human intestinal epithelial cells. Molecular & Cellular Proteomics: MCP. 2013;12:3935–47. doi:10.1074/mcp.M113.029066.

[36] Yu X, Jaatinen A, Rintahaka J, Hynonen U, Lyytinen O, Kant R, et al. Human gut-commensalic *Lactobacillus ruminis* ATCC 25644 displays sortase-assembled surface piliation: phenotypic characterization of its fimbrial operon through in silico predictive analysis and recombinant expression in *Lactococcus lactis*. PLoS One. 2015;10:e0145718. doi:10.1371/journal.pone.0145718.

[37] Lee YK, Salminen S. Handbook of Probiotics and Prebiotics: John Wiley & Sons, Inc., New Jersey; 2008. doi:10.1002/9780470432624

[38] Nishiyama K, Ueno S, Sugiyama M, Yamamoto Y, Mukai T. *Lactobacillus rhamnosus* GG SpaC pilin subunit binds to the carbohydrate moieties of intestinal glycoconjugates. Animal Science Journal. 2015. doi:10.1111/asj.12491.

[39] von Ossowski I, Reunanen J, Satokari R, Vesterlund S, Kankainen M, Huhtinen H, et al. Mucosal adhesion properties of the probiotic *Lactobacillus rhamnosus* GG SpaCBA and SpaFED pilin subunits. Applied and Environmental Microbiology. 2010;76:2049–57.

[40] Tripathi P, Beaussart A, Alsteens D, Dupres V, Claes I, von Ossowski I, et al. Adhesion and nanomechanics of pili from the probiotic *Lactobacillus rhamnosus* GG. ACS Nano. 2013;7:3685–97. doi:10.1021/nn400705u.

[41] Lebeer S, Claes I, Tytgat HL, Verhoeven TL, Marien E, von Ossowski I, et al. Functional analysis of *Lactobacillus rhamnosus* GG pili in relation to adhesion and immunomodulatory interactions with intestinal epithelial cells. Applied and Environmental Microbiology. 2012;78:185–93.

[42] von Ossowski I, Pietila TE, Rintahaka J, Nummenmaa E, Makinen VM, Reunanen J, et al. Using recombinant Lactococci as an approach to dissect the immunomodulating capacity of surface piliation in probiotic *Lactobacillus rhamnosus* GG. PLoS One. 2013;8:e64416. doi:10.1371/journal.pone.0064416.

[43] Vargas Garcia CE, Petrova M, Claes IJ, De Boeck I, Verhoeven TL, Dilissen E, et al. Piliation of *Lactobacillus rhamnosus* GG promotes adhesion, phagocytosis, and cytokine modulation in macrophages. Applied and Environmental Microbiology. 2015;81:2050–62. doi:10.1128/AEM.03949-14.

[44] Ganguli K, Collado MC, Rautava J, Lu L, Satokari R, von Ossowski I, et al. *Lactobacillus rhamnosus* GG and its SpaC pilus adhesin modulate inflammatory responsiveness and TLR-related gene expression in the fetal human gut. Pediatric Research. 2015;77:528–35. doi:10.1038/pr.2015.5.

[45] Ardita CS, Mercante JW, Kwon YM, Luo L, Crawford ME, Powell DN, et al. Epithelial adhesion mediated by pilin SpaC is required for *Lactobacillus rhamnosus* GG-induced cellular responses. Applied and Environmental Microbiology. 2014;80:5068–77. doi: 10.1128/AEM.01039-14.

[46] Kant R, Rintahaka J, Yu X, Sigvart-Mattila P, Paulin L, Mecklin JP, et al. A comparative pan-genome perspective of niche-adaptable cell-surface protein phenotypes in *Lactobacillus rhamnosus*. PLoS One. 2014;9:e102762. doi:10.1371/journal.pone.0102762.

[47] Guerin J, Bacharouche J, Burgain J, Lebeer S, Francius G, Borges F, et al. Pili of *Lactobacillus rhamnosus* GG mediate interaction with β-lactoglobulin. Food Hydrocolloids. 2016;58:35–41.

[48] Rintahaka J, Yu X, Kant R, Palva A, von Ossowski I. Phenotypical analysis of the *Lactobacillus rhamnosus* GG fimbrial spaFED operon: surface expression and functional

characterization of recombinant SpaFED pili in *Lactococcus lactis*. PLoS One. 2014;9:e113922. doi:10.1371/journal.pone.0113922.

[49] Fronzes R, Christie PJ, Waksman G. The structural biology of type IV secretion systems. Nature Reviews Microbiology. 2009;7:703–14. doi:10.1038/nrmicro2218.

[50] Waksman G, Hultgren SJ. Structural biology of the chaperone-usher pathway of pilus biogenesis. Nature Reviews Microbiology. 2009;7:765–74.

[51] Krishnan V, Gaspar AH, Ye N, Mandlik A, Ton-That H, Narayana SVL. An IgG-like domain in the minor pilin GBS52 of *Streptococcus agalactiae* mediates lung epithelial cell adhesion. Structure. 2007;15:893–903.

[52] Hilleringmann M, Ringler P, Muller SA, De Angelis G, Rappuoli R, Ferlenghi I, et al. Molecular architecture of *Streptococcus pneumoniae* TIGR4 pili. EMBO Journal. 2009;28:3921–30. doi:10.1038/emboj.2009.360.

[53] Singh D, von Ossowski I, Palva A, Krishnan V. Purification, crystallization and preliminary crystallographic analysis of the SpaA backbone-pilin subunit from probiotic *Lactobacillus rhamnosus* GG. Acta Crystallographica Section F, Structural Biology and Crystallization Communication. 2013;69:1182–5. doi:10.1107/S1744309113024676.

[54] Chaurasia P, von Ossowski I, Palva A, Krishnan V. Purification, crystallization and preliminary X-ray diffraction analysis of SpaD, a backbone-pilin subunit encoded by the fimbrial spaFED operon in *Lactobacillus rhamnosus* GG. Acta Crystallographica Section F, Structural Biology Communication. 2015;71:103–6. doi:10.1107/S2053230X14027216.

[55] Kant A, von Ossowski I, Palva A, Krishnan V. Crystallization and X-ray crystallographic analysis of the adhesive SpaC pilin subunit in the SpaCBA pilus of gut?adapted Lactobacillus rhamnosus GG. Protein & Peptide Letters. 2016;23:365-71. doi: 10.2174/0929866523666160106153055.

[56] Forde BM, Neville BA, O'Donnell MM, Riboulet-Bisson E, Claesson MJ, Coghlan A, et al. Genome sequences and comparative genomics of two *Lactobacillus ruminis* strains from the bovine and human intestinal tracts. Microbial Cell Factories. 2011;10 (Suppl. 1):S13. doi:10.1186/1475-2859-10-S1-S13.

[57] Broadbent JR, Neeno-Eckwall EC, Stahl B, Tandee K, Cai H, Morovic W, et al. Analysis of the *Lactobacillus casei* supragenome and its influence in species evolution and lifestyle adaptation. BMC Genomics. 2012;13:533. doi:10.1186/1471-2164-13-533.

[58] Douillard FP, Ribbera A, Jarvinen HM, Kant R, Pietila TE, Randazzo C, et al. Comparative genomic and functional analysis of *Lactobacillus casei* and *Lactobacillus rhamnosus* strains marketed as probiotics. Applied and Environmental Microbiology. 2013;79:1923–33. doi:10.1128/AEM.03467-12.

[59] Munoz-Provencio D, Rodriguez-Diaz J, Collado MC, Langella P, Bermudez-Humaran LG, Monedero V. Functional analysis of the *Lactobacillus casei* BL23 sortases. Applied and Environmental Microbiology. 2012;78:8684–93. doi:10.1128/AEM.02287-12.

[60] Toh H, Oshima K, Nakano A, Takahata M, Murakami M, Takaki T, et al. Genomic adaptation of the *Lactobacillus casei* group. PLoS One. 2013;8:e75073. doi:10.1371/journal.pone.0075073.

[61] Smokvina T, Wels M, Polka J, Chervaux C, Brisse S, Boekhorst J, et al. *Lactobacillus paracasei* comparative genomics: towards species pan-genome definition and exploitation of diversity. PLoS One. 2013;8:e68731. doi:10.1371/journal.pone.0068731.

[62] Aleksandrzak-Piekarczyk T, Koryszewska-Baginska A, Grynberg M, Nowak A, Cukrowska B, Kozakova H, et al. Genomic and functional characterization of the unusual pLOCK 0919 plasmid harboring the spaCBA pili cluster in *Lactobacillus casei* LOCK 0919. Genome Biology and Evolution. 2016;8:202–17. doi:10.1093/gbe/evv247.

[63] Dieye Y, Oxaran V, Ledue-Clier F, Alkhalaf W, Buist G, Juillard V, et al. Functionality of sortase A in *Lactococcus lactis*. Applied and Environmental Microbiology. 2010;76:7332–7. doi:10.1128/AEM.00928-10.

[64] Le DT, Tran TL, Duviau MP, Meyrand M, Guerardel Y, Castelain M, et al. Unraveling the role of surface mucus-binding protein and pili in muco-adhesion of *Lactococcus lactis*. PLoS One. 2013;8:e79850. doi:10.1371/journal.pone.0079850.

[65] Turroni F, Ribbera A, Foroni E, van Sinderen D, Ventura M. Human gut microbiota and bifidobacteria: from composition to functionality. Antonie van Leeuwenhoek. 2008;94:35–50. doi:10.1007/s10482-008-9232-4.

[66] Koenig JE, Spor A, Scalfone N, Fricker AD, Stombaugh J, Knight R, et al. Succession of microbial consortia in the developing infant gut microbiome. Proceedings of the National Academy of Sciences of the United States of America. 2011;108 (Suppl. 1): 4578–85. doi:10.1073/pnas.1000081107.

[67] Foroni E, Serafini F, Amidani D, Turroni F, He F, Bottacini F, et al. Genetic analysis and morphological identification of pilus-like structures in members of the genus *Bifidobacterium*. Microbial Cell Factories. 2011;10 (Suppl. 1):S16. doi:10.1186/1475-2859-10-S1-S16.

[68] Mishra A, Das A, Cisar JO, Ton-That H. Sortase-catalyzed assembly of distinct heteromeric fimbriae in *Actinomyces naeslundii*. Journal of Bacteriology. 2007;189:3156–65. doi: 10.1128/JB.01952-06.

[69] Mishra A, Wu C, Yang J, Cisar JO, Das A, Ton-That H. The *Actinomyces oris* type 2 fimbrial shaft FimA mediates co-aggregation with oral streptococci, adherence to red blood cells and biofilm development. Molecular Microbiology. 2010;77:841–54. doi: 10.1111/j.1365-2958.2010.07252.x.

[70] Budzik JM, Marraffini LA, Schneewind O. Assembly of pili on the surface of *Bacillus cereus* vegetative cells. Molecular Microbiology. 2007;66:495–510. doi:10.1111/j.1365-2958.2007.05939.x.

[71] Turroni F, Serafini F, Foroni E, Duranti S, O'Connell Motherway M, Taverniti V, et al. Role of sortase-dependent pili of *Bifidobacterium bifidum* PRL2010 in modulating bacterium-host interactions. Proceedings of the National Academy of Sciences of the United States of America. 2013;110:11151–6. doi:10.1073/pnas.1303897110.

[72] Kachlany SC, Planet PJ, DeSalle R, Fine DH, Figurski DH. Genes for tight adherence of *Actinobacillus actinomycetemcomitans*: from plaque to plague to pond scum. Trends in Microbiology. 2001;9:429–37.

[73] Burrows LL. *Pseudomonas aeruginosa* twitching motility: type IV pili in action. Annual Review of Microbiology. 2012;66:493–520. doi:10.1146/annurev-micro-092611-150055.

[74] Giltner CL, Nguyen Y, Burrows LL. Type IV pilin proteins: versatile molecular modules. Microbiology and Molecular Biology Reviews: MMBR. 2012;76:740–72. doi: 10.1128/MMBR.00035-12.

[75] Piepenbrink KH, Maldarelli GA, Martinez de la Pena CF, Dingle TC, Mulvey GL, Lee A, et al. Structural and evolutionary analyses show unique stabilization strategies in the type IV pili of *Clostridium difficile*. Structure. 2015;23:385–96. doi:10.1016/j.str.2014.11.018.

Chapter 7

Biosynthesis of Vitamins by Probiotic Bacteria

Qing Gu and Ping Li

Additional information is available at the end of the chapter

http://dx.doi.org/10.5772/63117

Abstract

Vitamins are important micronutrients that are often precursors to enzymes, which all living cells require to perform biochemical reactions. However, humans cannot produce many vitamins, so they have to be externally obtained. Using vitamin-producing microorganisms could be an organic and marketable solution to using pseudo-vitamins that are chemically produced, and could allow for the production of foods with higher levels of vitamins that could reduce unwanted side effects. Probiotic bacteria, as well as commensal bacteria found in the human gut, such as *Lactobacillus* and *Bifidobacterium*, can de novo synthesize and supply vitamins to human body. In humans, members of the gut microbiota are able to synthesize vitamin K, as well as most of the water-soluble B vitamins, such as cobalamin, folates, pyridoxine, riboflavin, and thiamine.

Keywords: probiotic, folate, riboflavin, cobalamin, biosynthesis

1. Introduction

Vitamins are typically categorized as fat-soluble vitamins, which includes vitamins A, D, E, and K, or as water-soluble vitamins, which includes vitamin C, biotin (vitamin H or B7), and a series of B vitamins—thiamin (B1), riboflavin (B2), niacin (B3), pantothenic acid (B5), pyridoxine (B6), folic acid (B11), and cobalamin (B12). While fat-soluble vitamins act as important elements of cell membranes, water-soluble vitamins serve as coenzymes that typically transport specific chemical groups [1]. Humans are incapable of synthesizing most vitamins and they consequently have to be obtained exogenously. The use of vitamin-producing microorganisms might represent a more natural and consumer-friendly alternative to fortification using chemically synthesized pseudo-vitamins.

The biochemical pathways involved in B-vitamin biosynthesis by food microorganisms were previously described in detail [2]. Many prokaryotes need water-soluble vitamins for nutritional purposes [3], but also typically need them for biosynthetic processes. The ability of particular microorganisms to produce B vitamins could supplant the expensive chemical production of these vitamins to enrich food or be improved for in situ fortification of fermented foods. Much research has been conducted in recent years to elucidate the biosynthetic pathways of these vitamins in a number of microorganisms.

Probiotic bacteria positively impact the immune system and the composition and functioning of the gut microbiota [4]. Furthermore, the production of vitamins has resulted in many healthy benefits to the host. Probiotic bacteria, mostly belonging to the genera *Lactobacillus* and *Bifidobacterium*, confer a number of health benefits, including vitamin production [5]. Probiotic bacteria, members of the gut microbiota, are able to synthesize vitamin K and most of the water-soluble B vitamins, such as biotin, cobalamin, folates, nicotinic acid, panthotenic acid, pyridoxine, riboflavin, and thiamine, in humans [6].

The production of B-vitamins, especially folate and riboflavin (B2), by probiotic bacteria has been extensively researched as described in a recent review [7, 8]. Several lactic acid bacteria (LAB) species (e.g., *Lactococcus lactis, Lactobacillus gasseri,* and *Lactobacillus reuteri*) and *Bifidobacterium* (e.g., *B. adolescentis*) produce these vitamins, often in large quantities, and are, therefore, often found in fermented foods [9, 10]. Moreover, increased vitamin biosynthesis has been obtained by metabolic engineering [11, 12]. Folate biosynthetic genes and riboflavin biosynthetic operon have been overexpressed in *L. lactis,* resulting in types that produce folate [12] or riboflavin [12] at higher rates. Sybesma et al. [13] modified the biosynthetic pathways of folate and riboflavin in *L. lactis*, resulting in the simultaneous overproduction of both vitamins, through directed mutagenesis and selection and metabolic engineering.

This review focused on riboflavin, folic acid, and cobalamin, three of the water-soluble B vitamins whose biosynthetic pathways were inextricably linked, briefly covering their physiological functions and dietary sources before concentrating on novel overproduction strategies in probiotics.

2. Riboflavin biosynthesis

In contrast to many plants, fungi, and bacteria, humans cannot produce riboflavin or vitamin B2, and thus require it as a dietary supplement. Riboflavin is available as a dietary source and is also produced by the microflora of the large intestine [6, 14]. Riboflavin (vitamin B2) plays an essential role in cellular metabolism, as it is the precursor of the coenzymes flavin mononucleotide (FMN) and flavin adenine dinucleotide (FAD), which both act as hydrogen carriers in many biological redox reactions.

Riboflavin is synthesized by many bacteria and its biosynthetic pathway has been studied extensively in *Bacillus subtilis* and *Escherichia coli*. Bacher et al. [15, 16] found that riboflavin biosynthesis requires the precursor's guanosine 5′-triphosphate (GTP) and ribulose 5-phosphate. The first step of the GTP-dependent branch of the biosynthetic pathway is encoded by ribA in *E. coli*. In *B. subtilis* it is also encoded by *rib*A but in this case RibA acts as a bifunctional enzyme that also catalyzes the configuration of 3,4-dihydroxy-2-butanone 4-phosphate from ribulose 5- phosphate [17]. The overexpression of RibA in *B. subtilis* produces 25% more riboflavin, indicating that this enzyme is rate-limiting in riboflavin biosynthesis [18]. However, in *Lactococcus lactis*, the overexpression of *ribA* did not lead to increased riboflavin production [12].

The ability of some bacteria and fungi to overproduce riboflavin has been harnessed for industrial production. Such commercial producers include the ascomycetes *Eremothecium ashbyii* and *Ashbya gossypii*. However, advantages were perceived in developing bacterial and yeast fermentations to avail of their high growth rates, and less costly and complex growth media. Currently, *A. gossypii*, *Candida famata*, and *B. subtilis* are exploited for riboflavin production, with riboflavin production levels reaching 15 g/L, 20 g/L, and 14 g/L, respectively [19–21]. In *A. gossypii*, metabolic engineering increased riboflavin production almost 10-fold [22]. *A. gossypii* has also been targeted as a microorganism to overproduce riboflavin using oil waste [23]. In the case of *B. subtilis*, high levels of riboflavin production were achieved as a result of exposure to purine analogues and the toxic riboflavin analogue roseoflavin, or by genetic engineering [19, 24].

It has been reported that fermentation of cow milk with *L. lactis* and *Propionibacterium freudenreichii* ssp. *shermanii* as starter cultures significantly increased the riboflavin content of milk. Since the riboflavin produced by starter cultures is largely in the free form, the bio-availability is expected to be better than the bio-availability of riboflavin in unprocessed milk [12, 25]. The food-grade fermentative LAB *L. lactis* also grows in the absence of riboflavin. On the basis of the genome sequence of *L. lactis* IL1403 [26], it seemed that all genes involved in riboflavin biosynthesis (*rib* genes) were present in this organism.

Species and/or strain-specific traits in LAB provided genetic information for riboflavin biosynthesis. Several of the sequenced members of LAB possessed similar abilities to produce riboflavin, as suggested by comparative genome analysis, but an interrupted *rib* operon was sometimes seen in certain strains. Deficient genetic information was usually related to the inability to produce riboflavin in LAB. For instance, the sequenced genome of *Lactobacillus plantarum* strain WCFS1 had an incomplete *rib* operon, which lacked the entire *rib*G and part of the *rib*B genes [27]. Further, this strain could not grow unless riboflavin was present [28]. However, several selected strains of *L. plantarum* contained the whole rib operon and could produce vitamin B2. The *L. plantarum* strain NCDO 1752, and the recently sequenced *L. plantarum* strain JDMI and *L. plantarum* strains, for example, were isolated from cereals-derived products [28, 29]. Furthermore, even in LAB strains that contained all *rib* genes, riboflavin production had to be confirmed by chemical analysis.

3. Folate biosynthesis by human gut commensals

Folic acid, also known as vitamin B11, is a dietary necessity for humans, because it is used in several metabolic reactions, such as the biosynthesis of the building blocks of DNA and RNA, the nucleotides. It is recommended that adults take 200 μg daily, but pregnant women are encouraged to take a double dose daily, as folic acid could thwart neural-tube defects in newborns [30]. Low folic acid has been linked to high homocysteine levels in the blood, which could lead to coronary diseases [31, 32]. It has also been shown to protect against some forms of cancer [33]. Folate is conspicuously absent in many food products and is considered an essential additive to the general diet.

Folates are comprised of a mono- or polyglutamyl conjugate and these compounds were named after the number of glutamyl residues (PteGlu*n*), where *n* denoted the total number of glutamyl residues. The folates act as enzyme co-substrates in one-carbon (C1) metabolism of amino acids and nucleotides, in which the fully reduced (tetrahydro-) form functions as an acceptor or donor of a single carbon unit [34]. Folic acid has played a significant role in the production of purines and pyrimidines, and, therefore, in DNA synthesis. Methionine synthase uses 5-methyltetrahydrofolate in the conversion of l-homocysteine to l-methionine [35]. A majority of the methionine formed is converted to S-adenosylmethionine, which is a common donor of methyl groups for DNA, RNA, hormones, neurotransmitters, membrane lipids, and proteins [36]. The folate molecule contains one pterin moiety, created from 6-hydroxymethyl-7,8-dihydropterin pyrophosphate (DHPPP), bound to para-aminobenzoic acid (pABA, vitamin B10). As such, de novo biosynthesis called for both the precursors, DHPPP and pABA. Plants and bacteria could make the latter from the pentose phosphate pathway. Erythrose 4-phosphate and phosphoenolpyruvate go through the shikimate pathway to become chorismate, which acts as a branching point toward the biosynthesis of aromatic amino acids and pABA. Chorismate is transformed via aminodeoxychorismate synthase into 4-amino-4-deoxychorismate. Subsequently, pyruvate is cleaved by 4-amino-4-deoxychorismate lyase to give pABA, which is ultimately necessary for folate biosynthesis. The biosynthesis of DHPPP proceeds via the conversion of GTP in four consecutive steps. The first step is catalyzed by GTP cyclohydrolase I and involves an extensive transformation of GTP, through Amadori rearrangement, to form a pterin ring structure. Following dephosphorylation, the pterin molecule undergoes aldolase and pyrophosphokinase reactions, which produce the activated pyrophosphorylated DHPPP.

Folate biosynthesis continues with the formation of a C–N bond joining DHPPP to pABA. This condensation reaction, catalyzed by dihydropteroate synthase, yields 7,8-dihydropteroate (DHP). DHP is glutamylated by dihydrofolate synthase, resulting in dihydrofolate (DHF). It is then reduced by DHF reductase to the biologically active cofactor tetrahydrofolate (THF) and subjected to the addition of multiple glutamate moieties by folylpolyglutamate synthase to yield THF-polyglutamate. Polyglutamilation may also take place before the occurrence of the reduction step, being catalyzed by DHF synthase or, in many bacteria, by a bifunctional enzyme that is responsible for both DHF synthase and folylpolyglutamate synthase activities [37].

However, although all available complete bifidobacterial genomes are expected to specify aminodeoxychorismate synthase, a gene specifying a putative 4-amino-4-deoxychorismate lyase can only be found on the genome of *B. adolescentis* ATCC15703 and *B. dentium* Bd1 [9], which are, thus, expected to accomplish de novo biosynthesis of pABA. In contrast, *B.*

animalis subsp. *lactis* does not appear to possess the entire pathway for DHPPP biosynthesis or the gene encoding dihydropteroate synthase. Thus, *B. animalis* subsp. *lactis* was predicted to be auxotrophic for folates or DHP, and would, therefore, be unable to complete folate biosynthesis, even if pABA was present.

Lactobacilli are also typical human gut commensals and were recently investigated to discover if they could serve as possible folate producers [38]. Lactobacilli from various fermented foods have been investigated as starter cultures for the manufacturing of folate-fortified dairy products, while lactobacilli isolated from the human gut have been explored as folate-producing probiotics [39–42]. The availability of genome sequences of various lactobacilli provided an important contribution to the genetics underlying folate biosynthesis in this group of microorganisms [38]. For example, lactobacilli did not appear to harbor the genetic determinants for de novo pABA synthesis, with the exception of *L. plantarum* WCFS1 [27], suggesting that the vast majority of lactobacilli were unable to synthesize folate in the absence of pABA.

Currently, the strains of *Lactobacillus* with the greatest relevance for the manufacturing of probiotics and functional foods belong to the species *L. acidophilus, L. casei, L. paracasei, L. plantarum, L. reuteri,* and *L. salivarius* [43]. Like *L. lactis,* these species harbor a folate biosynthesis cluster that includes the gene encoding dihydropteroate synthase and all of the genes for the biosynthesis of DHPPP, with the exception of alkaline phosphatase. In *L. lactis,* the dephosphorylation of dihydroneopterin triphosphate into the monophosphate was demonstrated to occur through an alternative route, involving a Nudix pyrophosphohydrolase [44]. Many lactobacilli contain various genes encoding putative Nudix enzymes, such as *mut*T genes for DNA repair. However, *Lactobacillus sakei, Lactobacillus helveticus,* and *Lactobacillus delbrueckii* have a homologue of the *L. lactis* gene in the *fol* cluster. In contrast, in *Lactobacillus fermentum, L. plantarum,* and *L. reuteri,* the *fol* cluster held the gene of a putative non-Nudix purine NTP pyrophosphatase, which could be responsible for hydrolyzing dihydroneopterin triphosphate in these species. As such, *L. plantarum, L. sakei, L. delbrueckii, L. reuteri, L. helveticus,* and *L. fermentum* were predicted to generate DHPPP and could also be folate producers if cultured with pABA present [37, 44].

4. Vitamin B12 biosynthesis

Vitamin B12, otherwise known as cobalamin, is the biggest and most intricate vitamin. Cobalamin describes a cluster of cobalt-containing compounds (corrinoids) that have a lower axial ligand, which holds the cobalt-coordinated nucleotide (5, 6-dimethylbenzimidazole) as a base. Although humans only use vitamin B12 for two enzymatic activities, it is still an important dietary supplement. (R)-methyl-malonyl-CoA mutase assists in the metabolism of propionyl-CoA, which compounds such as valine, thymine, methionine, and odd-chain fatty acids produce when broken down. This ado-cobalamin-dependent enzyme catalyzes the rearrangement of propionyl-CoA following its carboxylation and epimerization to succinyl-CoA, which then goes through the citric acid cycle. Methionine synthase needs vitamin B12 in the form of methylcobalamin. Using 5-methyltetrahydrofolate as a methyl donor, this enzyme methylates homocysteine to form methionine [45].

Humans cannot synthesize vitamin B12, and, thus must obtain it from organisms that can. Only a limited number of bacteria are known to produce vitamin B12, three of which—*Pseudomonas denitrificans*, *Bacillus megaterium*, and *Propionibacterium freudenreichii*—are used for commercial production [46–48].

Cobalamin has the most complex structure of all the vitamins synthesized by bacteria requiring about 30 genes for its biosynthesis. Most of the work in characterizing cobalamin biosynthesis has been performed in *Salmonella typhimurium* and *P. denitrificans*. Two different pathways exist for adenosylcobalamin (ado-cobalamin) biosynthesis: (1) an oxygen-dependent pathway, which is found in *P. denitrificans*, and (2) an anaerobic pathway, which has been identified in, among others, *S. typhimurium*, *P. freudenreichii* subsp. *Shermanii*, and *B. megaterium*. Every gene required in the anaerobic cobalamin biosynthesis was found on the genome of *S. sanguinis* [49].

Genes encoding enzymes contributing to the oxygen-dependent pathway have been given the prefix *cob*, while those involved in the oxygen-independent pathway have the prefix *cbi* [50]. Due to the early insertion of cobalt in the anaerobic pathway, the remaining intermediates are cobalto-complexes and therefore require enzymes with different substrate specificities than the intermediates in the aerobic pathway although many of the reactions catalyzed are similar. CobZ was identified in *Rhodobacter capsulatus*, which catalyzes a reaction similar to that advanced by CobG, but in a different way, as the two proteins did not display any primary sequence resemblance. CobZ was also found to have a flavin in the form of a non-covalently bound FAD, two Fe-S centers, and a b-type heme, which was not similar to CobG [51]. It was thought that the final step in the cobalamin biosynthetic pathway in *S. typhimurium* involved the dephosphorylation of adenosylcobalamin-5′-phosphate, which is catalyzed by CobC and challenges the pathway indicated where CobS catalyzes the condensation of a-ribazole and an Ado-GDP-cobinamide [52]. The gene that reduces cobalt in the aerobic pathway has yet to be identified, but two candidate genes were identified to encode this enzyme, named CobR [53].

LAB are traditionally known as auxotrophic for cobalamin and are generally used for the biological analysis of this vitamin. Recently, however, cobalamins were identified in *L. reuteri* as were some of the genes encoding enzymes for the biosynthesis of this vitamin [54]. The presence of a B12-dependent metabolic pathway that converts glycerol into propanediol most likely allowed this LAB to synthesize B12. The discovery of the biosynthetic genes could increase the production of B12 through metabolic engineering, and facilitate the transfer of the production pathway to other LAB.

L. reuteri CRL1098 was also found to metabolize glycerol in a B12-free medium, indicating that a LAB might also be able to make cobalamin [55]. Chromatographic analysis of the intracellular bacterial extract of *L. reuteri* CRL 1098 proved that this strain was able to produce a cobalamin-like compound with an absorption spectrum that was similar to that of standard cobalamin but had a distinct elution time, while cobalamin production was proved with different bioassays [55]. Genetic evidence of cobalamin biosynthesis by *L. reuteri* CRL 1098 was then achieved by using different molecular biology techniques, and it was found that at least 30 genes assisted the de novo synthesis of the vitamin. The genetic organization (*cob* and *cbi* genes) resembled that of *Salmonella enterica* and *Listeria innocua* [56].

The complete genome of *Lactobacillus sanfranciscensis* TMW 1.1304, isolated from industrial sourdough fermentation, was also recently sequenced [57]. The data showed that only one gene necessary to the cobalamine synthesis was encoded by the sequenced strain *L. sanfranciscensis* TMW1.1304. Conversely, growth experiments revealed that several *L. sanfranciscensis* strains grew on vitamin B12-free media, which implied that these strains could synthesize cobalamine de novo [57].

Other strains of genus *Lactobacilli* such as *Lactobacillus coryniformis* isolated from goat milk [58], *L. plantarum* isolated from *kanjika* or Japanese pickles [59, 60], *Lactobacillus rossiae* isolated from sourdough [61], and *Lactobacillus fermentum* CFR 2195 isolated from breast-fed healthy infants' fecal matter [62] were shown to produce cobalamin-type compounds. Moreover, the genetic and biochemical data suggested that cobalamin biosynthesis genes would be spread to *Lactobacillus buchneri*, *Lactobacillus hilgardii*, and *Lactobacillus brevis*, and also contain genes of the *cob-pdu* gene cluster [63]. Therefore, the possibility of various cobalamin-producing strains and species of LAB would benefit not only from future basic studies on cobalamin production, but also from its application in the development of vitamin B_{12}-contained fermented products.

5. Biosynthesis of other B-group vitamins

Thiamine (vitamin B1) is a coenzyme in the pentose phosphate pathway that is required to synthesize fatty acids, steroids, nucleic acids, and the aromatic amino acid precursors into various neurotransmitters and other bioactive compounds essential for brain function [64]. Beyond its role as a necessary cofactor in the folate cycle, vitamin B6 (pyridoxine) also plays an important role in amino acid metabolism, which makes it a rate-limiting cofactor in the synthesis of neurotransmitters such as dopamine, serotonin, gamma-aminobutyric acid (GABA), noradrenaline, and the hormone melatonin [64].

LAB fermentation in yogurt, cheese, and other fermented products was shown to result in increased levels of riboflavin, folate, vitamin B12, niacin, and pyridoxine [65, 66]. Soy fermentation with *Streptococcus thermophilus* ST5 and *Lactobacillus helveticus* R0052 or *Bifidobacterium longum* R0175 also caused a small increase in thiamine and pyridoxine concentration that was not statistically significant [67].

6. Biosynthesis of vitamin K

Vitamin K serves as a cofactor for the enzyme that converts specific glutamyl residues in a few proteins to g-carboxyglutamyl (Gla) residues, aiding in the process. Humans obtain the daily nutritional requirement for vitamin K through the dietary phylloquinone that exists in plants, and, to some extent, through bacterially produced polyisoprenyl-containing compounds called menaquinones created in the human gut [68]. LAB were examined for their ability to produce quinone compounds, as vitamin K occurred naturally in two forms, namely, K1 (phylloquinone) in green plants, and K2 (menaquinones) in animals and some bacteria [69].

7. Conclusions

The use of vitamin-producing strains provided a new perspective on the specific uses of probiotics. Many food-grade bacteria overproduce B vitamins, including riboflavin (vitamin B2), folate (vitamin B11), and cyanocobalamine (vitamin B12), which could allow them to organically enrich raw food materials like soy, milk, meat, and vegetables with B vitamins, preventing the need for additives. Thus, the food industry could take advantage of these novel and efficient vitamin-producing strains to add nutritional value to fermented products and save money in the process. Notably, vitamin metabolism pathways were shown in genes that specified the biosynthetic enzymes for riboflavin, cobalamin, and folate production. It is increasingly possible to identify potential vitamin-producing strains and interpret the intertwined mechanisms for their biosynthesis, because of the expanding availability of genome sequences, which could be used to expand the vitamin-producing capacities of the human gut.

Acknowledgements

This project was funded by the International Science & Technology Cooperation Program of China (2013DFA32330), the National Natural Science Foundation of China (No. 31071513, No. 31271821), the Natural Science Foundation of Zhejiang Province (No. LY16C200002), the National High Technology Research and Development Program ("863" Program) of China (2012AA022105B), the National Research Foundation for the Doctoral Program of Higher Education (20133326110005), and the Science Foundation of the Zhejiang Education Department (No. Y201534497).

Author details

Qing Gu* and Ping Li

*Address all correspondence to: guqing2002@hotmail.com

Key Laboratory for Food Microbial Technology of Zhejiang Province, College of Food Science and Biotechnology, Zhejiang Gongshang University, Hangzhou, China

References

[1] Baku TK, Dickerson JWT. *Vitamins in Human Health and Disease*. CAB International, Wallinford; 1996.

[2] LeBlanc JG, Laino JE, del Valle MJ, Vannini V, van Sinderen D, Taranto MP, de Valdez GF, de Giori GS, Sesma F. B-group vitamin production by lactic acid bacteria – current knowledge and potential applications. J Appl Microbiol. 2011;111:1297–1309. DOI: 10.1111/j.1365-2672.2011.05157.x

[3] Snell EE. From bacterial nutrition to enzyme structure: a personal odyssey. Annu Rev Biochem. 1993;62:1–27. DOI: 10.1146/annurev.bi.62.070193.000245

[4] Hill C, Guarner F, Reid G, Gibson GR, Merenstein DJ, Pot B, Morelli L, Canani RB, Flint HJ, Salminen S, Calder PC, Sanders ME. Expert consensus document. The International Scientific Association for Probiotics and Prebiotics consensus statement on the scope and appropriate use of the term probiotic. Nat Rev Gastroenterol Hepatol. 2014;11:506–514. DOI:10.1038/nrgastro.2014.66

[5] Kanmani P, Satish Kumar R, Yuvaraj N, Paari KA, Pattukumar V, Arul V. Probiotics and its functionally valuable products-a review. Crit Rev Food Sci Nutr. 2013;53:641–658. DOI: 10.1080/10408398.2011.553752

[6] Hill MJ. Intestinal flora and endogenous vitamin synthesis. Eur J Cancer Prev. 1997;6(Suppl 1):S43–S45. DOI: 10.1097/00008469-199703001-00009

[7] Burgess CM, Smid EJ, van Sinderen D. Bacterial vitamin B2, B11 and B12 overproduction: an overview. Int J Food Microbiol. 2009;133:1–7. DOI: 10.1016/j.ijfoodmicro.2009.04.012

[8] Rossi M, Amaretti A, Raimondi S. Folate production by probiotic bacteria. Nutrients. 2011;3:118–134. DOI: 10.3390/nu3010118

[9] Ventura M, Turroni F, Zomer A, Foroni E, Giubellini V, Bottacini F, Canchaya C, Claesson MJ, He F, Mantzourani M, Mulas L, Ferrarini A, Gao B, Delledonne M, Henrissat B, Coutinho P, Oggioni M, Gupta RS, Zhang Z, Beighton D, Fitzgerald GF, O'Toole PW, van Sinderen D. The *Bifidobacterium dentium* Bd1 genome sequence reflects its genetic adaptation to the human oral cavity. PLoS Genet. 2009;5:e1000785. DOI: 10.1371/journal.pgen.1000785

[10] Papagianni M. Metabolic engineering of lactic acid bacteria for the production of industrially important compounds. Comput Struct Biotechnol J. 2012;3:e201210003. DOI: 10.5936/csbj.201210003

[11] Hugenholtz J, Sybesma W, Groot MN, Wisselink W, Ladero V, Burgess K, van Sinderen D, Piard JC, Eggink G, Smid EJ, Savoy G, Sesma F, Jansen T, Hols P, Kleerebezem M. Metabolic engineering of lactic acid bacteria for the production of nutraceuticals. Antonie Van Leeuwenhoek. 2002;82:217–235.

[12] Burgess C, O' Connell-Motherway M, Sybesma W, Hugenholtz J, van Sinderen D. Riboflavin production in *Lactococcus lactis*: potential for in situ production of vitamin-enriched foods. Appl Environ Microbiol. 2004;70:5769–5777. DOI:10.1128/AEM.70.10.5769-5777.2004

[13] Sybesma W, Burgess C, StarrenburgM, van Sinderen D, Hugenholtz J. Multivitamin production in *Lactococcus lactis* using metabolic engineering. Metab Eng. 2004;6:109–115. DOI:10.1016/j.ymben.2003.11.002

[14] Wrong O, Edmonds C, Chadwich V. *The Large Intestine. Its Role in Mammalian Nutrition and Homeostasis*. Wiley & Sons, New York; 1981.

[15] Bacher A, Eberhardt S, Fischer M, Kis K, Richter G. Biosynthesis of vitamin b2 (riboflavin). Annu Rev Nutr. 2000;20:153–167. DOI: 10.1146/annurev.nutr.20.1.153

[16] Perkins JB, Pero J. Vitamin biosynthesis. In: Sonenshein A, Hoch J, Losick R., editors. *Bacillus subtilis and its Closest Relatives from Genes to Cells*. ASM Press, Washington, DC, USA; 2002. p. 271–286.

[17] Richter G, Ritz H, Katzenmeier G, Volk R, Kohnle A, Lottspeich F, Allendorf D, Bacher A. Biosynthesis of riboflavin: cloning, sequencing, mapping, and expression of the gene coding for GTP cyclohydrolase II in *Escherichia coli*. J Bacteriol. 1993;175:4045–4051. DOI: 0021-9193/93/134045-07$02.00/0

[18] Hümbelin M, Griesser V, Keller T, Schurter W, Haiker M, Hohmann H, Ritz H, Richter G, Bacher A, van Loon A. GTP cyclohydrolase II and 3,4-dihydroxy- 2-butanone 4-phosphate synthase are rate-limiting enzymes in riboflavin synthesis of an industrial *Bacillus subtilis* strain used for riboflavin production. J Ind Microbio Biotechnol. 1999;22:1–7. 10.1038/sj.jim.2900590

[19] Perkins J, Sloma A, Hermann T, Theriault K, Zachgo E, Erdenberger T, Hannett N, Chatterjee N, Williams II V, Rufo Jr. GA, Hatch R, Pero J. Genetic engineering of *Bacillus subtilis* for the commercial production of riboflavin. J Ind Microbiol Biotechnol. 1999;22:8–18. 10.1038/sj.jim.2900587

[20] Stahmann K, Revuelta J, Seulberger H. Three biotechnical processes using *Ashbya gossypii, Candida famata*, or *Bacillus subtilis* compete with chemical riboflavin production. Appl Microbiol Biotechnol. 2000;53:509–516. 10.1007/s002530051649

[21] Schallmey M, Singh A, Ward O. Developments in the use of *Bacillus* species for industrial production. Can J Microbiol. 2004;50:1–17. 10.1139/w03-076

[22] Jimenez A, Santos MA, Pompejus M, Revuelta JL. Metabolic engineering of the purine pathway for riboflavin production in *Ashbya gossypii*. Appl Environ Microbiol. 2005;71:5743–5751. doi:10.1128/AEM.71.10

[23] Park EY, Zhang JH, Tajima S, Dwiarti L. Isolation of *Ashbya gossypii* mutant for an improved riboflavin production targeting for biorefinery technology. J Appl Microbiol. 2007;103:468–476. DOI: 10.1111/j.1365-2672.2006.03264.x

[24] Perkins JB, Pero J, Sloma A. Riboflavin overproducing strains of bacteria. European patent EP0405370; 1991.

[25] Singh R, Deodhar AD. Relative bioavailability of riboflavin in cow's milk and fermented milk using rat bioassay. Int Dairy J. 1994;4:59–71. DOI:10.1016/0958-6946(94)90049-3

[26] Bolotin A, Wincker P, Mauger S, Jaillon O, Malarme K, Weissenbach J, Ehrlich SD, Sorokin A. The complete genome sequence of the lactic acid bacterium *Lactococcus lactis* ssp. *lactis* IL1403. Genome Res. 2001;11:731–753. DOI:10.1101/gr.169701

[27] Kleerebezem M, Boekhorst J, van Kranenburg R, Molenaar D, Kuipers OP, Leer R, Tarchini R, Peters SA, Sandbrink HM, Fiers MW, Stiekema W, Lankhorst RM, Bron PA, Hoffer SM, Groot MN, Kerkhoven R, de Vries M, Ursing B, de Vos WM, Siezen RJ. Complete genome sequence of *Lactobacillus plantarum* WCFS1. Proc Natl Acad Sci USA. 2003;100:1990–1995. DOI: 10.1073/pnas.0337704100

[28] Burgess CM, Smid EJ, Rutten G, van Sinderen D. A general method for selection of riboflavin-overproducing food grade micro-organisms. Microb Cell Factories. 2006;5:24. DOI: 10.1186/1475-2859-5-24

[29] Capozzi V, Menga V, Digesu AM, De Vita P, van Sinderen D, Cattivelli L, Fares C, Spano G. Biotechnological production of vitamin B2-enriched bread and pasta. J Agric Food Chem. 2011;59:8013–8020. DOI: 10.1021/jf201519h

[30] MRC Vitamin Study Research Group. Prevention of neural tube defects: results of the Medical Research Council vitamin study. Lancet. 1991;338:131–137. DOI: 10.1016/0140-6736(91)90133-A

[31] Boushey CJ, Beresford AA, Omenn GS, Moltulsky AG. A quantitative assessment of plasma homocysteine as a risk factor for vascular disease. J Am Med Assoc. 1995;274:1049–1057. DOI:10.1001/jama.1995.03530130055028

[32] Kamphuis MH, Geerlings MI, Grobbee DE, Kromhout D. Dietary intake of B(6-9-12) vitamins, serum homocysteine levels and their association with depressive symptoms: the Zutphen Elderly Study. Eur J Clin Nutr. 2008;62:939–945. DOI: 10.1038/sj.ejcn. 1602804

[33] Ames BN. Micronutrient deficiencies. A major cause of DNA damage. Ann NY Acad Sci. 1999;889:87–106. DOI: 10.1111/j.1749-6632.1999.tb08727.x

[34] Combs GF. *The Vitamins: Fundamental Aspects in Nutrition and Health*. Academic Press, San Diego; 1992.

[35] Brody T. Folic acid. In: Machlin LJ, editor. *Handbook of Vitamins*. Marcel Dekker Inc., New York; 1991. p. 453–489.

[36] Laiño JE, de Giori GS, LeBlanc JG. Folate production by lactic acid bacteria. In: Watson R, editor. *Bioactive Foods and Supplements in Health Promotion - Liver and Gastrointestinal*

Disease. Elsevier, Oxford, UK; 2013. p. 251–270. DOI:10.1016/B978-0-12-397154-8.00030-0

[37] De Crécy-Lagard V, El Yacoubi B, de la Garza RD, Noiriel A, Hanson AD. Comparative genomics of bacterial and plant folate synthesis and salvage: predictions and validations. BMC Genomics. 2007;8:245. DOI: 10.1186/1471-2164-8-245

[38] Kleerebezem M, Vaughan EE. Probiotic and gut lactobacilli and bifidobacteria: molecular approaches to study diversity and activity. Annu Rev Microbiol. 2009;63:269–290. DOI: 10.1146/annurev.micro.091208.073341

[39] Rao DR, Reddy AV, Pulusani SR, Cornwell PE. Biosynthesis and utilization of folic acid and vitamin B12 by lactic cultures in skim milk. J Dairy Sci. 1984;67:1169–1174. DOI: 10.3168/jds.S0022-0302(84)81419-8

[40] Wegkamp A, Starrenburg M, de Vos WM, Hugenholtz J, Sybesma W. Transformation of folate-consuming *Lactobacillus gasseri* into a folate producer. Appl Environ Microbiol. 2004;70:3146–3148. DOI: 10.1128/AEM.70.5.3146-3148.2004

[41] Santos F, Wegkamp A, de Vos WM, Smid EJ, Hugenholtz J. High-level folate production in fermented foods by the B12 producer *Lactobacillus reuteri* JCM1112. Appl Environ Microbiol. 2008;74:3291–3294. DOI: 10.1128/AEM.02719-07

[42] Laino JE, Leblanc JG, Savoy de Giori G. Production of natural folates by lactic acid bacteria starter cultures isolated from artisanal Argentinean yogurts. Can J Microbiol. 2012;58:581–588. DOI: 10.1139/w2012-026

[43] FAO/WHO. Health and nutritional properties of probiotics in food including powder milk with live lactic acid bacteria. In: *Report of a Joint FAO/WHO Expert Consultation on Evaluation of Health and Nutritional Properties of Probiotics in Food including Powder Milk with Live Lactic Acid Bacteria, Córdoba, Argentina*. WHO, Geneva, Switzerland; 2001. p. 1–34.

[44] Klaus SM, Wegkamp A, Sybesma W, Hugenholtz J, Gregory JF III, Hanson AD. A nudix enzyme removes pyrophosphate from dihydroneopterin triphosphate in the folate synthesis pathway of bacteria and plants. J Biol Chem. 2005;280:5274–5280. DOI: 10.1074/jbc.M413759200

[45] Ellenbogen L, Cooper BA. Vitamin B12. In: Machlin, L.J., editor *Handbook of Vitamins*. Marcel Dekker Inc., New York; 1991. p. 491–536.

[46] Warren MJ, Raux E, Schubert HL, Escalante-Semerena JC. The biosynthesis of adenosylcobalamin (vitamin B12). Nat Prod Rep. 2002;19:390–412. DOI: 10.1039/B108967F

[47] Warren MJ. Finding the final pieces of the vitamin B12 biosynthetic jigsaw. Proc Natl Acad Sci USA 2006;103:4799–4800. DOI: 10.1073/pnas.0601030103

[48] Escalante-Semerena JC. Conversion of cobinamide into adenosylcobamide in bacteria and archaea. J Bacteriol. 2007;189:4555–4560. DOI: 10.1128/JB.00503-07

[49] Xu P, Alves JM, Kitten T, Brown A, Chen Z, Ozaki LS, Manque P, Ge X, Serrano MG, Puiu D, Hendricks S, Wang Y, Chaplin MD, Akan D, Paik S, Peterson DL, Macrina FL, Buck GA. Genome of the opportunistic pathogen *Streptococcus sanguinis*. J Bacteriol. 2007;189:3166–3175. DOI: 10.1128/JB.01808-06

[50] Martens JH, Barg H,Warren MJ, Jahn D. Microbial production of vitamin B12. Appl Microbiol Biotechnol. 2002;58:275–285. DOI: 10.1007/s00253-001-0902-7

[51] McGoldrick HM, Roessner CA, Raux E, Lawrence AD, McLean KJ, Munro AW, Santabarbara S, Rigby SE, Heathcote P, Scott AI, Warren MJ. Identification and characterization of a novel vitamin B12 (cobalamin) biosynthetic enzyme (CobZ) from *Rhodobacter capsulatus*, containing flavin, heme, and Fe–S cofactors. J Biol Chem. 2005;280:1086–1094. DOI: 10.1074/jbc.M411884200

[52] Zayas CL, Escalante-Semerena JC. Reassessment of the late steps of coenzyme B12 synthesis in *Salmonella enterica*: evidence that dephosphorylation of adenosylcobalamin- 5′-phosphate by the CobC phosphatase is the last step of the pathway. J Bacteriol. 2007;189:2210–2218. DOI: 10.1128/JB.01665-06

[53] Heldt D, Lawrence AD, Lindenmeyer M, Deery E, Heathcote P, Rigby SE, Warren MJ. Aerobic synthesis of vitamin B12: ring contraction and cobalt chelation. Biochem Soc Trans. 2005;33:815–819. DOI: 10.1042/BST0330815

[54] Kleerebezem M, Hugenholtz J. Metabolic pathway engineering in lactic acid bacteria. Curr Opin Biotechnol. 2003;14:232–237. DOI:10.1016/S0958-1669(03)00033-8

[55] Taranto MP, Vera JL, Hugenholtz J, de Valdez GF and Sesma F. *Lactobacillus reuteri* CRL1098 produces cobalamin. J Bacteriol. 2003;185:5643–5647. DOI: 10.1128/JB. 185.18.5643-5647.2003

[56] Santos F, Vera JL, Lamosa P, de Valdez GF, de Vos WM, Santos H, Sesma F and Hugenholtz J. Pseudovitamin B(12) is the corrinoid produced by *Lactobacillus reuteri* CRL1098 under anaerobic conditions. FEBS Lett. 2007;581:4865–4870. DOI: 10.1016/ j.febslet.2007.09.012

[57] Vogel RF, Pavlovic M, Ehrmann MA, Wiezer A, Liesegang H, Offschanka S, Voget S, Angelov A, Böcker G, Liebl W. Genomic analysis reveals *Lactobacillus sanfranciscensis* as stable element in traditional sourdoughs. Microb Cell Factories. 2011;10:S6. DOI: 10.1186/1475-2859-10-S1-S6

[58] Martin R, Olivares M, Marin ML, Xaus J, Fernandez L, Rodriguez JM. Characterization of a reuterin-producing *Lactobacillus coryniformis* strain isolated from a goat's milk cheese. Int J Food Microbiol. 2005;104:267–277. DOI: 10.1016/j.ijfoodmicro.2005.03.007

[59] Madhu AN, Giribhattanavar P, Narayan MS, Prapulla SG. Probiotic lactic acid bacterium from kanjika as a potential source of vitamin B12: evidence from LC-MS, immunological and microbiological techniques. Biotechnol Lett. 2010;32:503–506. DOI: 10.1007/s10529-009-0176-1

[60] Masuda M, Ide M, Utsumi H, Niiro T, Shimamura Y, Murata M. Production potency of folate, vitamin B(12), and thiamine by lactic acid bacteria isolated from Japanese pickles. Biosci Biotechnol Biochem. 2012;76:2061–2067. DOI: 10.1271/bbb.120414

[61] De Angelis M, Bottacini F, Fosso B, Kelleher P, Calasso M, Di Cagno R, Ventura M, Picardi E, van Sinderen D, Gobbetti M. *Lactobacillus rossiae*, a vitamin B12 producer, represents a metabolically versatile species within the Genus *Lactobacillus*. PLoS One. 2014;9:e107232. DOI: 10.1371/journal.pone.0107232

[62] Basavanna G, Prapulla SG. Evaluation of functional aspects of *Lactobacillus fermentum* CFR 2195 isolated from breast fed healthy infants' fecal matter. J Food Sci Technol. 2013;50:360–366. DOI: 10.1007/s13197-011-0345-9

[63] Capozzi V, Russo P, Duenas MT, Lopez P, Spano G. Lactic acid bacteria producing B-group vitamins: a great potential for functional cereals products. Appl Microbiol Biotechnol. 2012;96:1383–1394. DOI: 10.1007/s00253-012-4440-2

[64] Kerns JC, Arundel C, Chawla LS. Thiamin deficiency in people with obesity. Adv Nutr Int Rev J. 2015;6:147–153. DOI: 10.3945/an.114.007526

[65] Shahani K, Chandan RC. Nutritional and healthful aspects of cultured and culture-containing dairy foods. J Dairy Sci. 1979;62:1685–1694. DOI:10.3168/jds.S0022-0302(79)83481-5

[66] Alm L. Effect of fermentation on B-vitamin content of milk in Sweden. J Dairy Sci. 1982;65:353–359. DOI: 10.3168/jds.S0022-0302(82)82199-1

[67] Champagne CP, Tompkins TA, Buckley ND, Green-Johnson JM. Effect of fermentation by pure and mixed cultures of *Streptococcus thermophilus* and *Lactobacillus helveticus* on isoflavone and B-vitamin content of a fermented soy beverage. Food Microbiol. 2010;27:968–972. DOI: 10.1016/j.fm.2010.06.003

[68] Suttie JW. The importance of menaquinones in human nutrition. Annu Rev Nutr. 1995;15:399–417. DOI: 10.1146/annurev.nu.15.070195.002151

[69] Morishita T, Tamura N, Makino T, Kudo S. Production of menaquinones by lactic acid bacteria. J Dairy Sci. 1999;82:1897–1903. DOI:10.3168/jds.S0022-0302(99)75424-X

Chapter 8

Bioactive Compounds of Lactic Acid Bacteria. Case Study: Evaluation of Antimicrobial Activity of Bacteriocin-producing Lactobacilli Isolated from Native Ecological Niches of Ecuador

Gabriela N. Tenea and Lucia Yépez

Additional information is available at the end of the chapter

http://dx.doi.org/10.5772/63112

Abstract

Food preservation through natural methods represents one of the concerns worldwide to solve economic losses due to microbial decomposition of raw materials and foodstuffs. However, public concern over the emergence of strains resistant to many antibiotics, particularly pathogens such as *E. coli* and *Salmonella* sp. draw much attention as new challenge in food industry is to find new alternative quality-control methods of food products. In Ecuador, the lack of quality control, bad storage condition, and insufficient preservation against spoilage bacteria had at higher extent repercussions on food safety and security. The most frequent pathogens detected in fresh meat and drinks along with traditional local food products, represent a serious problem producing sizable food damage and associated diseases. The capacity of lactobacilli to inhibit pathogens has been recently exploited to prevent microbial spoilage. Here we briefly review the principal biopeptides (i.e., bacteriocins) of lactic acid bacteria, their main mode of action, the classification, and its biotechnological applications. Moreover, we discussed the preliminary results on the evaluation of antimicrobial activity of some native lactic acid bacteria isolated from microbiota of Ecuador against frequent contaminants found in the local market.

Keywords: lactic acid bacteria, biopreservation, bacteriocins, food pathogens, probiotic

1. Introduction

Lactic acid bacteria (LAB) are among the most favorable microorganisms known for their probiotic properties and for the ability to produce antimicrobial compounds (i.e., bacteriocin, organic acids, diacetyl, hydrogen peroxide) with inhibitory action of harmful bacteria growth along with their critical role in food protection and health maintenance [1–3].

Nowadays, one of the biggest issues faced by the food-processing industry is contamination with pathogens caused by poor maintenance and unhygienic sanitary behavior and insufficient attention to the handling and preservation, contributing greatly to decrease the quality of products and also increase consummators foodborne illness in the population [4–6]. Thus, the preservation through natural methods represents one of the main concerns at the global level to solve economic losses due to microbial decomposition of raw materials and foodstuffs.

With concomitant expansion of the research, commercial, food industry and medical sectors, the field of biopreservation using probiotic bacteria is developing rapidly with accumulation of many data about their benefits. The complete genome sequencing as well as the identification of functional properties will further contribute to the reinforcement of most powerful products with improved biotechnological characteristics. Although many bacteria produce antimicrobial substances, the benefits of those produced by LAB is of particular interest because of their Generally Recognized as Safe (GRAS) status, which acts as natural biopreservative and natural flavor enhancers [3, 7–9]. Hence, the majority of antimicrobial peptide-producing LAB are ideally suited to food applications. Therefore, the production of bacteriocins by LAB is not only advantageous to the bacteria themselves but could also be exploited as a tool of food industry to control undesirable bacteria in a natural manner, and be allowable to the consumer.

As the main source of knowing LAB is represented by the human microflora and fermented milk products, it would be more valuable to search for other sources of probiotic microorganism, which might possess powerful properties and beneficial for either human health or food preservation. During the last decade, extensive progress has been made with respect to the isolation of LAB with highly antimicrobial properties as well as comprehension of bacteriocin structure and function, regulation, and immunity. Further investigations may help to develop new methods for food preservation by direct comparisons between strains bacteriocin producers and non-produced isogenic strains. In this context, bacteriocin of LAB would offer several benefits such as the use reduction of chemical compounds in food preservation. In this chapter, we will briefly review the main information about the role of bacteriocin of LAB in food preservation, their classification and mode of action along with their biotechnological benefits. Moreover, we shall present the preliminary results on the evaluation of antimicrobial activity of some native lactic acid bacteria isolated from microbiota of Ecuador against frequent contaminants found in the local food market.

2. Bacteriocins of lactic acid bacteria and their biotechnological applications

Antimicrobial heterogeneous compounds (i.e., bacteriocine) are ribosomally synthesized polypeptide or low-molecular-weight proteins (composed of 20–60 amino acid residues), which, in case of LAB, are generally recognized as safe compounds [9]. They bind to the receptor of the target cell, and their mode of action included pore formation, degradation of cellular DNA, disruption through specific cleavage of 16S rRNA, and inhibition of peptidoglycan synthesis [10, 11]. Bacteriocins being proteinaceous agents differ from most antibiotics because they are rapidly digested by proteases in the digestive tract.

2.1. Types of bacteriocins

More than three hundred different bacteriocins have been described for the genera *Lactobacillus, Lactococcus, Leuconostoc, Pediococcus,* and *Enterococcus*. These peptides are colorless, odorless, and tasteless, and according to their molecular mass, thermo stability, enzymatic, and sensitivity, the presence of posttranslational modified amino acids and their mode of action are classified into four major groups [10–13].

Bacteriocins of Class I: They, known as lantibiotics, are small peptides of <5 kDa, heat stable that acting on the membrane structure, and contain the thio-ester amino acids lanthionine and methyllanthionine as well as other modified amino acids such as dehydrated serine and threonine. From this class, the most studied bacteriocin is nisin produced by *Lactococcus lactis* subsp. *lactis* and discovered since 1928 as being the first bioactive compound used in food system as biopreservative [12]. According to their structural similarities, the lantibiotics were divided into two subclasses. *Subclass Ia,* comprising positively charged peptides (i.e., nisin), generally acts by forming pores in the cytoplasmic membrane of the target species. *Subclass Ib* are peptides either negatively charged or no net charged, more rigid in their structure which exert their action by interfering with enzymatic reactions of sensitive bacteria. The most studied bacteriocins of class I are Nisin Z and Q, Enterocin W, and Nukacin ISK-1 [14–16].

Bacteriocins of Class II: They, known as non-lantibiotics, are heat-stable bacteriocins of variable molecular weight, <10 kDa, containing in their composition regular amino acids. This class was subdivided into four subclasses. *Subclass IIa,* comprising Pediocin PA-1 and Sakacin P, are known for their antimicrobial activity against *Listeria*. Members of pediocin-like peptides have a high degree of homology (40–60%), particularly at the N-terminal domain, containing "pediocine box" or homologous region YGNGVXCXXXXCXV, with two residues of cysteine forming a disulfide bridge. Other known bacteriocins of *subclass IIa* are Enterocin NKR-5-3C [17, 18], Enterocin A [15], Munditicin [19], and Leucocin A [15]. *Subclass IIb,* comprising distinct peptides with little or no activity, refers to two-component bacteriocins that require two peptides to work synergistically. In this group are enclosed Lactacin F and Lactococcin G. *Subclass IIc* are small peptides, heat stable, and transported by leader peptides, comprising Diverginin A and Acidocin B. *Subclass IId* includes sec-dependent bacteriocins, and leaderless bacteriocins are Lacticin Q [20], Z [21], Weissellicin Y and M [22], and Leucocin Q and N [15].

Bacteriocins of Class III: They are larger peptides, about 430 kDa, heat liable comprising Helveticins J and V, Acidofilicin A, and Lactacins A and B.

Bacteriocins of Class IV: They contain modified peptides with either lipid or carbohydrate components, or they form large complexes with other chemical moieties, lipids, or carbohydrates.

Regardless of many biotechnological applications, *nisin* remain the only commercial bacteriocin approved by World Health Organization Expert Committee on Food Additives and by the US Food and Drug for its use in food industry [23]. Nisin is a 34 amino acid long peptide of 5-kDa molecular weight, and its synthesis is a complex mechanism involving processes of transcription, transduction, posttranscriptional modifications, secretion, and signs of transduction [24]. There are two forms of nisin, A and Z known for their action against *Bacillus* and *Clostridium* in processed cheese. Its lethal activity is close related with two important properties, cationic and hydrophobicity. However, small-size bacteriocins are active at different ranges of pH (i.e., from 3.0 up to 9.0), and their high isoelectric point allows the interaction with the anionic surface at the bacterial membrane at physiological pH values. Another feature is heat stability related to the monosulfide and disulfide intramolecular bonds, which maintain stable the secondary structure by reduction of the possible unfolded structures. This property explains the high resistance to autoclaving conditions of some LAB bacteriocins [25]. For example, Helveticin J is inhibited after 1- to 15-min incubation at 60–100°C, but can be easily recovered from bacterial culture. On the other hand, nisin has higher antimicrobial activity at pH of 2.0–4.0, and has heated stability at 100°C for 10 min of incubation while at pH 7.0 it is inactivated making this bacteriocin useful for food preservation [25].

Early studies showed that bacteriocins overcome different functions of the living cells, such as transcription, translation, and replication, due to their variation in the chemical structure, but most of them are acting by forming membrane channels or pores that destroy the energy of sensitive cells [25]. Regarding their mode of action, it has been shown that they are effective against Gram-positive bacteria and might be inefficient to inhibit Gram-negative organisms [24, 26–28]. Have been proposed numerous mechanisms of action such as the inhibition of spore germination as well as inactivation of anionic carriers through the formation of selective and non-selective pores and alteration of enzymatic activity [26, 27]. The effect on sensitive cells could be bactericidal or bacteriostatic depending on the dosage, degree of purification, and physiological state on the indicator cells along with experimental working conditions [24]. They bind to the cell cytoplasmic membrane with harmful effects in different ways. *Subclass Ia* bacteriocins are associated electrostatically with the negatively charged membrane phospholipids, which allowed the interaction with the cytoplasmic membrane of the target cell generating unspecific ionic channels. Inhibitory activity of *subclass IIa* is related to the presence of the sequence YGNGV at their N-terminus region. According to previous studies, some non-lanthionine bacteriocins are more active at the lower pH [24, 26]. In case of *subclass IIc*, the mechanism of action is controlled by the presence or absence of intramolecular disulfide bonds. For example, in case of lactococcin A, a bacteriocine without cysteine residues, the activity is related to the pore formation on sensitive cell membranes, while, in cerein 7/8, activity decreases the osmolarity of growth culture suggesting that this bacteriocin acts at the membrane level [25].

2.2. Genetics and biotechnological potential of LAB bacteriocins

Recent studies showed that almost all genetic determinants of bacteriocins are clustered in *operons* or *regulons* and its production is controlled by the presence of extrachromosomal elements such as plasmids [25]. Genes encoding for bacteriocins are located on the chromosome (e.g., subtilin), plasmids (e.g., divergicin A), or transposons (e.g., nisin). In general, lantibiotic operons are more complex than non-lantibiotic ones because they need additional genes encoding enzymes for posttranscriptional modifications. In case of nicin, the genetic determinants are located on the conjugative transposon Tn5276 within the bacterial chromosome. Gene *nisA* has been sequenced and found as been part of a polycistronic operon [24]. Other genes presented in the nisin operon are *nisB, nisI, nisR,* and *nisP. NisB* contains several putative transmembrane helical regions and appears to bind to artificial phospholipid vesicles suggesting that the nisin synthesis occurs at the cytoplasmic region, while *nisP* appears to be involved in the regulation of nisin biosynthesis. Another bacteriocin, lacticin 481, produced by *Lactococcus lactis* had the genes on the transposon Tn5721 located on a 70-kb plasmid [24].

Most of the genetically characterized class II bacteriocin gene clusters are composed of three gene modules: a module that includes the structural and immunity genes, a transport gene module, and a regulatory gene module. The structural gene for the bacteriocin is cotranscribed with the corresponding immunity gene located downstream, although there are exceptions to this genetic organization. For example, in case of the non-lantibiotic bacteriocin, carnobacteriocin BM1 produced by *Carnobacterium piscicola,* while its structural gene is located on the bacterial chromosome, its expression is dependent on the presence of a 61-kb plasmid, which carries some of the genes required for the export and the immunity.

Pediocin-like bacteriocins of *subclass IIa* have a very complex structure, containing double-glycine leader peptide, and are transported by ABC transporter. Among this class, few bacteriocins pediocin such as PA-1, AcH, and sakacin A were most characterized [5]. Pediocin PA-1 and pediocin AcH were produced by strains of *Pediococcus acidilactici,* possessing plasmids with sizes 9.4 and 8.9 kb respectively, and Sakakin A was determined by a 60-kb *Lactobacillus sakei* plasmid.

Although the expression of bacteriocin genes is regulated by external induction factors, bacteriocins' production depends upon environmental conditions (temperature, pH, etc.). Their use in food preservation offers several benefits: among them, it reduces the use of chemical preservatives and decreases the elongation of heated treatments. Bacteriocins can be produced *in situ* by the inoculation of the producer strain or can be produced *ex situ* and added to the food as antimicrobial additives. However, the composition of the food matrix and the interaction with other preservation factors affect its production and its activity.

In food industry, numerous control measurements to prevent or minimize pathogen contamination, including good manufacturing practices, effective sanitation, and hygiene measures, have been developed [29]. Nevertheless, despite these safety measures, foodborne outbreaks do occur frequently with particular concern on consumers health. Among food pathogens, *L. monocytogenes* is extremely strong, surviving refrigeration temperatures and high salt concentration. Other pathogens such as *Salmonella* sp. and *E. coli* are also frequently detected in processed or fresh foods. Nowadays, many investigations are focused on discovering novel bacteriocins for controlling the undesirable bacteria in food products [25, 29]. There is a need to attract consumer attention to natural substances rather than conventional synthesis of chemical one as protector against pathogens. As probiotics has been accepted in the market for their beneficial properties, and in the same way, the bacteriocin-producing probiotic strains should become attractive especially to natural food preservation.

Continued research on bacteriocins will undoubtedly lead to our increased understanding, and with the emergence of new bacteriocins, new potential biopreservatives.

3. Antimicrobial activity of LAB strains isolated from native microbiota of Ecuador

The presence of pathogens in many food products has become a serious problem worldwide. During the last decade, several laboratories have worked towards the identification of novel probiotic strains with better performance benefits such as novel attractive alternative antimicrobial methods to conventional ones [30–36].

Ecuador is known as country with large diversity of native unexploited resources. Some regions were included recently in the governmental policy as important resources to be exploited as reservoirs of unknown microorganisms that could become as potential areas of highly interest for biotechnology research, food sovereignty, and security. The lack of quality control, bad storage condition, and lack of preservation against spoilage bacteria had effect on food safety and security. Among the most food pathogens worldwide due to the considerable human rates of illness reported, *Salmonella* and *E. coli* remain the wide species detected in the local food market in Ecuador. Most produced traditional foods, such as mote (a fermented maize dish), handmade chees, and milk containing drinks, maintained in defective storage conditions appear to pose significant number of pathogens; therefore, the risk of developing diseases associated with food born pathogens is elevated. In this context, the aforementioned problems identifying new alternatives for food biopreservation have become an attractive approach to be considered. Some native wild plants and fruits derived have been recently screened for the presence of probiotic LAB [37]. Preliminary investigation reveled the presence of LAB showing probiotic potential (submitted manuscript). Probiotic bacteria, although not a new concept, draw the attention of the scientific community for their highly potential to act as natural food preservative. However, in this study, we present the results on the antimicrobial activity of ten LAB strains to select those with promising potential in biopreservation. A preliminary characterization of the bacteriocin of selected LAB is also described.

4. Materials and methods

4.1. Bacteria and sampling source of isolation

Sampling material consisting of native fruits and flowers has been collected without no specific ethic permits. The reservation was located on subtropical humid mesothermal region of Santo Domingo de Los Tsachilas Provence at 43 km away from Quito, the capital city. At the location, the GPS points have been recorded and the location map was designed using the ArcGIS software (a complete platform of GIS to create, analyze, store, and disseminate geographic data, models, and maps) in order to track each sample in case of cross-contamination. Approximately ten grams of wild orange, immature and mature berries, guayusa, strawberry, achiote and flower inflorescence (*Heliconia* sp., *Fucsia* sp., *Bromelia* sp.) collected aseptically were transferred in Erlenmeyer flasks (500 ml) containing sterile water (100 ml) and incubated statically for up to 5 days at the room temperature. MRS agar [38] plates were used for the inoculation, the samples were incubated under anaerobic conditions at 37°C for 72 h, and isolated individual colonies were randomly selected and purified by replating on same medium. The purified colonies (>100 colonies/each sample) were Gram stained and tested for the mobility, indole production, catalase production, spore formation, and production of gas from glucose. Cells morphology and colonial characteristics on MRS agar were examined, and based on these results the colonies were preliminary classified as follows: (i) presumptive lactococci, gram positive, coccal morphology, catalase negative, non-motile, and gas production from glucose, and (ii) gram positive, with morphological aspect of rods, catalase negative, non-motile, with and without production of gas from glucose, and presumptive lactobacilli, stored at −80°C in 20% glycerol. Moreover, the API 50CH strips (Biomerieux, Marcy l'Etoile France, cat # 50300) were used for the metabolic characterization of the each isolate and tentatively identified at genus level. Furthermore, the isolates selected for their probiotic performance (bile tolerance, survival under acidic conditions, antibiotic tolerance, and salt tolerance) were analyzed for their antimicrobial activity. As reference strain, *Lactobacillus fermentum* CNCM 1-2998 (API50CH, 80% identity) recuperated from an available commercial probiotic Lacteol Forte (Axcan Pharma, France) has been used.

4.2. Pathogens isolation

Food products consisting of chicken and cheese were purchased from the local market, and standard bacterial culture media were used to screen and isolate the contaminants. However, *Salmonella* sp. and *Escherichia coli* were identified in each food sample. The isolated and purified bacterial cultures were further purified and used as indicator strain.

4.3. Antimicrobial activity of selected isolates

Antimicrobial activity was performed against both *E. coli* and *Salmonella* sp., using agar well diffusion method under anaerobic conditions [1]. The LAB isolates were grown in MRS broth at 37°C for 16 h, and the supernatants were collected by centrifugation at 13000×*g* for 20 min sterilized using 0.22 μm porosity filter. The indicator strains (100 μl) grown in broth medium

(7 log CFU/ml) were mixed with 1.5 ml of soft MRS agar (0.75%), were overlaid on the nutrient agar plates, and incubated at 37°C for 2 h. The cell-free supernatant (100 μl) was spotted onto the wells (7 mm) made on overlaid agar, incubated at 37°C, and subsequently examined for inhibition zones at different intervals of time (18–24–36–48 h). The experiments were run in triplicate, and the mean values of zone of inhibition were estimated. We considered that the isolates had higher inhibitory activity when the diameter of zone of inhibition was higher than >15 mm, intermediary activity when the zone of inhibition was 10–15 mm, and lower activity when the diameter of zone of inhibition was lower than 7 mm.

4.4. The effect of different pH, heat, and detergents on antimicrobial activity

The pH of supernatant was adjusted to 3.0, 4.0, and 7.0 and then kept at room temperature for 4 h. To test heat sensitivity, 100 μl of culture supernatant was heated for 30 min at 30, 45, 60, 75, and 90°C. Residual activity of each isolate for different pHs and temperature was determined by the agar well diffusion method as described above for both indicator strains. The resistant culture supernatants were further heated for 10, 30, and 60 min at 100°C. Another batch of cell-free supernatants treated with 1, 2 and 5% Triton X-100 (BDH Chemicals Ltd, Poole, England) and the same concentration of EDTA (Merck) were incubated for 30 min at 30°C. The activity was measured using agar well diffusion method [1].

4.5. Effect of chloroform on antimicrobial activity

To test the effect of chloroform on inhibitory activity, the culture supernatant of each sample was mixed with an equal volume of chloroform and kept at room temperature for 4 h before antimicrobial activity testing.

4.6. Statistical analysis

Statistical analysis was carried out by one-way analysis of variance, the means were separated by Tukey post-hoc test, and the results were considered statistically significant at the $p < 0.05$ level (SPSS version 10.0.6, USA).

5. Results and discussions

5.1. Screening of LAB isolates

Regardless of numerous probiotic strains presented in the market, there is an ongoing need for the improvement of LAB strains to be used as starter cultures or to develop new natural method for biopreservation; thus, LAB isolated from their natural environment (e.g., native fruits, flowers) might possess unusual characteristics including phenotypic differences and intraspecific variability compared to the known ones. In this investigation, we assumed that acid-tolerant bacteria might be detected as the fermentation of raw material reached at about pH 3.5. **Figure 1** shows the distribution of biological material used as source of initial screening of LAB.

However, preliminary phenotypic analysis suggested the relatedness of the bacterial isolates from wild-type fruits and mature inflorescence of several tropical flowers (>100 colonies/sample) with LAB, which were affiliated to two larger groups: *Lactococcus* (54%) and *Lactobacilli* (46%) genera. Furthermore, carbohydrate profiles conducted on ten randomly selected isolates related to each type of biological material (sample of origin) assigned the selected isolates as follows: UTNFa38, UTNFa40, and UTNFa41 were identified as *Lactococcus lactis* ssp. *lactis*, with identity of 90–99%, the isolate UTNFa37, as *Lactobacillus collinoides* (99%), UTNFa39, as *Lactobacillus brevis* 3 with 98% identity, while UTNFa19 and UTNFa23 were identified as *Lactobacillus paracasei* ssp. *paracasei* 1 with 99.7 and 98.2%, respectively. The isolates UTNFa33 and UTNFa17.2 were identified as *Lactobacillus paracasei* ssp. *paracasei* 3 with 99.6 and 97.9% identity, and UTNFa8.2 was identified as *Lactobacillus pentosus* with 98.3%. **Table 1** presents the classification of isolates on the basis of morphological, physiological and metabolic properties. Similar to our study, numerous lactobacilli species (i.e., *L. paracasei, L. pentosus)* were identified in different fruits and vegetables [39].

Strain code	Cell form/cellular arrangement	Specie assignation	% of identity based on API 50 CHL
UTNFa19	Coccus/single	*Lactobacillus paracasei* ssp. *paracasei 1*	99.70
UTNFa38	Bacilli/rods/single	*Lactococcus lactis* ssp. *lactis*	98.00
UTNFa17.2	Bacilli/rods/single	*Lactobacillus paracasei* ssp. *paracasei 3*	97.90
UTNFa23	Bacilli/rods/single	*Lactobacillus paracasei* ssp. *paracasei 1*	98.20
UTNFa8.2	Bacilli/rods/single	*Lactobacillus pentosus*	98.30
UTNFa33	Bacilli/rods/single	*Lactobacillus paracasei* ssp. *paracasei 1*	99.60
UTNFa39	Bacilli/rods/single	*Lactobacillus brevis 3*	98.00
UTNFa40	Coccus/single	*Lactococcus lactis* ssp. *lactis*	90.00
UTNFa41	Coccus/single	*Lactococcus lactis* ssp. *lactis*	99.00
UTNFa37	Bacilli/rods/single	*Lactobacillus collinoides*	99.00

Table 1. Classification of LAB isolates.

The antimicrobial activity of the selected strains was evaluated against two Selected foodborn pathogens using agar-well assay. The zone of inhibition was easily visualized, and the mean value of the inhibition zone was determined. The cell-free supernatants were considered as crude bacteriocin. Among tested isolates, most of them showed elevated inhibitory activity for both pathogen tested. Nonetheless, results from enzyme inactivation analysis demonstrated that antimicrobial activity was lost or unstable after treatment with proteolytic enzymes such proteinase K and trypsin, whereas catalase treatment did not affect the activity of antimicrobial substance produced by the tested isolates, confirming its protein status. The sensitivity of the found substance to proteolytic enzymes is a proof of its proteinaceous nature, which allows considering as bacteriocin.

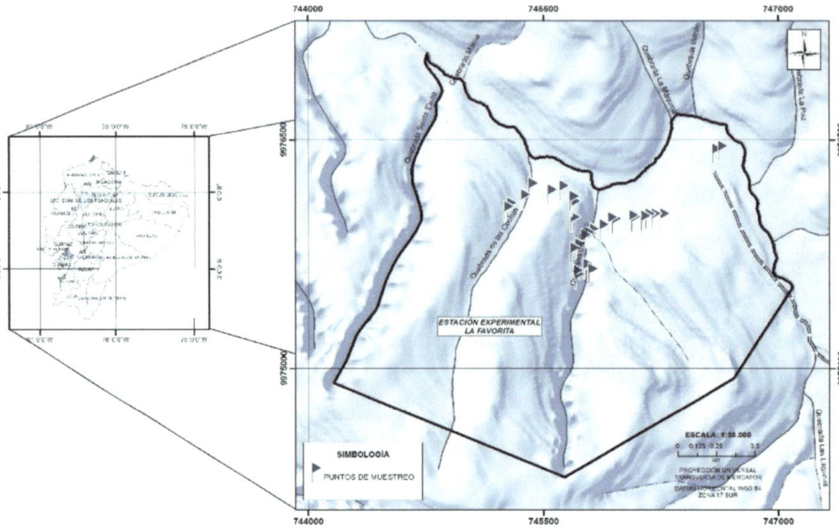

Figure 1. Origin of sampling (geographical distribution according with ArcGIS software).

5.2. Effect of pH on inhibitory activity

The antimicrobial effect exerted by LAB strains is related to the production of lactic acid, reduction of pH, and inhibitory compounds [39], has attracted much attention, and attributed as important selection criteria of a probiotic microorganism [2, 33]. An elevated antimicrobial activity against both food pathogens was observed at the pH 3.0 with the mean range value of inhibition zone 15.25 mm (±0.5) of the supernatant of tested isolates. In **Figure 2A**, we showed the mean value of inhibition zone displayed by each isolate at different pH towards *Salmonella* sp. Although at the pH 4.0 no significant difference between the mean values of inhibition zone was recorded, the mean range of inhibition zone was 13.58 mm (±1.24) for *E. coli* and 12.09 mm (±2.04) for *Salmonella* sp., after 48 h of incubation. With the increase of the pH, we observed a gradually reduction of the antimicrobial activity as no activity was recorded at the pH 7.0 for all selected isolates as well as the reference probiotic. **Figure 2B** showed the clear inhibition zone of two isolates UTNFa40 and UTNFa41 at the pH 3.0 and 4.0, and no zone formation at pH 7.0.

Overall all selected isolates, in particular two isolates, UTNFa40 and UTNFa41, displayed elevated inhibitory activity in comparison with the reference strain. Of course, the efficiency and the nature of this antimicrobial activity have to be investigated. Recent studies showed the importance of bacteriocin produced by the *Lactobacillus pentosus* ST712BZ strain isolated from boza in the preservation of beverage products [3]. In other investigation, *L. pentosus*, a bile-resistant strain, displayed bacteriocin activity against a wide range of spoilage and pathogen bacteria [32]. In agreement with the studies, we showed that the isolate UTNFa8.2

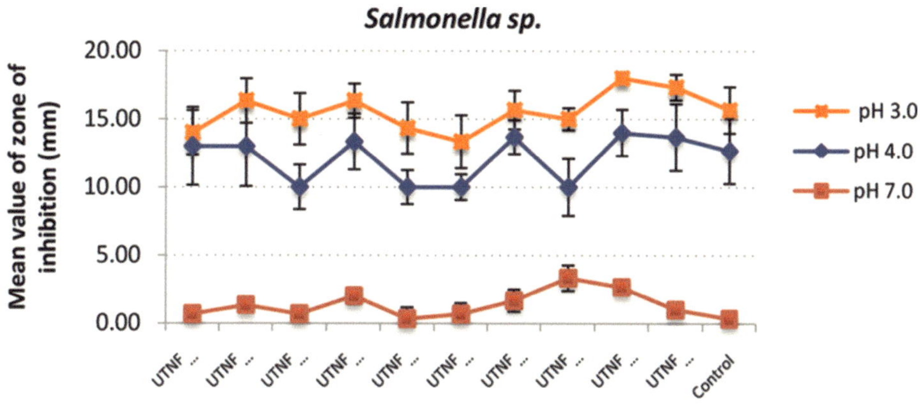

A.

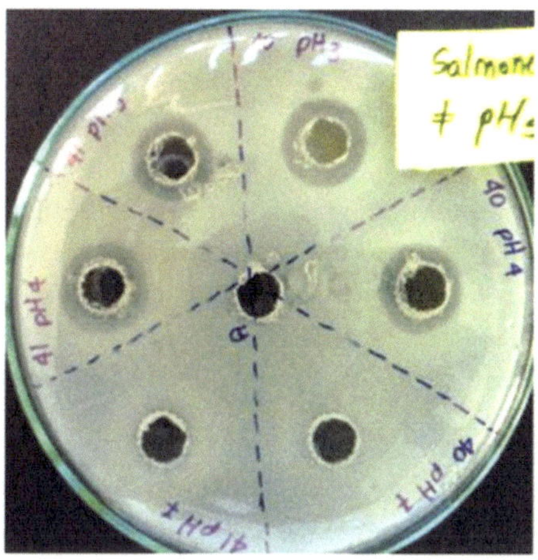

B.

Figure 2. Antimicrobial activity towards *Salmonella* sp. (A) Mean value of zone of inhibition in mm recorded at tested pHs (bars represent the means ± SD). (B) The visualized clear zone of inhibition at pH 3.0, 4.0, and 7.0 of UTNFa41 and UTNFa40.

assigned as *L. pentosus*, a bile, and acid-resistant strain displayed elevated antimicrobial activity, which will further allow us to explore its biotechnological properties.

5.3. Effect of the heat, detergents, and chloroform on inhibitory activity

The inhibitory activity was not significantly reduced in case of the heat treatment. The mean value of zone on inhibition varied at the incubation temperature of 30°C from 19 mm (±2.34) towards *Salmonella* sp. and, respectively, from 20.18 mm (±3.72) towards *E. coli*. At the 60°C, it varies from 16.33 mm (±2.92) towards *Salmonella* sp. and from 17.5 mm (±3.17) towards *E. coli*, and at the 75°C it varies from 14.83 mm (±3.05) towards *Salmonella* and from 15.5 mm (±3.27) in case of *E. coli*. The increase of temperature of 90°C showed a reduction of the inhibition zone was observed for both pathogens. **Figure 3** shows the mean values of the inhibition zone recorded after 30-min incubation at different temperature. At 100°C, after 30 min of incubation, two isolates were resistant and maintain its inhibitory activity.

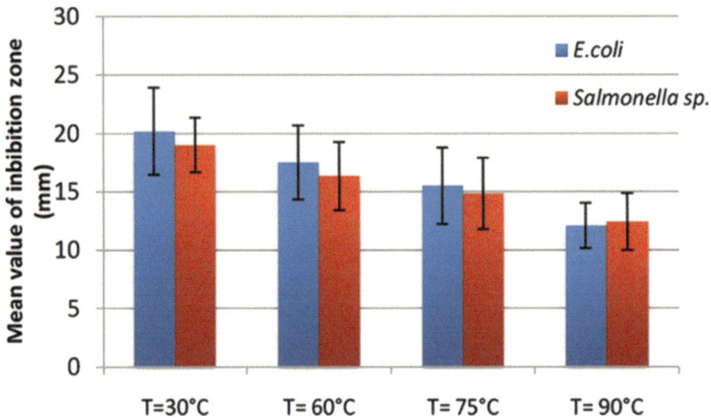

Figure 3. Mean values of zone of inhibition at different temperature of cell-free supernatant towards *E. coli* and *Salmonella* sp. (bars represent the means ± SD).

The heat stability could be an advantage when the strains are intended to be used as biopreservative of processed foods. Similarly, Todorov and col., showed that some bacteriocins remain stable after incubation at 100°C for 120 min [34]. In other study, bacteriocin-like substance of *Lactobacillus fermentum* KN02 was strongly influenced by the pH and temperature. The strain has the maximum productivity at the pH 2.0 and was resistant to heat at 100°C [40].

Due to their resistance to temperature and low pH, the bacteriocins would be digested by human and animal peptidases, thus avoiding resistance and problems associated with the presence of residues in feed and food [35]. However, at the treatment of the selected cell-free supernatants with Triton-X 100 and EDTA, an increase in the inhibitory activity was recorded. An increase with 5% of both Triton-X 100 and EDTA results in an increase of inhibitory activity for some of the isolates. For example, **Figure 4** shows the mean values of the zone of inhibition recorded towards *E. coli* and *Salmonella* sp. after the treatment with 1, 2 and 5% Triton-X 100 for each strain tested. Similar studies showed that the heat does not have any effect on cell-free supernatants activity as well as no effect on the inhibitory activity of the bacteriocins of *Lactobacillus sakei* isolated from the fermented meat was observed after the treatment with several detergents including EDTA and Triton-X 100 [35].

On the contrary, in our study, we observed an increase in the concentration of either EDTA or Triton-X 100, and the inhibitory activity was elevated for most of the isolates. **Figure 5A** shows the inhibitory activity towards *Salmonella* sp. by the appearance of the clear zone after treatment of cell-free supernatant with different concentration of EDTA. In **Figure 5B**, the effect of EDTA on antimicrobial activity towards *Salmonella* is shown. We observed an increase in the inhibitory activity with the increase of the concentration of EDTA. However, a positive effect of detergents in the antimicrobial activity of each isolate has been detected.

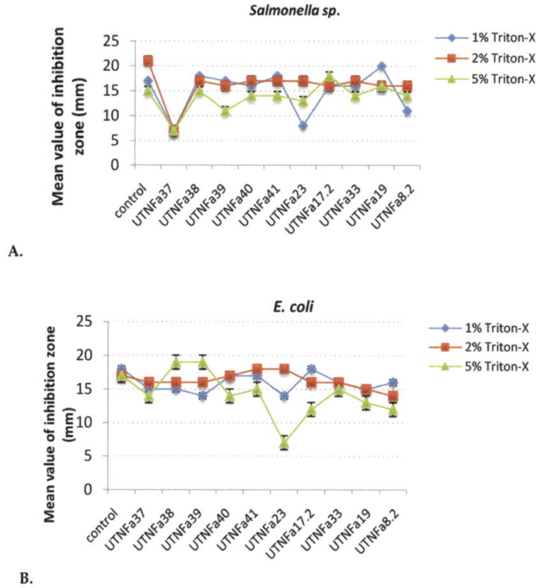

Figure 4. The inhibition activity of the isolated strains towards *Salmonella* sp. (A) and *E. coli* (B) after the treatment with Triton-X 100.

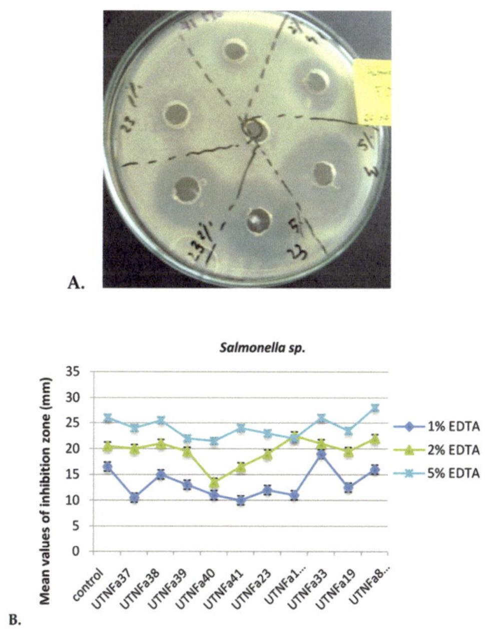

Figure 5. (A) The appearance of the clear inhibition zone at different concentration of EDTA of isolates UTNFa23 and UTNFa41 towards *Salmonella* sp. (B). The antimicrobial activity recorded as mean value of inhibition zone of LAB after the treatment with 1, 2, 5% EDTA towards *Salmonella* sp.

The antimicrobial activity of most of the isolates was lost in case of chloroform treatment of the cell-free supernatants. Among analyzed strains, the isolate UTNFa38 and isolate UTNFa41 remained active towards *E. coli* as well as *Salmonella* sp., after the treatment with chloroform. The mean value of inhibition zone was 10 mm for UTNFa38 and respectively, 11 mm for UTNFa41 towards *E. coli,* while the mean value of inhibition zone was 9 mm for UTNFa38 and 12 mm for UTNFa41, towards *Salmonella* sp. The resistance to chloroform treatment and boiling demonstrates the nature of *low-molecular, non-lipid-containing bacteriocins*. Eight isolates were identified as lipid-containing bacteriocins because of their sensitivity to chloroform. Similar studies showed the broad spectrum of inhibitory activity of *Lactobacillus paracasei* subsp. *paracasei* isolated from natural homemade cheese [41]. Besides several *Lactobacillus* strains from different species, the bacteriocin from *L. paracasei* ssp. *paracasei* also inhibits the growth of various pathogenic bacteria such as *Streptococcus, Staphylococcus, Shigella, Listeria,* and *Pseudomonas*.

The stability of crude cell supernatant of each selected LAB to different conditions reflects that these compounds would remain effective in the processing of foods [42]. Recent investigation showed the broad spectrum of inhibitory activity towards *Pseudomonas* of some bacilli isolated from onion and fresh-cut salads [43]. In other work, it has been demonstrated the antimicrobial activity against spoilage pathogens of some LAB isolated from mango pulp [44]. The six isolated strains had inhibitory effects on sensitive bacteria including *E. coli,* demonstrating the potential of usage of this compound as a preservative in mango or fruit pulp industry. In similar work, several LAB isolated from foods and spoilage halotolerant bacteria isolated from charqui, a Brazilian fermented, salted meat product. The bacteriocin of *Lactococcus lactis* subsp. *lactis* (*L. lactis* 69) inhibited, *in vitro, Listeria monocytogenes, S. aureus* [45]. In our study, the resulted data revealed a wide spectrum of inhibitory activity against two food pathogens of some LAB isolated from natural microbiota of Ecuador, and shall further characterize and determine its molecular size and mode of action, as well as its effectiveness as a biopreservative in different food products as such or in combination with other methods.

6. Conclusions

Bacteriocins produced by genera *Lactobacillus* or other genera have been reported. Nevertheless, the studies in the field of natural food biopreservation are conducted to an increasing extent. As consumers are more concern about the food quality along with their refusal of chemical additives, there is a growing demand for alternative antimicrobial treatments and bioactive compounds such as bacteriocins from lactic acid bacteria are well-accepted natural means of selective microbial inhibition.

However, characterization of specific microbiota would further contribute substantially to gain better knowledge for the improvement of current commercial probiotic strains. The studies conducted up to date indicate that interest on bacteriocins will be high. Thus, all the studies carried out on novel bacteriocins are important to propose new alternatives in food preservation.

http://dx.doi.org/10.5772/63112

Acknowledgements

The Technical University of the North, Ibarra Republic of Ecuador research Grant No. 01388, financed the work. GNT was sponsored by the Prometeo Project of the Secretary for Higher Education, Science, Technology and Innovation (SENESCYT). The authors would like to thank Dr. Miguel Naranjo Toro for his technical support.

Author details

Gabriela N. Tenea* and Lucia Yépez

*Address all correspondence to: gntenea@utn.edu.ec; gtenea@hotmail.com

Faculty of Engineering in Agricultural and Environmental Sciences, Technical University of the North, Av. 17 de Julio s-21 y José María Córdova. Ibarra, Barrio El Olivo, Ecuador

References

[1] Ehrmann MA, Kurzak P, Bauer J, Vogel RF. Characterization of lactobacilli towards their use as probiotic adjuncts in poultry. J Appl Microbiol. 2002;92:966–975. doi: 10.1046/j.1365-2672.2002.01608.x.

[2] Tesfaye A. Antagonism and primary in vitro probiotic evaluation of lactic acid bacteria (LAB) recovered from ergo. ARPN J Agric Biol Sci. 2014;9(7):240–245. ISSN 1990-6145.

[3] Todorov SD, Dicks LMT. Bacteriocin production by *Lactobacillus pentosus* St712bz isolated from boza. Braz J Microbiol. 2007;38:166–172. ISSN 1517-8283.

[4] Hernandez D, Cardell E, Zarate V. Antimicrobial activity of lactic acid bacteria isolated from Tenerife cheese: initial characterization of plantaricin TF711, a bacteriocin-like substance produced by *Lactobacillus plantarum* TF711. J Appl Microbiol 2005;99:77–84. doi:10.1111/j.1365-2672.2005.02576.x.

[5] Todorov SD, Vaz-Velho M, Gambossy de Melo Franco BD, Holzapfel WH. Partial characterization of a bacteriocins produced by three strains of *Lactobacillus sakei* isolated from salpicao, a fermented meat product from North-West of Portugal. Food Control. 2013;30:111–121. doi:10.1016/j.foodcont.2012.07.022.

[6] Enan G, Al-Mohammadi AR, El-Didamony G, Mahmoud EF, Haliem A, Zakaria A. Antimicrobial activity of *Enterococcus faecium* NM2 Isolated from Urine: purification, characterization and bactericidal action of enterocin NM2. Asian J Appl Sci. 2014;7:621–634. doi:10.3923/ajaps.2014.621.634.

[7] Longdet IY, Kutdhik RJ, Nwoyeocha IG. The probiotic efficacy of *Lactobacillus casei* from human breast milk against Shigellosis in Albino rats. Adv Biotechnol Chem Proc. 2011;1:12–16. doi:10.5772/2825.

[8] Mirnejad R, Vahdati AR, Erfani M, Piranfar V. The antimicrobial effect of *Lactobacillus casei* culture supernatant against multiple drug resistant clinical isolates of *Shigella sonnei* and *Shigella flexneri* in vitro. Iran Red Crescent Med J. 2013;15(2):122–126. doi: 10.5812/ircmj.7454.

[9] Soumya TV, Reshma J, Surya J. Characterization of bacteriocin produced by *Lactobacillus* sp and optimization of cultural conditions. IJSRP. 2012;2(12). ISSN 2250-3153.

[10] Deegana LH, Cottera PD, Hilla C, Ross P. Bacteriocins: biological tools for biopreservation and shelf-life extension. Int Dairy J. 2006;16:1058–1071. doi:10.1016/j.idairyj.2005.10.026.

[11] Murua A, Todorov SD, Vieira ADS, Martinez RCR, Cenci, A, Franco BDGM. Isolation and identification of bacteriocinogenic strain of *Lactobacillus plantarum* with potential beneficial properties from donkey milk. J Appl Microbiol. 2013;14:17931809. doi: 10.1111/jam.12190.

[12] Gürakan GC. Biopreservation by lactic acid bacteria. In Metabolism and Applications of Lactic acid bacteria. Editor: Barbaros Ozer. Published by Research Signpost, India. 2007:15–31. ISBN: 978-81-308-0203-9.

[13] Klaenhammer TR. Bacteriocins of lactic acid bacteria. Biochimie. 1988;70:337–349. doi: 10.1016/0300-9084(88)90206-4.

[14] Matsusaki H, Endo N, Sonomoto K, Ishizaki A. Lantibiotic nisin Z fermentative production by *Lactococcus lactis* IO-1: relationship between production of the lantibiotic and lactate and cell growth. Appl Microbiol Biotechnol. 1996;45:36–40. doi:10.1007/s002530050645.

[15] Sawa N, Wilaipun P, Kinoshita S, Zendo T, Leelawatcharamas V, Nakayama J, Sonomoto K. Isolation and characterization of enterocin W, a novel two-peptide lantibiotic produced by *Enterococcus faecalis* NKR-4-1. Appl Environ Microbiol. 2012;78:900–903. doi:10.1128/AEM.06497-11.

[16] Sashihara T, Kimura H, Higuchi T, Adachi A, Matsusaki H, Sonomoto K, Ishizaki A. A novel lantibiotic, nukacin ISK-1, of *Staphylococcus warneri* ISK-1: cloning of the structural gene and identification of the structure. Biosci Biotechnol Biochem. 2000;64:2420–2428. doi:10.1271/bbb.64.2420.

[17] Himeno K, Fujita K, Zendo T, Wilaipun P, Ishibashi N, Masuda Y, Yoneyama F, Leelawatcharamas V, Nakayama J, Sonomoto K. Identification of enterocin NKR-5-3C, a novel class IIa bacteriocin produced by a multiple bacteriocin producer, *Enterococcus faecium* NKR-5-3. Biosci Biotechnol Biochem. 2012;76:1245–1247. doi:10.1271/bbb.120089.

[18] Ishibashi N, Himeno K, Fujita K, Masuda Y, Perez RH, Zendo T, Wilaipun P, Leelawatcharamas V, Nakayama J, Sonomoto K. Purification and characterization of multiple bacteriocins and an inducing peptide produced by Enterococcus faecium NKR-5-3 from Thai fermented fish. Biosci Biotechnol Biochem. 2012;76:947–953. doi: 10.1271/bbb.110972.

[19] Zendo T, Eungruttanagorn N, Fujioka S, Tashiro Y, Nomura K, Sera Y, Kobayashi G, Nakayama J, Ishizaki A, Sonomoto K. Identification and production of a bacteriocin from *Enterococcus mundtii* QU2 isolated from soybean. J Appl Microbiol. 2005;99:1181–1190. doi:10.1111/j.1365-2672.2005.02704.x.

[20] Fujita K, Ichimasa S, Zendo T, Koga S, Yoneyama F, Nakayama J, Sonomoto K. Structural analysis and characterization of lacticin Q, a novel bacteriocin belonging to a new family of unmodified bacteriocins of Gram-positive bacteria. Appl Environ Microbiol. 2007;73:2871–2877. doi:10.1128/AEM.02286-06.

[21] Iwatani S, Zendo T, Yoneyama F, Nakayama J, Sonomoto K. Characterization and structure analysis of a novel bacteriocin, lacticin Z, produced by *Lactococcus lactis* QU 14. Biosci Biotechnol Biochem. 2007;71:1984–1992. doi:10.1271/bbb.70169.

[22] Masuda Y, Zendo T, Sawa N, Perez RH, Nakayama J, Sonomoto K. Characterization and identification of weissellicin Y and weissellicin M, novel bacteriocins produced by *Weissella hellenica* QU 13. J Appl Microbiol. 2012;112:99–108. doi:10.1111/j.1365-2672.2011.05180.x.

[23] Perez RH, Zendo T, Sonomoto K. Novel bacteriocins from lactic acid bacteria (LAB): various structures and applications, Perez et al. Microb Cell Factories. 2014;13(Suppl 1):S3.

[24] Parada JL, Caron Ricoy C, Bianchi P, Medeiros A, Soccol CR. Bacteriocins from lactic acid bacteria: purification, properties and use as biopreservatives. Braz Arch Biol Technol. 2007;50(3):521–542. ISSN 1516-8913.

[25] Oscariz JC, Pisabarro AG. Classification and mode of action of membrane-active bacteriocins produced by gram-positive bacteria. Int Microbiol. 2001;4:13–19. doi: 10.1007/s101230100003.

[26] Abee T. Pore-forming bacteriocins of gram-positive bacteria and self-protection mechanisms of producer organisms. FEMS Microbiol Lett. 1995;129:1–10. doi: 10.1111/j.1574-6968.1995.tb07548.x.

[27] Abee T, Krockel L, Hill C. Bacteriocins: mode of actions and potentials in food preservation and control of food poisoning. Int J Food Microbiol. 1995;28:169–185. doi: 10.1016/0168-1605(95)00055-0.

[28] Ennahar S, Sashihara T, Sonomoto K, Ishizaki A. Class IIa bacteriocins: biosynthesis, structure and activity. FEMS Microbiol Rev. 2001;24:85–106. doi:10.1111/j.1574-6976.2000.tb00534.x.

[29] Adak GK, Long SM, O'Brian SJ. Trends in indigenous foodborne disease and deaths, England and Wales. Gut. 2002;51:832–841. doi:10.1136/gut.51.6.832.

[30] Choi HJ, Cheigh CI, Kim SB, Pyun YR. Production of a nisin-like bacteriocin by *Lactococcus lactis* subsp. lactis A164 isolated from Kimchi. J Appl Microbiol. 2000;88:563–571. doi:10.1046/j.1365-2672.2000.00976.x.

[31] Danielsen M, Wind A. Susceptibility of *Lactobacillus* spp. to antimicrobial agents. Int J Food Microbiol. 2003;82:1–1. doi:10.1016/S0168-1605(02)00254-4.

[32] Enan G, Al-Mohammadi AR, El-Didamony G, Mahmoud EF, Haliem A, Zakaria A. Antimicrobial activity of *Enterococcus faecium* NM2 Isolated from Urine: purification, characterization and bactericidal action of enterocin NM2. Asian J Appl Sci. 2014;7:621–634. doi:10.3923/ajaps.2014.621.634.

[33] Longdet IY, Kutdhik RJ, Nwoyeocha IG. The probiotic efficacy of *Lactobacillus casei* from human breast milk against Shigellosis in Albino rats. Adv Biotechnol Chem Proc. 2011;1:12–16.

[34] Nes IF, Johnsborg O. Exploration of antimicrobial potential of LAB by genomics. Curr Opin Biotechnol. 2004;15(2):100–4. doi:10.1016/j.copbio.2004.02.001.

[35] Todorov SD, Rachman C, Fourrier A, Dicks LMT, van Reenen CA, Prevost, H, et al. Characterization of a bacteriocins produced by *Lactobacillus sakei* R1333 isolated from smoked salmon. Anaerobe. 2011;17(1):23–31. doi:10.1016/j.anaerobe.2010.01.004.

[36] Todorov SD, Vaz-Velho M, Gambossy de Melo, Franco BD, Holzapfel WH. Partial characterization of a bacteriocin produced by three strains of *Lactobacillus sakei* isolated from salpicao, a fermented meat product from North-West of Portugal. Food Control. 2013;30:111–121. doi:10.1016/j.foodcont.2012.07.022.

[37] Yepez L, Tenea GN. Genetic diversity of lactic acid bacteria strains towards their potential probiotic application. Rom Biotechnol Lett. 2015;20(2):10191–10199. ISSN 2248-3942.

[38] De Man JC, Rogosa M, Sharpe E. A medium for the cultivation of lactobacilli. J Appl Bacteriol. 1960;23:130–155. doi:10.1111/j.1365-2672.1960.tb00188.x.

[39] Maldonado-Barragan A, Caballero-Guerrero B, Lucena-Padros H, Ruiz-Barba JL. Genome sequence of Lactobacillus pentosus IG1, a strain isolated from Spanish-style green olive fermentations. J Bacteriol. 2011;193(19):5605. doi:10.1128/JB.05736-11.

[40] Nithya K, Senbagam D, Senthilkumar B, Udhayashree N, Gurusamy R. Characterization of bacteriocin-producing lactic acid bacteria and its application as a food preservative. Afr J Microbiol Res. 2012;6 (6):1138–1146. doi:10.5897/AJMR11.1214.

[41] Tolinački M, Kojić M, Lozo J, Terzić-Vidojević A, Topisirović L, Fira D. Characterization of the bacteriocin-producing strain *Lactobacillus paracasei* subsp. paracasei Bgub9. Arch Biol Sci Belgrade. 2010;62(4):889–899. doi:10.2298/ABS1004889T.

[42] Osmanagaoglu O. Detection and characterization of Leucocin OZ, a new anti-listerial bacteriocin produced by *Leuconostoc carnosum* with a broad spectrum of activity. Food Control. 2007;18:118–123. doi:10.1016/j.foodcont.2005.08.015.

[43] Sharpe VD. Biopreservation of fresh-cut salads using bacteriocinogenic lactic acid bacteria isolated from commercial produce. Dalhousie University, Halifax, NS, Canada, Master thesis. 2009.

[44] Ravi V, Prabhu M, Subramanyam D. Isolation of bacteriocin producing bacteria from mango pulp and its antimicrobial activity. J Microbiol Biotechnol Res. 2011;1(2):54–63. http://scholarsresearchlibrary.com/archive.html.

[45] Biscola V, Todorov SD, Capuano VSC, Abriouel H, Gálvez A, Franco BDGM. Isolation and characterization of a nisin-like bacteriocin produced by a *Lactococcus lactis* strain isolated from charqui, a Brazilian fermented, salted and dried meat product. Meat Sci. 2013;93:607–613.

Chapter 9

Fructosyltransferase Sources, Production, and Applications for Prebiotics Production

Mariela R. Michel, Rosa M. Rodríguez-Jasso,
Cristóbal N. Aguilar, Silvia M. Gonzalez-Herrera,
Adriana C. Flores- Gallegos and
Raúl Rodríguez-Herrera

Additional information is available at the end of the chapter

http://dx.doi.org/10.5772/62827

Abstract

Fructooligosaccharides (FOS) are considered prebiotic compounds and are found in different vegetables and fruits but at low concentrations. FOS are produced by enzymatic transformation of sucrose using fructosyltransferase (FTase). Development of new production methods and search for FTase with high activity and stability for FOS production Is an actual research topic. In this article is discussed the most recent advances on FTase and its applications. Different microorganisms have been tested under various fermentation systems in order to identify and characterize new genes codifying for FTase. Some of these genes have been isolated from bacteria, fungi, and plants, with a wide range of percentages of identity but retaining the eight highly conserved motifs of the hydrolase family 32 glycoside. Therefore, this article presents an overview of the most recent advances on FTase and its applications.

Keywords: Enzyme production, Fructooliogosacarides, Fructosyltransferase, 1-kestose, 1-nystose, 1-β-fructofuranosyl nystose

1. Introduction

At the present time, there is a growing consumer demand for healthier and calorie-controlled foods. For this reason, food industry has developed different alternatives for sweeteners, and among them is the fructooligosaccharides (FOS). Use of these compounds offers multiple health advantages. FOS are fructose oligomers with a terminal glucosyl unit and a general formula of GFn; where typical values of *n* are 2–4 and are composed of sugars units such as 1-kestose, 1-nystose, and 1- β -fructofuranosyl nystose, which can be found in different fruits and vegetables, but in very low concentrations to exert a beneficial effect on health. In addition, its production is limited by seasonal conditions [1]. FOS cannot be hydrolyzed by the gastrointestinal enzymes and are recognized as prebiotic which selectively stimulate growth and/or activity of bifidobacteria and lactobacilli, microorganisms that promote benefits to human health [2, 3].

FOS can be produced by the action of different types of enzymes with transfructosylation activity (i.e., fructosyltransferase—FTase [EC 2.4.1.9] and/or β-fructofuranosidase—FFases [EC 3.2.1.26]). These enzymes are obtained from different plants and microorganisms [4]. The reaction mechanism of FTase depends on enzyme source [5]. Most of these enzymes have been isolated from different fungal strains such as: *Aureobasidium* spp., *Aspergillus* spp., *Penicillium* spp., and *Fusarium* spp. [6]. However, different FTases from bacterial (*Bacillus macerans, Lactobacillus reuteri,* and *Zymomonas mobilis*) species have been also reported [7].

2. FTase: an overview

FOS can be synthesized in nature by the catalytic action of enzymes with transfructosylating activity. They are classified as 1^F-FTases (E.C. 2.4.1.9, E.C. 2.4.1. 99, and E.C. 2.4.1.100), or β -FFases (, E.C. 3.2.1.26). FTase catalyzes the transfer of a fructosyl group to a molecule of sucrose or a FOS when a FOS with a chain longer by one fructosyl unit is formed [8]. This enzyme also mediates polymerization reactions, where degree of polymerization (DP) decreases to the maximum by transferring fructosyl units from higher molecular mass fructans [9]. The reaction mechanism of the FTases depends on the enzyme source. In plants and some microorganisms, a series of enzymes act together, whereas a single enzyme works in most of the microorganisms [10].

The FTase that converts sucrose to the shortest β (2–1) linked fructan 1-kestose is called sucrose: sucrose 1-FTase (1-SST) [11]. It is reported that, FTase differs in molecular weight and properties depending on its origin [12]. Properties of FTases can change according to the microorganism and culture medium composition, especially the carbon source, which can play a role as an inductor [1]. FTase can be produced intra- and/or extracellular by different microorganisms, including bacteria and fungi. Despite the large number of microbial FTase producers, only some of them have the potential for industrial application and have been used in several studies about FOS production [1]. The transfructosylating activity is responsible for FOS production from sucrose, although quantitative differences exist because of the microbial strains [13].

FTase has been produced using both solid and liquid fermentation, and FOS obtained by these fermentations have been reported. Factors affecting FOS by fermentation were mentioned, such as temperature, pH, and substrate concentration [14, 15]. FTase has a temperature optimum between 50 and 60°C, and the optimal pH is between 4.5 and 6.5 [1, 8].

http://dx.doi.org/10.5772/62827

2.1. Mechanism of action

The reaction mechanism depends on the enzyme source and purity. The accepted mechanism is a type disproportionate reaction where FTase catalyzes the transfer of a fructosyl moiety of a sucrose or fructooligosacharide donor to another sucrose or FOS acceptor to provide a superior FOS [1]. The reaction mechanism has been expressed as follows:

$$GFn + GF_n GF_{n+1} GF_{n-1} n = 1 - 3$$

where GF is sucrose or FOS n is the number of fructosyl units.

3. Microbial and plant FTases

Several fungal strains, especially those from *Aspergillus* genus, are known to produce extracellular or intracellular FTase. The microbial FTase (Ftase; E.C. 2.4.1.9) catalyses formation of FOS from sucrose; FTases obtained from microorganisms are single enzymes with both transferase and hydrolase activities [12]. Some of the fungi reported as FTase producers are the following: *Aspergillus niger* ATCC 20611 [13], *A. niger* strain AN 166 [16], *Aspergillus foetidus* [17], *Aspergillus oryzae* CFR 202 [15, 18–20], *Aureobasidium pullulans* CFR 77 [18], *A. oryzae* KB [21], and *Aspergillus awamori* GHRTS [22]. Some of these fungal strains have the capacity to produce two types of FTases (Table 1). The enzymatic activity is different because it depends on carbon source and type of microorganism. The FFase with a high transfructosylating activity has been studied extensively in *A. niger* because this fungal specie is used for industrial production of FOS. *A. niger* AS0023 produces two types of FFases, and one of the enzymes has high transfructosylating activity [24].

Source	FTase Activity	Temperature	Reference
Aspergillus niger YZ59	Recombinant Ftase 1020 U/ml	55°C	[23]
Aspergillus awamori GHRTS	6120 U/gds	30°C	[22]
Aspergillus oryzae CFR 202	16.5 U/ml/min	30°C	[19]
Aspergillus niger	107.87 U/mL	30°C	[16]

Table 1. Microbial FTases produced by filamentous fungi, its activity, and fermentation temperature of the maximum enzyme activity reached.

Bacterial strains have been reported to produce different inulinases, but reports on enzymes able to produce FOS are scarce from bacterial strains. Someone bacteria mentioned to produce these enzymes are the following: *B. macerans, L. reuteri,* and *Z. mobilis* [7].

The FTases obtained from plants have other amino acid composition that is different from microbial FTases such as sucrose: sucrose 1-FTase (1-SST) and fructan: fructan 1-FTase (1-FFT).

Plants such as *Cichorium intybus* and *Helianthus tuberosus* produce high levels of FTases such as 1-SST, (EC. 2.4.1.99) [10]. In 1995, Ftase were isolated and purified from barley (*Hordeum vulgare*) [25].

4. Structure of FTase

According to the Protein Data Bank (PDB) of Research Collaborators for Structural Bioinformatics (RCSB) data base, the crystal dimensional structure of FTase from *Aspergillus japonicus* comprises 632 residues that fold into two domains, with a N-terminal five-blade-propeller (residues 21–468), and a C-terminal sandwich domain (480–653), which are linked by a 9-residue short-helix (469–479) [26].

5. FTases properties

5.1. Factors affecting FTase activity

Fructosyltransferase (FTase) participates on FOS/fructan production by catalyzing the transfer of a fructose unit from one sucrose/fructan to another [26]. This enzyme has been included in the glycoside hydrolase family 32 (GH32) and has been isolated from different sources, and the optimal conditions for the enzyme activity have been reported (Table 2). The optimal temperature reported for FTase enzyme activity ranges from 52 to 65°C, while the optimal pH varies widely from 4.5 to 8.0 [27, 28]. There are different reports mentioned about the chemical reagents and amino acids that positively affect FTase activity [29, 30]. On the other hand, there is a controversy in the use of detergents—some authors mention that these compounds enhance FTase activity [29], and in contrast there are others who mention that these compounds negatively affect FTase activity [27].

Source	Temperature	pH	Positive effect	Observation	References
Aspergillus sp.	52 °C	4.5	FeSO4, Fe2+, Fe2+ Ca2+	Intra- and extracellular	[27]
Marine *Aspergillus niger*	65°C	8.0		Intracellular	[28]
Aspergillus aculeatus	60°C	5.0–7.0	Dithiothreitol, 2-mercaptoethanol, sodium dodecylsulphate, Tween 80		[29]
Penicillium purpurogenum	55 °C	5.5	Leucine induced slightly extracellular production	Intra- and extracellular	[30, 31]

Table 2. Optimal conditions for FTase activity from different microbial sources.

5.2. Carbon and nitrogen sources

Different reports mentioned that the preferred carbon source to produce FTase is sucrose. Patil and Butle [31] indicated that *Syncephalastrum recemosum Cohn* preferred sucrose to produce FTase. Similarly, Dhake and Patil [30] employing *Penicillium purpurogenum* found that the best carbon source for FTase production was sucrose. The complete hydrolysis of this carbohydrate was reported by Kumar *et al.* [28] who used a marine *A. niger* strain to degrade sucrose, and the product consisted entirely of D-fructose, although different products from sucrose hydrolysis have been reported depending on the FTase enzyme origin. A recombinant FTase from timothy (*Phleum pratense* L.) and expressed in *Pichia pastoris* produced linear β (2, 6)-linked levans from sucrose [32]. While recombinant FTase from *L. reuteri* for sucrose hydrolysis was used, large amounts of FOS with _(231)-linked fructosyl units, plus a high-molecular-weight fructan polymer (>107) with _-(231) linkages (an inulin) were found [33]. Amount of sucrose in the fermentation reactor may alter the final product. Ghazi *et al.* [29] found that FTase from *A. aculeatus* at elevated sucrose concentrations showed a high transferase/hydrolase ratio. The *k*cat and *K*m values for transfructosylating and hydrolytic activities vary. Ghazi *et al.* [29] modified sucrose using a microbial FTase and found transfructosylating activity of 1.62 ± 0.09 × 104 s − 1 for *k*cat and 0.53 ± 0.05 M for *K*m, whereas for hydrolytic activity, the *k*cat and *K*m values were 775 ± 25 s − 1 and 27 ± 3 mM, respectively. On the other hand, the best nitrogen source to produce FTase by *S. recemosum Cohn* is ammonium nitrate [31].

5.3. FTase biochemical properties

Biochemical properties of FTase may change depending on its origin. Ghazi *et al.* [29] reported a dimeric glycoprotein with 20% of carbohydrate content and a molecular mass of around 135 kDa from *A. aculeatus.* In contrast, a FTase from *A. foetidus* was found as extensively glycosylated, with a probable active form of a dimer of identical subunits and an apparent mass of 180 kDa [34]. On the other hand, a FTase which catalyze formation and extension of P-2, 6-linked fructans in barley (*H. vulgare* L.) was mentioned to occur in two closely similar isoforms having both of them two subunits with masses of 49 and 23 kDa [25].

Chuankhayan *et al.* [26] sequenced a recombinant FTase from *Aspergillus japonica.* In this case, they found that this enzyme comprises two domains with an N-terminal catalytic domain containing a five-blade-propeller-fold linked to a C-terminal-sandwich domain. In addition, the same authors reported four substrate-binding subsites (1–3) in the catalytic pocket with shapes and characters distinct from those of clan GH-J enzymes; in this step, they used different FTase mutants. The residue Asp-60 was proposed for nucleophile, Asp-191 for transition-state stabilizer, and Glu-292 for general acid/base catalyst, which govern the binding of the terminal fructose at the 1 subsite and the catalytic reaction. Although to define the 1 subsite for FTase preference of fructosyl and glucosyl, moieties are needed, the residues Ile-143, Arg-190, Glu-292, Glu-318, and His-332 combine the hydrophobic Phe-118 and Tyr-369. On the one hand, to define the _2 subsite for raffinose, Ile-143 and Gln-327 are required, on the other hand, Tyr-404 and Glu-405 are needed to define the 2 and 3 subsites for inulin-type substrates with higher structural flexibilities.

6. FTases gene organization

Genome sequence of different microorganisms and vegetables has allowed identification of some enzymes, development of new products, improvement of strains, and increase of process efficiency. There are some reports of isolation and cloning of the FTase gene. The genes coding for FTase have been isolated from bacteria, fungi, and plants, with a wide range of percentages of identity but retaining the eight highly conserved motifs of hydrolyses family 32 glycoside [35]. Fungal FTase genes have been isolated mainly from *Aspergillus* strains (Table 3), although there are reports about Ftase genes from other fungal genera [37].

Source	Enzyme	Bp	Intron	Size	Molecular weight	Amino acids	References
Aspergillus oryzae N74	FTase	1620	172–224		57 kDa	525	[35]
Aspergillus foetidus	FTase			1.6 kb	59.1 kDa	537	[34]
Aspergillus niger	FTase			1.9 kb	76 kDa		[36]

Table 3. Characteristics of different FTase genes and its enzyme.

The gene that encodes *A. oryzae* N74 FTase accounts for a 525 amino acids protein of 57 kDa, with a signal peptide of 17 amino acids. Alignment of genomic and mRNA sequence from *A. oryzae* N74 strain showed the presence of a 52 bp intron located between 172 and 224 bp [35]. Other authors mentioned that the FTasa was partially purified using a three-step procedure involving anion exchange chromatography, hydrophobic interaction, and ultrafiltration. The *A. sydowi* IAM 2544 FTase gene was expressed in conidia; the gene encodes a protein with a calculated molecular mass of 75 kDa and comprises 682 amino acids [38]. Genes of *Aspergillus* FTases are more homogeneous with a size ranging from 1.6 kb to 2 kb and coding for enzymes about 500–600 amino acids long.

7. Fructooligosaccharides

FOS is a common name for fructose oligomers and corresponds to complex carbohydrates which are nondigestible oligosaccharide food ingredients and are fermentable by the gut microbiota. For this reason, they can be classified as prebiotics, and its commercial production has increased in response to a growing consumer demand for the so-called "health foods" [16, 39]. FOS are mainly composed of 1-kestose (GF2), 1-nystose (GF3), and 1- β-fructofuranosyl nystose (GF4), in which 1–3 fructosyl units (F) are bound at the β (2–1) status of sucrose molecule (GF) (Figure 1) [4].

http://dx.doi.org/10.5772/62827

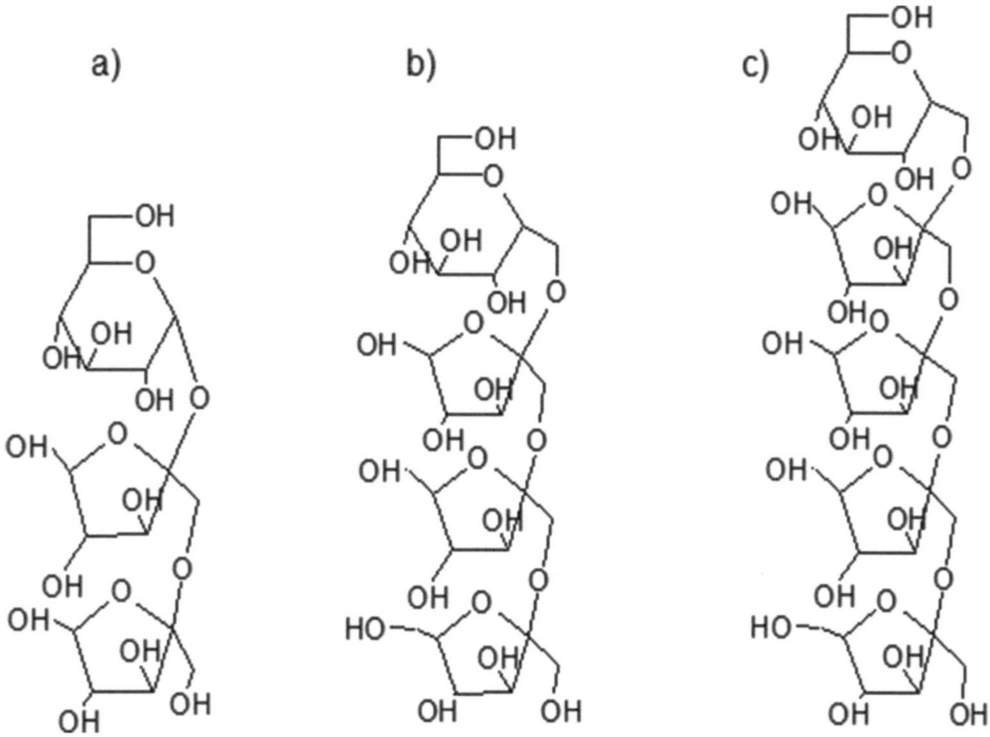

Figure 1. Chemical structures of the most common FOS, where (a) 1-kestose, (b) 1- nystose, and (c) 1-β fructofuranosyl nystose.

FOS can be found in several vegetal sources such as tomato, onion, barley, garlic, Jerusalem artichoke, banana, rye, honey, sugar beet, to name a few; however, FOS concentration in these sources is low, and mass production are limited by seasonal conditions [3, 4]. At the industrial level, FOS are mainly produced from the disaccharide sucrose by action of different microbial enzymes with transfructosylating activity such as FTase (EC 2.4.1.9) and/or β-fructofuranosidase (EC 3.2.1.26), [4]. Moreover, FOS compounds have received a generally recognized as safe status (GRAS) from the Food and Drug Administration (FDA) and has been consumed because of the several benefits of FOS to human health such as calorie-free and noncariogenic sweeteners, stimulate bifidobacteria growth, and activation of the immune system; have been claimed to contribute to the prevention of colon cancer and reduce the levels of serum cholesterol, phospholipids, and triglycerides; also promote calcium and magnesium absorption in animals and the human gut [14, 19, 22, 40, 41].

Dominguez *et al.* [7] reported that FOS have low sweetness intensity as they are only about one-third as sweet as sucrose, they supply small quantities of power, about 0–3 kcal/g sugar substitute. Other authors mentioned that FOS are about 0.4–0.6 times sweeter than sucrose and are considered as noncariogenic since no compounds are produced when polyglucanes are passing through the mouth [37]. These last properties are very useful in types of foods in which sucrose use is limited because of its high sweetness [7].

7.1. FOS production

Production of FOS has received particular attention in recent years, so there is necessity for the development of new enzymatic systems [42]. FOS represent one of the major classes of bifidogenic oligosaccharides in terms of production volume. Kestose and nystose are the main prebiotic compounds, which can be principally produced by hydrolysis of inulin or by transfructosylation of sucrose [24]. The enzymes that are potentially useful for high production of FOS were reported about three decades ago. Hidaka *et al.* [13] reported an *A. niger* enzyme with transfructosylating activity which reached a maximum FOS conversion of 55–60% (w/w) based on total sugars, and this enzyme was successively used for industrial production of FOS. Almost at the same time, McCleary *et al.* [43] investigated the other *A. niger* enzyme with transfructosylating activity, which could compete with other enzymes for industrial production of FOS because of its considerably high activity. Chien *et al.* [39] mentioned a FOS production process using *A. japonicus* enzymes, while Antosova *et al.* [44] reported a FOS production process using enzymes from *A. pullulans* CCY 27-1-1194.

8. Use of FTAse for FOS production

FOS have demonstrated important properties for improving human health, thus they have attracted an increased interest mainly as ingredients for food applications. They contribute to 10% of the natural sweeteners, and their demand has risen rapidly (about 15% per year) in the last 15 years [45]. Consequently, establishing sustainable and economically viable industrial process for the production of FOS with high yields and productivities is strongly desirable [46]. These can be manufactured by three methods: (1) extraction from inulin-rich plant materials, (2) by enzymatic synthesis from sucrose, and (3) by enzymatic degradation of inulin [45, 47]. Most of the FOS marketed as food ingredients/nutritional supplements are synthesized either from sucrose by the action of FTases [48, 49] or by enzymatic degradation of inulin [50, 51]. In this section, we will discuss the production of FOS through FTase.

Commercial production of FOS was first developed using enzymatic fructosyl transfer on sucrose by Hidaka *et al.* [52], and since then, β-fructofuranosidase has been isolated especially from fungi: *A. niger* [13, 53], *A. japonicus* [54, 55], *A. oryzae* [21, 56], *A. pullulans* [57, 58], and *Fusarium oxysporum* [59].

Nowadays, to reduce cost, enzyme immobilization techniques have been applied. Fungal β-fructofuranosidase has been covalently immobilized onto inorganic supports such as porous glass or porous silica [54, 60]. *Aspergillus* FTase was immobilized in methacrylamide-based polymeric beads and various linocellulosic materials to produce FOS from sucrose [55]. Ganaie *et al.* [49] evaluated immobilization of *Aspergillus flavus* FTase with sodium alginate and chitosan forming gel bead for continuous production of FOS, showing that recycling efficiency of alginate beads was more successful as compared to chitosan beads. In addition, formation of FOS by FTase entrapped alginate beads was higher than by chitosan beads in 36 h of enzyme-substrate reaction according to HPLC analysis (66.75 and 42.79%, respectively).

However, it has been observed that enzymes immobilized on a porous support decrease apparently its enzymatic activity because of diffusion resistance. Instead, the use of magnetic nanoparticles is proposed, which offers (a) a higher specific surface area that permits binding of a larger amount of enzyme, (b) relatively low mass transfer resistance and (c) selective separation from a reaction mixture by application of a magnetic field [61, 62]. Chen *et al.* [63] evaluated that β-fructofuranosidase from *A. japonicus* was immobilized in Fe_3O_4-CS nanoparticles, retaining up to 88% of its activity. The recovery of enzyme activity was inversely proportional to enzyme concentration. The main oligosaccharide products were 1-kestose and nystose. After 10 days, it was observed that the consumption of sucrose appear to have stopped because of the accumulation of glucose, which inhibited transfructosylating reactions [64]. The immobilized enzyme can easily be recovered by applying a magnetic field and reused it for FOS production.

Another alternative for FOS production is the use of solid-state fermentation (SSF). Most investigations on FOS production are based on submerged fermentation systems, but SSF is attractive because of low capital cost and low demand of water, generating less wastewater as a consequence. Besides, higher productivities and yields could be obtained at industrial scale [14]. Mussatto *et al.* [46] evaluated the economic and environmental impact of three different fermentation processes for FOS production: (1) submerged fermentation of sucrose solution by *A. japonicus* using free cells (FCF) or (2) using immobilized cells in corn cobs (ICF), and (3) SSF using coffee silver-skin as support material and nutrient source (SSF). In this study, an annual productivity goal of 200 t was established. Based on parameters such as productivity, product concentrations, yields, and thermo-physical data, SSF was the most attractive process with higher annual productivity of FOS (232.6 t) and purity (98.6%) against 148.9 t and 96.6% for FCF and 158.3 t and 98.4% for ICF. The SSF also produced greater amounts of the shorter chain FOS (GF2 and GF3), which have more prebiotic activity and stronger sweetness [65]. Although, the three processes are economically feasible, SSF has the highest potential to be implemented on an industrial scale not only because of productivity and purity but also because of the lowest payback time, wastewater generation, carbon footprint, and highest annual profit.

9. Properties of FOS

General structure of FOS can be depicted as GFn, where "*n*" is the number of fructosyl units (F) that are bound by β (2→1) position of sucrose with the last one attached to a terminal glucose (G) [51]. FOS produced from sucrose have lower DP (DP◎4) than those from inulin (DP > 9) [47]. This is relevant because DP plays an important role in the gut fermentation of FOS. The short-chain FOSs are fermented by the bacteria present in the proximal colon, while the long-chain FOS are fermented in distal colon [66]. Structurally, FOSs produced from sucrose are kestose (GF2), nystose (GF3), and 1-β-fructofuranosyl nystose (GF4).

FOSs contain several qualities that make its usage possible as an alternative sweetener in the food market. They are water soluble and one-third as sweet as sucrose [67]. However, their viscosity and thermal stability is higher than sucrose. They are stable in a pH range from 4.0 to 7.0 and can be refrigerated for a period of one year. Their high moisture-retaining capacity provides prevention of excessive drying besides controlling microbial contamination owing their low water interacting activity [68].

They can be considered as noncariogenic sugar substitutes in confectionary, gums, and drinks since they cannot serve as a substrate of *Streptococcus mutans, Lactobacillus acidophilus,* and other bacteria to form insoluble β-glucans implicated in plaque formation, which causes dental cavities [69]. As FOSs possess β-configuration in anomeric carbon, C_2 in the fructose monomers, they are nondigestible by human digestive enzymes which are mostly specific for α-glycosidic bonds and therefore, are not utilized as energy source in the body [70]. Consequently, they are safe for consumption by diabetics [65, 71, 72].

10. FOS as prebiotic

The most widely used definition for prebiotic is "nondigestible food ingredient that beneficially affects host's health by selectively stimulating the growth and/or activity of one or a limited number of bacteria in the colon" [73]. In 2004, the definition was updated, and it was defined as "selectively fermented ingredients that allow specific changes, both in the composition and/or activity in the gastrointestinal microbiota that confers benefits upon host well-being and health" [74]. According to this, prebiotics are a major part of the functional foods and among them, the FOS are in focus due to their functional properties and economical potential [65, 75].

A prebiotic must fulfill three criteria: (1) no hydrolysis or absorption in the upper part of the digestive system, (2) selective substrate for one or more desired bacteria species in the colon and stimulation of that species regarding growth and activation and (3) able to positively influence the numeric proportion of different bacteria species in the colon [76]. FOS selectively stimulates the growth of *Bifidobacteria* and *Lactobacillus* sp. in the colon, and these bacteria show commensalism association in the host body. These colon-specific anaerobic bacterial groups degrade FOS producing short-chain fatty acids (SCFA) such as acetate (C2), propionate (C3), and butyrate (C4), decreasing colon pH and subsequently enhancing the absorption of mineral ions (Ca^{2+} and Mg^{2+}) and nutrients in the host body [77, 78].

Many Bifidobacteria and *Lactobacillus* sp. are resistant to acidic pH, but it is harmful to those antagonist bacteria in colon like *Clostridium* sp. [79]. Furthermore, compared with other anaerobes in the gastrointestinal tract, lactobacilli and bifidobacteria have enzymes with lower activities, such as β-glucosidase, β-glucuronidase, urease, azoreductase, and nitrate reductase, which are involved in the formation of mutagens and carcinogens [80].

Antiinflammatory and antitumorigenic roles of SCFA have been reported [81, 82]. As a result of the prebiotic function, a decrease in inflammatory markers such as phagocytosis and interleukin (IL)-6 production by increasing CD^{3+}, CD^{4+}, and CD^{8+} populations has been observed [83]. In case of antitumorigenic roles, especially in the context of colon cancer, the action mechanism is yet unclear [80]. However, it is known that butyrate has an important role on DNA methylation thus modifying gene expression so it may directly enhance cell proliferation of normal cells, but suppress cell proliferation of transformed cells. Furthermore, in the presence of butyrate, apoptosis may be enhanced in transformed cells but inhibited in normal cells [84]. Thus, the regular intake of FOS as a part of diet could help to improve health and over all well-being by providing resistance against the intestinal/extra intestinal pathogens, enhancing the growth of the colon microbiota which have metabolic activities and biochemical processes with a tremendous influence in human host [85].

11. Applications of FOS

FOS are components of functional food that are becoming popular in the society because they have a potential for enhancing flavor quality and physicochemical properties of food products, besides FOS offer various benefits for human health and are also of industrial interest [34]. FOS are used in different food applications and other areas because of its positive impact on human health, physical performance, or state of mind [12], and the most relevant uses in food formulations are the following: beverages (fruit drinks, coffee, cocoa, tea, soda, health drinks, and alcoholic beverages), dairy products (fermented milk, instant powders, powdered milk, and ice cream), also in light jam products and confectionary [86].

12. Functional foods

The growing interest of consumers in the relationship between nutrition and health has increased demand among the population for food products that improve or benefit their health beyond basic nutrition [87, 88]. Because of this demand, both the academic community and the food industry have focused on developing products that meet these characteristics, which are now called functional foods.

The term "functional foods" was first coined in Japan after a group of scientists and nutritionists conducted numerous studies and defined them as "Food for specified health uses" (FoSHU) [89]. Though there is a great number of definitions, Doyon and Labrecque [90] identified four key concepts after reviewing more than 20 definitions: (a) health benefits, (b) the nature of the food, (c) level of function, and (d) consumption pattern. The definition of functional food has evolved, and the latest is that proposed by the European Commission for concerted action Functional Food Science in Europe (FUFOSE) that mentions that "a food can be regarded as 'functional' if it is satisfactorily demonstrated to beneficially effect one or more target functions in the body, beyond adequate nutritional effects, in a way that is relevant to either an improved state of health and well-being and/or reduction of risk of disease. Functional foods must remain as food and they must demonstrate their effects in amounts that can normally be expected to be consumed in the diet: they are not pills or capsules, but part of a normal food pattern" [91, 92].

The challenges for the food industry are great so that the biological value of the functional ingredient is not disturbed and sensory characteristics of the food are acceptable [93]. According to various investigations, the success and acceptance of these foods is influenced by factors such as clarity and understanding of the information about nutrition and health benefits that are provided to consumers, especially in elderly consumers [87].

Experts recognize that there are scientific evidence on the effectiveness of various functional foods, which can be useful to balance a poor diet or assist in avoiding health problems in some cases [94]. In general, the consumers' attitude towards functional foods is positive and have great potential in the food industry.

13. Applications of FOS in food formulations

FOS are ingredients that have been applied in a variety of food matrices, their prebiotic potential has been proven, and its technological properties allow easy incorporation into foods, mainly those that are probiotics [95]. The FOS have comparable glucose syrups and sugar properties and proved approximately a 30–50% sweetness compared with sugar table. Therefore, their application has a dual benefit: (1) as a substitute for sugar and (2) for their prebiotic properties [96].

Akalin and Erisir [97] evaluated the effect of supplementation of oligofructose or inulin in symbiotic ice cream, in the rheological properties and probiotics survival. They found that the survival rate of the probiotics during storage at 30, 40, and 90 days was better with oligofructose. The FOS were evaluated in cookies and Quicks bread and found that consumers had preference equal to or greater for products supplemented with FOS [96, 98]. Although the FOS are easy to incorporate into foods such as yogurt, processing conditions such as acidity and temperature should be considered since they have reported low prebiotic activities under acidic conditions and high thermal processing times [95].

New applications in different food matrices are being evaluated. Valencia *et al.* [99] supplemented a creamy milk chocolate dessert with FOS and probiotics. They found positive results in the consumer acceptability test and in the survival probiotics. Moreover, in a cooked ham, FOS as substitutes of dextrose were added; the appearance of the ham did not change and the addition of FOS in ham transformed it into a healthier product [100].

There is an innovative trend in the FOS application in different types of food and, undoubtedly, to maximize the benefits that can confer the FOS, factors as type of food matrix, processing conditions, and added amount should be considered.

14. Future trends

Because of the importance of this enzyme in the modern industry, it is important to relate a set of FTases from different organisms to allow the identification of features that could be used for the identification and classification of new FTases, and also it is necessary to improve the

http://dx.doi.org/10.5772/62827

conditions and costs of FTases production process. Further studies of gene sequencing will allow distinguishing among the set of FTase and β FFase enzymes.

15. Conclusions

The studies on production and application of FOS are of high interest for food industry because of several health benefits and biofunctional properties that these compounds provide. FOS can be synthesizing from precursors such as sucrose using FTase enzymes. These enzymes can be obtained from different microorganisms (bacteria and fungi) and plants. The main disadvantage of this production is the low yields of enzymatic activity and FOS. Thus, search for new microbial sources of FTase enzymes is a very important research topic as well as studies about the evolution of FTase genes from different sources, and relate their function with the nucleotide sequence using functional genomics studies.

Acknowledgements

This project was financially supported by the Universidad Autónoma de Coahuila. MRMM would like to thank the financial support received from CONACYT during her master's degree.

Author details

Mariela R. Michel[1], Rosa M. Rodríguez-Jasso[1], Cristóbal N. Aguilar[1], Silvia M. Gonzalez-Herrera[2], Adriana C. Flores- Gallegos[1] and Raúl Rodríguez-Herrera[1*]

*Address all correspondence to: raul.rodriguez@uadec.edu.mx

1 Department of Food Research, Autonomous University of Coahuila, Saltillo, Mexico.

2 Division of Postgraduate Studies, Durango Institute of Technology, Durango, Mexico

References

[1] Maiorano A. E., Piccoli R. M., Da Silva E. S., De Andrade Rodrigues M. F. Microbial production of fructosyltransferases for synthesis of prebiotics. *Biotechnology Letters.* 2008; 30:1867–1877. DOI:10.1007/s10529-008-9793-3.

[2] Antošová M., Illeová V., Vandáková M., Družkovská A., Polakovič M. Chromatographic separation and kinetic properties of fructosyltransferase from *Aureobasidium pullulans*. *Journal of Biotechnology*, 2008; 135:58–63. DOI:10.1016/j.jbiotec.2008.02.016.

[3] Mussatto S. I., Prata M. B., Rodrigues L. R., Teixeira J. A. Production of fructooligosaccharides and β-fructofuranosidase by batch and repeated batch fermentation with immobilized cells of Penicillium expansum. *European Food Research and Technology*. 2012; 235:13–22. DOI:10.1007/s00217-012-1728-5.

[4] Mussatto S. I., Aguilar C. N., Rodrigues L. R., Teixeira J. A. Colonization of *Aspergillus japonicus* on synthetic materials and application to the production of fructooligosaccharides. *Carbohydrate Research*. 2009; 344:795–800. DOI:10.1016/j.carres.2009.01.025.

[5] Sánchez O. F., Rodriguez A. M., Silva E., Caicedo L. A. Sucrose biotransformation to fructooligosaccharides by *Aspergillus* sp. N74 Free Cells. *Food and Bioprocess Technology*. 2008; 3:662–673. DOI:10.1007/s11947-008-0121-7.

[6] Dominguez A., Nobre C., Rodrigues L. R., Peres A. M., Torres D., Rocha I., Teixeira J. New improved method for fructooligosaccharides production by *Aureobasidium pullulans*. *Carbohydrate Polymers*. 2012; 89:1174–1179. DOI:10.1016/j.carbpol.2012.03.091.

[7] Dominguez A. L., Rodrigues L. R., Lima N. M., Teixeira J. A. An overview of the recent developments on fructooligosaccharide production and applications. *Food and Bioprocess Technology*. 2013; 7:324–337. DOI:10.1007/s11947-013-1221-6.

[8] Antošová M., Polakovič M. Fructosyltransferases: the enzymes catalyzing production of fructooligosaccharides. *Chemical Papers*. 2001; 55:350–358.

[9] Koops A. J., Jonker H. H. Purification and Characterization of the enzymes of fructan biosynthesis in tubers of *Helianthus Fuberbsus* Colombia. *Plant Physiology*. 1996; 110:1167–1175.

[10] Edelman J., Jefford T. G. The mechanisim of fructosan metabolism in higher plants as exemplified in *Helianthus tuberosus*. *New Phytologist*.1968;67:517–531. DOI:10.1111/j.1469-8137.1968.tb05480.x.

[11] Altenbach D., Rudiño-Pinera E., Olvera C., Boller T., Wiemken A., Ritsema T. An acceptor-substrate binding site determining glycosyl transfer emerges from mutant analysis of a plant vacuolar invertase and a fructosyltransferase. *Plant Molecular Biology*. 2009; 69:47–56. DOI:10.1007/s11103-008-9404-7.

[12] Sangeetha P. T., Ramesh M. N., Prapulla S. G. Recent trends in the microbial production, analysis and application of Fructooligosaccharides. *Trends in Food Science and Technology*. 2005; 16:442–457. DOI:10.1016/j.tifs.2005.05.003

[13] Hidaka H., Hirayama M., Sumi N. A Fructooligosaccharide-producing enzyme from. *Agricultural and Biological Chemistry*. 1988; 52:1181–1187.

[14] Mussatto S. I., Teixeira J. A. Increase in the fructooligosaccharides yield and productivity by solid-state fermentation with *Aspergillus japonicus* using agro-industrial residues as support and nutrient source. *Biochemical Engineering Journal*. 2010; 53:154–157. DOI:10.1016/j.bej.2010.09.012

[15] Sangeetha P. T., Ramesh M. N., Prapulla S. G. Production of fructosyl transferase by *Aspergillus oryzae* CFR 202 in solid-state fermentation using agricultural by-products. *Applied Microbiology and Biotechnology*. 2004; 65:530–537. DOI:10.1007/s00253-004-1618-2

[16] La Rotta C. E., Ospina S. A., López-Munguía A. Production and characterization of crude enzimatic extracts with fructosyl transferase activity. *Revista Colombiana de Ciencias Químico-Farmacéuticas*. 1998; 27:53–56 (in Spanish).

[17] Wang X. D., Rakshit S. K. Improved extracellular transferase enzyme production by *Aspergillus foetidus* for synthesis of isooligosaccharides. *Bioprocess Engineering*. 1999; 20: 429–434.

[18] Sangeetha P. T., Ramesh M. N., Prapulla S. G. Production of fructo-oligosaccharides by fructosyl transferase from *Aspergillus oryzae* CFR 202 and *Aureobasidium pullulans* CFR 77. *Process Biochemistry*. 2004; 39:755–760. DOI:10.1016/S0032-9592(03)00186-9

[19] Sangeetha P. T., Ramesh M. N., Prapulla S. G. Fructooligosaccharide production using fructosyl transferase obtained from recycling culture of *Aspergillus oryzae* CFR 202. *Process Biochemistry*. 2005; 40:1085–1088. DOI:10.1016/j.procbio.2004.03.009

[20] Sangeetha P. T., Ramesh M. N., Prapulla S. G. Maximization of fructooligosaccharide production by two stage continuous process and its scale up. *Journal of Food Engineering*. 2005; 68:57–64. DOI:10.1016/j.jfoodeng.2004.05.022.

[21] MasahiroKurakake, OgawaKenji, SugieMotoki, A. T., Kouji Sugiura, T. Komaki. Two types of fructofuranosidases from *Aspergillus oryzae* KB. *Journal of Agricultural and Food Chemistry*. 2008; 56:591–596.

[22] Sathish T., Prakasham R. S. Intensification of fructosyltransferases and fructo-oligosaccharides production in solid state fermentation by *Aspergillus awamori* GHRTS. *Indian Journal of Microbiology*. 2013; 53:337–342. DOI:10.1007/s12088-013-0380-5.

[23] Yang H., Wang Y., Zhang L., Shen W. Heterologous expression and enzymatic characterization of fructosyltransferase from *Aspergillus niger* in *Pichia pastoris*. *New Biotechnology*. 2015; 00:1–7. DOI:10.1016/j.nbt.2015.04.005.

[24] Yoshikawa J., Amachi S., Shinoyama H., Fujii T. Multiple◎β-fructofuranosidases by *Aureobasidium pullulans* DSM2404 and their roles in fructooligosaccharide production. *FEMS Microbiology Letters*. 2006; 265:159–163. DOI:10.1111/j.1574-6968.2006.00488.x

[25] Sprenger N., Bortlik K., Brandt A., Boller T., Wiemken A. Purification, cloning, and functional expression of sucrose: fructan 6-fructosyltransferase, a key enzyme of fructan synthesis in barley. *Proceedings of the National Academy of Sciences*. 1995; 92:11652–11656.

[26] Chuankhayan P., Hsieh C. Y., Huang Y. C., Hsieh Y. Y., Guan H. H., Hsieh Y. C., Chen C. J. Crystal structures of *Aspergillus japonicus* fructosyltransferase complex with donor/

acceptor substrates reveal complete subsites in the active site for catalysis. *Journal of Biological Chemistry*. 2010; 285:23251–23264. DOI:10.1074/jbc.M110.113027.

[27] ArtheeR., VijilaK. Study on fructosyltransferase enzyme from *Aspergillus* sp. in fructooligosaccharides production. *Research Journal of Recent Sciences*. 2014; 3:147–153.

[28] AmrendraKumar, Vaishnavi .R, Saravanakumar .,A K. S.A. and, Tank S. K. Biotransformation of sucrose by using thermostable and alkaline fructosyltransferase enzyme isolated. *International Journal of Science, Environment*. 2014; 3:708–713.

[29] Ghazi I., Fernandez-Arrojo L., Garcia-Arellano H., Ferrer M., Ballesteros A., Plou F. J. Purification and kinetic characterization of a fructosyltransferase from *Aspergillus aculeatus*. *Journal of Biotechnology*. 2007; 128:204–211. DOI:10.1016/j.jbiotec.2006.09.017.

[30] Dhake,A. B., Patil M. B. Effect of substrate feeding on production of fructosyltransferase by *Penicillium purpurogenum*. *Brazilian Journal of Microbiology*. 2007; 38:194–199. DOI: 10.1590/S1517-83822007000200002.

[31] Patil M. B., ButleA.. Fructosyltransferase production by indigenously isolated *Syncephalastrum racemosum* Cohn. *Journal of Global Biosciences*. 2014; 3:597–603.

[32] Tamura K. I., Kawakami A., Sanada Y., Tase K., Komatsu T., Yoshida M. Cloning and functional analysis of a fructosyltransferase cDNA for synthesis of highly polymerized levans in timothy (*Phleum pratense* L.). *Journal of Experimental Botany*. 2009; 60:893–905. DOI:10.1093/jxb/ern337.

[33] Van Hijum S. a F. T., Van Geel-Schutten G. H., Rahaoui H. Van der Maarel M. J. E. C., Dijkhuizen, L. Characterization of a novel fructosyltransferase from *Lactobacillus reuteri* that synthesizes high-molecular-weight inulin and inulin oligosaccharides. *Applied and Environmental Microbiology*. 2002; 68:4390–4398. DOI:10.1128/AEM.68.9.4390-4398.2002.

[34] Rehm J., Willmitzer L., Heyer A. G. Production of 1-kestose in transgenic yeast expressing a fructosyltransferase from *Aspergillus foetidus*. *Journal of Bacteriology*. 1998; 180:1305–1310.

[35] Rodríguez M. A, Sánchez O. F., Alméciga-Díaz C. J. Gene cloning and enzyme structure modeling of the *Aspergillus oryzae* N74 fructosyltransferase. *Molecular Biology Reports*. 2011; 38:1151–1161. DOI:10.1007/s11033-010-0213-0.

[36] Goosen C., Yuan X.-L., van Munster J. M., Ram A. F. J., van der Maarel M. J. E. C., Dijkhuizen L. Molecular and biochemical characterization of a novel intracellular invertase from *Aspergillus niger* with transfructosylating activity. *Eukaryotic Cell*. 2007; 6: 674–681. DOI:10.1128/EC.00361-06.

[37] Alméciga-Díaz C. J., Gutierrez Á. M., Bahamon I., Rodríguez A., Rodríguez M. A, Sánchez O. F. Computational analysis of the fructosyltransferase enzymes in plants, fungi and bacteria. *Gene*. 2011; 484:26–34. DOI:10.1016/j.gene.2011.05.024.

[38] Heyer A. G., Wendenburg R. Gene cloning and functional characterization by heterologous expression of the fructosyltransferase of *Aspergillus sydowi* IAM 2544. *Applied and Environmental Microbiology*. 2001; 67:363–370. DOI:10.1128/AEM.67.1.363.

[39] Chien C.-S., Lee W.-C., Lin T.-J. Immobilization of *Aspergillus japonicus* by entrapping cells in gluten for production of fructooligosaccharides. *Enzyme and Microbial Technology*. 2001; 29:252–257. DOI:10.1016/S0141-0229(01)00384-2.

[40] Mussatto S. I., Ballesteros L. F., Martins S., Maltos D. A. F., Aguilar C. N., Teixeira J. A. Maximization of fructooligosaccharides and β-fructofuranosidase production by *Aspergillus japonicus* under solid-state fermentation conditions. *Food and Bioprocess Technology*. 2013; 6:2128–2134. DOI:10.1007/s11947-012-0873-y.

[41] Silva J. B. Da, Fai A. E. C., dos Santos R., Basso L. C., Pastore G. M. Parameters evaluation of fructooligosaccharides production by sucrose biotransformation using an osmophilic *Aureobasium pullulans* strain. *Procedia Food Science*. 2011; 1:1547–1552. DOI: 10.1016/j.profoo.2011.09.229.

[42] L'Hocine, L., Wang Z., Jiang B., Xu S. Purification and partial characterization of fructosyltransferase and invertase from *Aspergillus niger* AS0023. *Journal of Biotechnology*. 2000; 81:73–84. DOI:10.1016/S0168-1656(00)00277-7.

[43] McCleary B. V., Gibson T. S., Sheehan H., Casey A., Horgan L., O'Flaherty, J. Purification, properties, and industrial significance of transglucosidase from *Aspergillus niger*. *Carbohydrate Research*. 1989; 185:147–162.

[44] Antosova M., Polakovic M., Slovinská M., Madlová A., Illeová V., Bales V. Effect of sucrose concentration and cultivation time on batch production of fructosyltransferase by *Aureobasidium pullulans* CCY 27-1-1194. *Hemical Papers-Slovak Academy of Sciences*. 2003; 56:394–399.

[45] Panesar P.S., Bali V., Kumari S., Babbar N., Oberoi H.S. Prebiotics. In: G.S. Brar (Ed.), *Biotransformation of Waste Biomass into High Value Biochemicals*. Springer. Ney York, USA, 2014; 504 pp.

[46] Mussatto S. I., Aguiar L. M., Marinha M. I., Jorge R. C., Ferreira E. C. Economic analysis and environmental impact assessment of three different fermentation processes for fructooligosaccharides production. *Bioresource Technology*. 2015; 198:673–681. DOI: 10.1016/j.biortech.2015.09.060.

[47] Rastall R.A. Functional oligosaccharides: application and manufacture. *Annual Review of Food Science and Technology*. 2010; 1:305–339.

[48] Bali V., Panesar P.S., Bera M.B., Panesar R. Fructo-oligosaccharides: production, purification and potential applications. *Critical Reviews in Food Science and Nutrition*. 2015; 55:1475–1490.

[49] Ganaie M. A., Rawat H. K., Wani O. A., Gupta U. S., Kango N. Immobilization of fructosyltransferase by chitosan and alginate for efficient production of fructooligosaccharides. *Process Biochemistry*. 2014; 49:840–844. DOI:10.1016/j.procbio.2014.01.026.

[50] Mutanda T., Mokoena M. P., Olaniran, A. O., Wilhelmi, B. S., Whiteley, C. G. Microbial enzymatic production and applications of short-chain fructooligosaccharides and inulooligosaccharides: Recent advances and current perspectives. *Journal of Industrial Microbiology and Biotechnology*. 2014; 41:893–906. DOI:10.1007/s10295-014-1452-1.

[51] Singh R. S., Singh R. P. Production of fructooligosaccharides from inulin by endoinulinases and their prebiotic potential. *Food Technology and Biotechnology*. 2010; 48: 435–450.

[52] Hidaka,H., Eida,T., Tokunaga,T., Tashiro,Y. Effects of fructooligosaccharides on intestinal flora and human health. *Bifidobacteria and Microflora*. 1986; 5:37–50.

[53] Nguyen,Q.D., Rezessy-Szabo,J.M., Bhat,M.K. Purification and some properties of b-fructofuranosidase from *Aspergillus niger* IMI303386. *Process Biochemistry*. 2005; 40:2461–2466.

[54] Hayashi,S., Matsuzaki,K., Takasaki,Y., Ueno,H., Imada,K. Production of b-fructofuranosidase by *Aspergillus japonicus*. *World Journal of Microbiology and Biotechnology*. 1992; 8:155–159.

[55] Mussatto,S.I., Aguilar,C.N., Rodrigues,L.R., Teixeira,J.A. Fructooligosaccharides and b-fructofuranosidase production by *Aspergillus japonicus* immobilized on lignocellulosic materials. *Journal of Molecular Catalisis B: Enzymatic*. 2009; 59:76–81.

[56] Chang,C.T., Lin,Y.Y., Tang,M.S., Lin,C.F. Purification and properties of betafructofuranosidase from *Aspergillus oryzae* ATCC 76080. *Biochemistry and Molecular Biology International*. 1994; 32:269–277.

[57] Jung,K.H., Lim,J.Y., Yoo,S.J., Lee,J.H., Yoo,M.Y. Production of fructosyltransferase from *Aureobasidium pullulans*. *Biotechnology Letters*. 1987; 9:703–708.

[58] Yoshikawa,J., Amachi,S., Shinoyama,H., Fujii,T. Purification and some properties of b-fructofuranosidase I formed by *Aureobasidium pullulans* DSM 2404. *Journal Bioscience and Bioengineering*. 2007; 103:491–493.

[59] Nishizawa,M., Maruyama,Y., Nakamura,M. Purification and characterization of invertase isozyme from *Fusarium oxysporum*. *Agricultural and Biological Chemistry*. 1980; 44:489–498.

[60] Ortega-Muñoz,M., Morales-Sanfrutos,J., Megia-Fernandez,F., Lopez-Jaramillo,F. J., Hernandez-Mateo,F., Santoyo-Gonzalez,F. Vinyl sulfone functionalized silica: a ready to use pre-activated material for immobilization of biomolecules. *Journal of Materials Chemistry*. 2010; 20:7189–7196.

[61] Halling,P.J., Dunnill,P. Magnetic supports for immobilized enzymes and bioaffinity adsorbents. *Enzyme and Microbial Technology*.1980; 2: 2–10.

[62] Kim,J., Grate,J.W., Wang,P. Nanostructures for enzyme stabilization. *Chemical Engineering Science*. 2006; 61:1017–1026.

[63] Chen S. C., Sheu D. C., Duan K. J. Production of fructooligosaccharides using β-fructofuranosidase immobilized onto chitosan-coated magnetic nanoparticles. *Journal of the Taiwan Institute of Chemical Engineers*. 2014; 45:1105–1110. DOI:10.1016/j.jtice.2013.10.003.

[64] Duan,K. J., Chen,J.S., Sheu,D.C. Kinetic studies and mathematical model for enzymatic production of fructooligosaccharides from sucrose. *Enzyme and Microbial Technology*. 1994; 16:334–339.

[65] Yun J. W. Fructooligosaccharides—occurrence, preparation, and application. *Enzyme and Microbial Technology*. 1996; 19:107–117. DOI:10.1016/0141-0229(95)00188-3.

[66] Meyer D., Stasse-Wolthuis M. The bifidogenic effect of inulin and oligofructose and its consequences for gut health. *European Journal of Clinical Nutrition*, 63:1277–1289. DOI: 10.1038/ejcn.2009.64.

[67] Salinas M. A., Perotti N. A. Production of fructosyltransferase by *Aureobasidium* sp. ATCC 20524 in batch and two-step batch cultures. *Journal of India Industrial Microbiology Biotechnology*. 2009; 36:39–43.

[68] Crittenden R. G., Playne M. J. Production, properties and applications of food-grade oligosaccharides. *Trends in Food Science and Technology*. 1996; 7: 353–361.

[69] Oku T. Special physiological functions of newly developed mono-and oligosaccharides. In: Goldberg (Ed.), *Functional Foods: Designer Foods, Pharmafoods, Nutraceuticals. Chapman &Hall, Ney York, USA*. pp. 202–218.

[70] Kaur N., Gupta A. K. Applications of inulin and oligofructose in health and nutrition. *Journal of Biosciences*. 2002; 27:703–714. DOI:10.1007/BF02708379.

[71] Rycroft C. E., Jones M. R., Gibson G. R., Rastall R. A. A comparative in vitro evaluation of the fermentation properties of prebiotic oligosaccharides. *Journal of Applied Microbiology*. 2001; 91:878–887. DOI:10.1046/j.1365-2672.2001.01446.x.

[72] Villegas B., Costell E. Flow behaviour of inulin-milk beverages. Influence of inulin average chain length and of milk fat content. *International Dairy Journal*. 2007; 17:776–781. DOI:10.1016/j.idairyj.2006.09.007.

[73] Gibson,G. R., Roberfroid,M. B. Dietary modulation of the human colonic microbiota: introducing the concept of prebiotics. *Journal of Nutrition*. 1995; 125:1401–1412.

[74] Gibson G. R., Probert, H. M., Loo, J. Van, Rastall R. A, Roberfroid M. B. Dietary modulation of the human colonic microbiota: updating the concept of prebiotics. *Nutrition Research Reviews*. 2004; 17:259–275. DOI:10.1079/NRR200479.

[75] Flores-Gallegos A. C., Contreras-Esquivel J. C., Morlett-Chavez J. A, Aguilar C. N., Rodriguez-Herrera R. Comparative study of fungal strains for thermostable inulinase production. *Journal of Bioscience and Bioengineering*. 2015; 119:421–426. DOI:10.1016/j.jbiosc.2014.09.020.

[76] Kovács Z., Benjamins E., Grau K., Rehman A.U., Ebrahimi M., and Czermak P. Recent developments in manufacturing oligosaccharides with prebiotic functions. *Advances in Biochemical Engineering Biotechnology*. 2014; 143:257–295.

[77] Scholz-Ahrens K.E., Ade P., Marten B., Weber P., Timm W., Asil Y., Glüer C., Schrezenmeir J. Mint: Prebiotics, probiotics, and synbiotics affect mineral absorption, bone mineral content and bone structure. *Journal Nutrition*. 2007; 137:838S–8346S.

[78] Tazoe H., Otomo Y., Kaji I., Tanaka R., Karaki S.I., Kuwahara A. Roles of short-chain fatty acids receptors, GPR41 and GPR43 on colonic functions. *Journal of Physiology and Pharmacology*. 2008; 59:251–262.

[79] Sangeetha P. T., Ramesh M. N., Prapulla S. G. Microbial production of fructooligosaccharides. *Asian Journal of Microbiology Biotechnology Environmental Sciences*. 2003; 5:313–331.

[80] Pool-Zobel B.L., Neudecker C., Domizlaff I., Ji S., Schillinger U., Rumney C., Moretti M., Vilarini I., Scassellati S.R., Rowland I. *Lactobacillus*- and *Bifidobacterium*-mediated antigenotoxicity in the colon of rats. *Nutrition and Cancer*. 1996; 26:365–380.

[81] Alva-Murillo N., Ochoa-Zarzosa A., Lopez-Meza J.E. Short chain fatty acids (propionic and hexanoic) decrease *Staphylococcus aureus* internalization into bovine mammary epithelial cells and modulate antimicrobial peptide expression. *Veterinary Microbiology*. 2012; 155:324–331.

[82] Tan J., Mckenzie C., Potamitis M., Thorburn A. N., Mackey C. R., Macia L. The role of short-chain fatty acids in health and disease. *Advances in Immunology*. 2014; 121:91–119.

[83] Guigoz Y., Rochat F., Perruisseau-Carrier G., Rochat I., Schiffrin E. J. Effects of oligosaccharide on the faecal flora and non-specific immune system in elderly people. *Nutrition Research*. 2002; 22:13–25. DOI:10.1016/S0271-5317(01)00354-2.

[84] Hass R., Busche R., Luciano L., Reale E., Engelhardt W. Lack of butyrate is associated with induction of bax and subsequent apoptosis in the proximal colon of guinea pig. *Gastroenterology*. 1997; 112:875–881.

[85] Peshev D., den Ende W. V. Fructans: prebiotics and immunomodulators. *Journal of Functional Foods*. 2014; 8:348–357.

[86] Mussatto S. I., Mancilha I. M. Non-digestible oligosaccharides: a review. *Carbohydrate Polymers*. 2007; 68:587–597. DOI:10.1016/j.carbpol.2006.12.011.

[87] Vella M.N.; Stratton L.M.; Sheeshka J.; Duncan A.M. Functional food awareness and perceptions in relation to information sources in older adults. *Nutrition Journal*. 2014; 13:1–25.

[88] Abdel-Salam A.M. Functional food: hopefulness to good health. American *Journal of Food Technology*. 2010; 5:86–99.

[89] Shimizu M. Functional food in Japan: current status and future of gut-modulating food. *Journal of Food and Drug Analysis*. 2012; 20:213–216.

[90] Doyon M.; Labrecque J. A. Functional foods: a conceptual definition. *British Food Journal*. 2008; 110:1133–1149.

[91] Diplock A., Aggett P., Ashwell M., Bornet F., Fern E., Roberfroid M. Scientific concepts of functional foods in Europe: consensus document. *British Journal of Nutrition*. 1999; 9:1–27.

[92] Ozen A. E., Pons A., Tur J. A. Worldwide consumption of functional foods: A systematic review. *Nutrition Reviews*. 2012; 70:472–481.

[93] Spence J. T. Challenges related to the composition of functional foods. *Journal of Food Composition and Analysis*. 2006; 19:S4–S6.

[94] Crowe K. M., Francis C. Position of the academy of nutrition and dietetics: functional foods. *Journal of the Academy of Nutrition and Dietetics*. 2013; 113:1096–1103.

[95] Vega R., Zuniga-Hansen M. E. The effect of processing conditions on the stability of fructooligosaccharides in acidic food products. *Food Chemistry*. 2015; 173:784–789.

[96] Handa C., Goomer S., Siddhu A. Physicochemical properties and sensory evaluation of fructoligosaccharide enriched cookies. *Journal of Food Science And Technology*. 2012; 49:192–199.

[97] Akalın A. S., Erişir D. Effects of inulin and oligofructose on the rheological characteristics and probiotic culture survival in low fat probiotic Ice cream. *Journal of Food Science*. 2008; 73:M184-M188.

[98] Rößle C., Ktenioudaki A., Gallagher E. Inulin and oligofructose as fat and sugar substitutes in quick breads (scones): a mixture design approach. *European Food Research and Technology*. 2011; 233:167–181.

[99] Valencia M.S., Salgado S.M., Andrade S.A.C., Padilha V.M., Livera A.V.S., Stamford T.L.M. Development of creamy milk chocolate dessert added with fructooligosaccharide and *Lactobacillus paracasei* subsp. *Paracasei* LBC 81. LWT—*Food Science and Technology*. 2016; 69:104–109.

[100] Resconi V.C., Keenan D.F., Barahona M., Guerrero L., Kerry J.P., Hamill R.M. Rice starch and fructo-oligosaccharides as substitutes for phosphate and dextrose in whole muscle cooked hams: sensory analysis and consumer preferences. *LWT—Food Science and Technology*. 2016; 66:284–292.

Chapter 10

Antimicrobial Effect of Probiotics against Common Pathogens

Sabina Fijan

Additional information is available at the end of the chapter

http://dx.doi.org/10.5772/63141

Abstract

The antimicrobial or antagonistic activity of probiotics is an important property that includes the production of antimicrobial compounds, competitive exclusion of pathogens, enhancement of the intestinal barrier function and others. There are many methods to ascertain probiotic properties, including various *in vitro* and *in vivo* methods. The *in vivo* methods include various modifications of the spot-on lawn assay, agar well diffusion assay (AWDA), co-culturing methods, usage of cell lines and others. In many cases *in vitro* antagonist activity is observed, but in real settings it is not observed. The *in vivo* methods mainly used are animal models; however, their use is being restricted according to the European legislation OJ L136. The justification of animal models is also questionable as the results of studies on animals do not predict the same results for humans. The use of replacement alternative methods, for example incorporating human cells and tissues, avoids such confounding variables. Most important studies are double-blinded randomized clinical trials; however, these studies are difficult to perform as it is not easy to achieve uniform conditions. There is a clear need for more elaborate assays that would better represent the complex interactions between the probiotics and the final host. This complex situation is a challenge for scientists.

Keywords: antimicrobial effect, *in vitro* methods, *in vivo* methods, pathogens, probiotics

1. Introduction

Throughout the history of microbiology, most human studies have been focused on the disease-causing organisms found on or in people; whilst fewer studies have examined the benefits of the resident bacteria. However, we are surrounded by beneficial microorganisms that live in or on the human body. The intestinal microbiota is very well adapted, exceptionally stable and very specific for each individual. In normal conditions of stable functioning of the digestive system, neutral and beneficial microorganisms dominate. It is estimated that there are 100 trillion microorganisms in the intestine of a human adult and this is 10 times larger than the number of cells in the human body [1, 2]. However, the balance of the intestinal microbiota is negatively influenced by modern lifestyle, leading to increased numbers of pathogenic microorganisms that disrupt microbial balance and cause a reverse from beneficial to harmful functioning. In such cases, the external support with probiotics is very welcome and supported by several scientific studies [3].

According to the Food and Agriculture Organisation of the United Nations (FAO) and the World Health Organisation (WHO), probiotics are defined as live microorganisms, which when administered in adequate amounts confer a health benefit on the host [4, 5]. The most common probiotic bacteria are certain strains from the genera *Lactobacillus* (i.e., *L. rhamnosus, L. acidophilus, L. plantarum, L. casei, L. delbrueckii subsp. Bulgaricus,* etc.) and *Bifidobacterium* (i.e., *B. infantis, B. animalis* subsp. *lactis, B. longum,* etc.). Other probiotic bacteria include *Pediococcus acidilactici, Lactococcus lactis* subsp. *lactis, Leuconostoc mesenteroides, Bacillus subtilis, Enterococcus faecium, Streptococcus thermophilus, Escherichia coli* Nissle 1917, etc. Certain yeasts such as *Saccharomyces boulardii* are also probiotics [6, 7].

Probiotics together with other beneficial microbes are commensals of the gut and differ from pathogenic bacteria in the terms of their actions on immune cells in the gut as they do not stimulate the proliferation of mononuclear cells or trigger an inflammatory action [8]. Regardless of whether the probiotics are used for human or animal consumption, there are several characteristics that a probiotic must achieve. Some of the important characteristics of probiotics include the following: a probiotic must be generally required as safe (GRAS); a probiotic should exhibit bile and acid tolerance in order to survive the path from the oral cavity to the small intestine where it lives, multiplies and excretes beneficial nutrients and molecules; a probiotic should have the ability to adhere to mucus and/or epithelial cells, and/or other surfaces; a probiotic should be susceptible to antibiotics; a probiotic should exhibit antimicrobial activity against pathogens [3, 5, 9, 10]. Although it is accepted that probiotics must be of human origin [4, 5], many authors have found that some strains that are not normally isolated from human have shown to be effective [11, 12], which negates this requirement. As noted above, one of the important attributes of probiotics is their antimicrobial effect against pathogens by maintaining the homeostasis of the intestinal flora. Assessing the antimicrobial effect of various probiotics against pathogenic microorganisms is the guiding concept of this chapter. This chapter reviews the principles and results from various authors of different methods for determining the antimicrobial or antagonistic effect of probiotics against potential pathogens.

2. Antimicrobial or antagonistic properties of probiotics

In literature both the terms "antimicrobial" and "antagonistic" are found to determine the ability of one species to inhibit the growth of another species. According to the online Encyclopaedia Britannica, "antagonism" refers to an "association between organisms in which one benefits at the expense of the other,." However, this encyclopaedia does not include the adverb "antimicrobial." On the other hand, it contains "antimicrobial agent" that refers to "a large variety of chemical compounds that are used to destroy microorganisms or to prevent their development.." The online Merriam Webster dictionary defines "antimicrobial" as "destroying or inhibiting the growth of microorganisms and especially pathogenic microorganisms" and "antagonistic" as "showing dislike or opposition: showing antagonism."

This antimicrobial/antagonistic ability is especially important for probiotics as one of the functional beneficial requirements of probiotics is a broad antimicrobial spectrum as well as antagonism against pathogenic bacteria with strong antimicrobial activity. The antagonistic activity of one microorganism against another can be caused by competitive exclusion, immune modulation, stimulation of host defence systems, production of organic acids or hydrogen peroxide that lower pH, production of antimicrobials such as bacteriocins, antioxidants, production of signalling molecules that trigger changes in gene expression [13–15]. Antimicrobial substances produced by beneficial microorganisms are known to include lactic acid, acetic acid, formic acid, phenyllactic acid, benzoic acid as well as other organic acids, short chain fatty acids, hydrogen peroxide, carbon dioxide, acetaldehyde, acetoin, diacetyl, bacteriocins and bacteriocins-like inhibitory substances and others [10, 16, 17]. The most common bacteriocins include lacticin, lactocin, pediocin, pisciolin, enterocin, reuterin, plantaricin, enterolysin and nisin [18, 19].

3. Methods

3.1. Methods of literature research

A literature overview of three databases was conducted using the two following keywords: "probiotic" and "antimicrobial" between the years 1980 and 2016. The search yielded 2882, 1017, and 6200 publications in PubMed, Web of Science, and Science Direct databases, respectively (**Figure 1**).

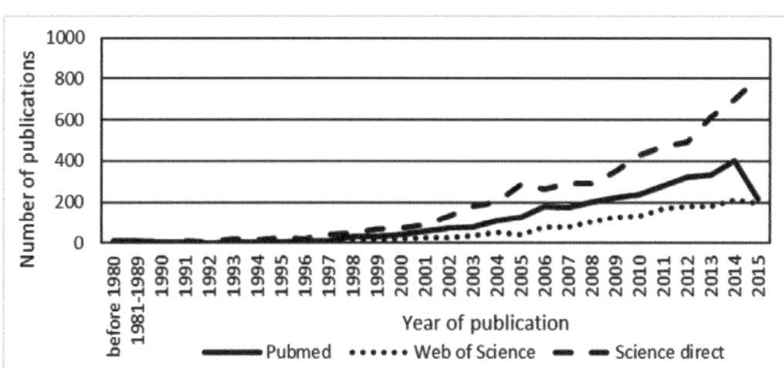

Figure 1. Results of the publications in PubMed, Web of Science and Science Direct databases using keywords: "probiotic" and "antimicrobial" between the years 1980 and 2015.

All three databases showed great increase in the number of publications in the past 10 years. The highest results were obtained via Science Direct due to the fact that this database includes various journals and books from the area of food and dairy sciences, the area of probiotics for animals as well as the area of human probiotics. PubMed on the other hand contains only research of probiotics for humans. Also, the programs for keyword searching for each chosen database seem to differ among each other thus yielding very different numbers of publications in journals, chapters and conference proceedings. The research on the methods for determining the antimicrobial effect of strain-specific probiotics was conducted by adding an additional keyword aside "probiotic." This keyword described the various investigated methods for determining the antimicrobial/antagonistic activity of probiotics (i.e., spot-on lawn, agar spot, agar well diffusion, paper disc, co-culturing, *in vivo*). Of course, it was not possible to screen every single article therefore only a selection of the most recent or relevant were used.

3.2. *In vitro* methods for determining the antimicrobial/antagonistic effect of probiotics against other microorganisms

3.2.1. Spot-on lawn antimicrobial assay/agar spot antimicrobial assay

The spot-on lawn antimicrobial assay has been described by several authors. Several modifications of the method have been made. Also various other expressions are used such as agar spot assay, critical dilution assay and deferred antagonism assay [10, 16, 20–22].

One of the simplest published principles of the spot-on lawn antimicrobial assay (**Figure 2a**) consists of the following steps: different nutrients, selective or differential media, are prepared and various chosen indicator microorganisms or pathogens at different initial concentrations are either inoculated in a confluent manner after hardening of agar or are mixed with the agar in liquid state and poured into the plate. Different dilutions of aliquots of the investigated probiotic or cell-free supernatant with bacteriocins are then spotted onto the media already inoculated with chosen indicator microorganisms [20, 23, 24].

After incubation, the antimicrobial activity is expressed either as inhibition zone or as arbitrary units (AU/mL). The zone of inhibition is noted either as the diameter or the area of the inhibition zone. The critical dilution is noted as the last dilution that produces a zone of inhibition larger than 6 mm. Arbitrary units are defined as the reciprocal of the highest dilution at which the growth of the indicator microorganism or pathogen is inhibited and are calculated as $(1000/a) \times D$ in AU/mL, where a is the aliquot of cell-free supernatant added to well in μL and D is the dilution factor [22, 24].

A modification is the agar spot antimicrobial assay (**Figure 2b**) and consists of the following steps: MRS agar or other specified agar is prepared and the probiotic bacteria or test cultures (few μL) are spotted on. These agars are then incubated to develop spots. Next, the indicator bacteria (pathogenic species, spoilage species and other probiotic species) are mixed into specific soft agar (0.7%) and poured over a plate. The plates are then incubated aerobically or anaerobically and the inhibition zones are read. A clear zone of more than 1 mm around the spot is considered as positive [25]. A third modification is the spot-on lawn antimicrobial assay with wells (**Figure 2c**), which consists of the following steps: chosen nutrients, selective or differential media, are prepared. Wells (6 mL, 7 mm or other dimensions) are bored in each plate and the bottom of the wells is sealed with agar. Aliquots of active cultures at different dilutions are pipetted into the wells. The plates are left at room temperature to allow migration and settling of the test cultures. The samples are then incubated for 3 h at 37°C and the plates are then overlaid with agar seeded with indicator pathogenic microorganisms (or other indicator organisms) and incubated at suitable incubation conditions. After incubation, the antimicrobial activity is expressed either as inhibition zone or as arbitrary units (AU/mL) [16].

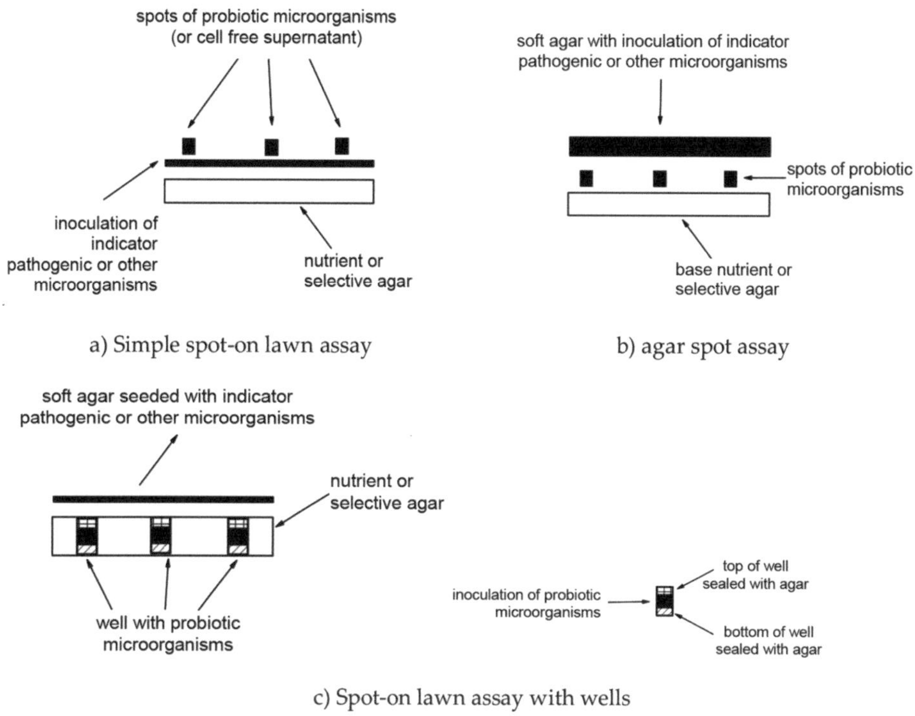

Figure 2. Schemes of different versions of spot-on lawn/agar spot assays: (a) simple spot-on lawn assay, (b) agar spot assay and (c) spot-on lawn assay with wells.

The fourth modification is the cross streak assay [26] where each probiotic strain is streaked in three parallel lines onto agar using a 1-mL loop. Once these lines have dried, test pathogenic strains are streaked perpendicular to these initial strains in the same fashion, giving three possible zones of inhibition for each combination of strains. It was assumed that when there is inhibition, it is caused by the tester probiotic strain hindering the growth of the second-streaked (indicator) strain.

3.2.2. *Agar well diffusion assay/paper disc assay*

The agar well diffusion assay (AWDA) (**Figure 3a**) is used for determining the antagonistic effects of cell-free supernatants. The general principle of agar well diffusion assay consists of the following steps: different nutrients, selective or differential media, are prepared. The plates are inoculated with the chosen indicator microorganism. The 6-mm or 7-mm wells are bored in each plate. Aliquots of different dilutions of cell-free supernatants are pipetted into the wells. After incubation, the antimicrobial activity is expressed either as inhibition zone or as arbitrary units (AU/mL) [20, 22]. The paper disc assay (**Figure 3b**) is a modification where instead of making wells, discs measuring 6 mm are absorbed with aliquots of cell-free supernatant and placed on the agar inoculated with indicator strains. After incubation, the inhibition zone is evaluated based on the clear zone around the paper disc [23].

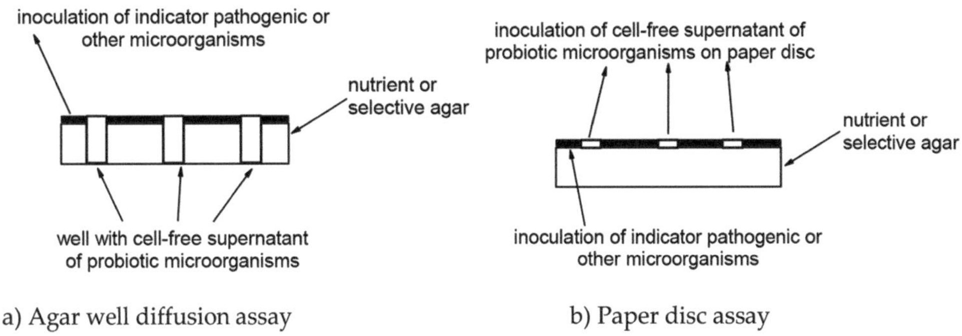

Figure 3. Scheme of the agar well diffusion assay and paper disc assay: (a) agar well diffusion assay and (b) paper disc assay.

3.2.3. Co-culturing assays for determining the antimicrobial activity

Determining the antimicrobial activity of probiotics against common pathogens is also possible with the co-culturing assay. This method includes the following steps: preparation of incubation media (i.e., nutrient broth, reconstituted skim milk, sterilized milk, yogurt, whey, etc.). Aliquots of pathogenic and probiotics microorganisms are inoculated into the incubation media. The samples are mixed well and incubated. After incubation, the population of pathogenic bacteria are counted on appropriate agars. Values are usually expressed as log cfu/mL [14–16, 27, 28].

The microtitre plate assay is a version of the co-culturing assay that includes the following steps: cell-free supernatant of active probiotic or other investigated microorganism is prepared and divided into several parts that undergo different conditions (i.e., NaOH added to neutralize pH, left acidic, heated, etc.). Pathogenic microorganisms are cultured and added to appropriate broth. The microtitre plate is used to prepare mixes of probiotics/cell-free supernatants and pathogenic microorganisms and incubated at suitable incubation conditions. Before and after incubation, the optical density at 620 nm is measured and the suppressive activity is calculated as a percentage of inhibition of pathogen growth [15].

Another important type of co-culturing assay is using cell lines. As several important mechanisms underlying the beneficial effects of probiotics include the effects of probiotic properties on specific tissues, particularly on the intestine, the evaluation of probiotic effects on human intestinal cell lines *in vitro* is meaningful as these cells mimic the systemic environment of an organism and are used as a biological matrix alternative to *in vivo* tests. In fact, *in vitro* evidence is particularly important considering that the EU directives tend to discourage *in vivo* experiments on animals [29]. Several different cell lines have been used, such as HT-29 cell line from human colon [29], IPEC-J2 porcine neonatal jejunal cell line [30], Vero African green monkey kidney epithelial cell line [31], Caco-2 colon adenocarcinoma cell line [32], HIEC-6 normal epithelial small intestine cell line [33], BALB/c3T3 murine embryonal fibroblast cell line [29] and many others. Cells are routinely grown in Dubelco's modified Eagles' medium (DMEM), McCoy's 5a medium or other medium and seeded in well plates or microtitre plates that are incubated at 37°C for 24 h in 1 mL medium in 5% CO_2. Probiotic and pathogenic microorganisms are then added and the cell viability is determined after incubation.

3.3. *In vivo* methods for determining the antimicrobial/antagonistic effect of probiotics against other microorganisms

For *in vivo* testing, randomized double blind, placebo-controlled human trials should be undertaken to establish the efficacy of the probiotic product. The consultation recognized that there is a need for human studies in which adequate numbers of subjects are enrolled to achieve statistical significance. In order to ascertain that a given probiotic can prevent or treat a specific pathogen infection, a clinical study must be designed to verify exposure to the said pathogen (preventive study) or that the infecting microorganism is that specific pathogen (treatment study). If the goal is to apply probiotics in general to prevent or treat a number of infectious gastroenteritis or urogenital conditions, the study design must define the clinical presentation, symptoms and signs of infection, and include appropriate controls [4].

However, many scientists have reverted to *in vivo* animal studies. The animal models do not necessarily provide scientifically appropriate and relevant results for human, due to obvious species-specific differences in anatomy, biochemistry, physiology, pharmacokinetics and toxic responses. Especially, in medicine and pharmacy, the "safety testing" on animals led to thousands of deaths worldwide due to the evidence that animal tests are not only worthless, but they are also dangerously unpredictable. The use of replacement alternative methods, especially incorporating human cells and tissues, avoids such confounding variables [32].

The European legislation OJ L136 of 08.06.2000 includes the 3Rs regulation that results in important reduction of studies on animal models and consists of the following. *Reduction*: using alternative methods for obtaining comparable levels of information from the use of fewer animals in scientific procedure or for obtaining more information from the same number of animals. *Refinement*: using alternatives methods that alleviate or minimise potential pain, suffering and distress, and which enhance animal wellbeing. *Replacement*: using alternative methods that permit a given purpose to be achieved without conducting experiments or other scientific procedures on animals [32].

The *in vivo* animal model antimicrobial study is described as follows: briefly, all animal models include at least two groups under controlled settings. One group receives chosen probiotic and pathogen (treated infected group) and the other receives only the pathogen (untreated infected group). The observed difference includes the exanimation of faeces as well as the examination of different cells after scarifying the animals (spleens, lymph nodes, blood, liver, colon, cecum, etc.). Animals used in these studies include mice, rats, chicks, rabbits, pigs, Fish and even worms [30, 34–37]. Work is done under accordance with the guidelines of the European convention for the protection of vertebrate animals used for experimental and other scientific purposes (Directive 86/609/EEC).

4. Recent results of *in vitro* antimicrobial/antagonistic assays for various probiotic strains

The following section contains results of the antimicrobial/antagonistic assays for various probiotic strains or strains with probiotic-like properties against various potential pathogens, spoilage microorganisms, or other probiotic microorganisms. The results reported using different assays (spot-on lawn/agar spot, agar well diffusion/paper disc, co-culturing, micro-titre plate and cell line assays) are published by various authors stated in the text and some of the individual procedures are briefly explained.

4.1. Recent results of selected spot-on lawn/agar spot antimicrobial assays

The antimicrobial activity of *Lactobacillus plantarum* EM against seven potential pathogens using the spot-on-lawn assay was conducted by Choi and Chang [10]. The following nutrient and selective media were used: Luria-Bertani agar for *E. coli* O157:H7 ATCC 43895, *P. aeruginosa* ATCC 27853, *S. enterica* serovar Typhi ATCC 19430, nutrient agar supplemented with 2% NaCl for *V. parahaemolyticus* ATCC 17802 and tryptic soy agar for *B. cereus* KCTC 3624, *M. luteus* ATCC 15307 and *S. aureus* ATCC 29123. All potential pathogenic bacteria had an initial inoculum of 6 log cfu/mL. An aliquot of 10 μL of *L. plantarum* EM was spotted onto each plate. The plates were incubated aerobically at 37°C. After incubation the arbitrary units (AU/mL) were determined. *L. plantarum* EM exhibited strong antimicrobial activity against the seven chosen potential pathogenic bacteria. The strongest activity was noted against *V. parahaemolyticus*, ATCC 17802 (25600 units) and the weakest activity was noted for *S. aureus*, ATCC 29123 (200 units). As one of the most important requirements of probiotics is a broad antimicrobial spectrum, the authors found that *L. plantarum* EM fulfilled the beneficial requirements of probiotics [10].

In another research [24], screening for bacteriocins using the spot-on lawn method was used. One hundred and fifty lactic acid bacteria were isolated from samples of traditional fermented Vietnamese pork. The isolate named *L. plantarum* KL-1 was found to produce bacteriocins, effective against various Gram-positive and Gram-negative bacteria. The test was conducted by preparing two layers of soft agar (0.8% agar). The first layers were poured into the plate; then the top layer, which included 5 mL of soft agar together with 10 μL (about 10^7 cfu/mL) of freshly grown test bacterial strains, was added. The Gram-positive strains included *S. aureus* TISTR 118, *E. faecalis* JCM 5803, *E. faecalis* TISTR 888, *L. lactis* subsp. *cremoris* TISTR1344, *L. mesenteroides* JCM 6124, *L. mesenteroides* TISTR 942, *L. sakei* subsp. *sakei* JCM 1157, *L. sakei* TISTR 890, *L. plantarum* ATCC 14917, *L. inoccua* ATCC 33090, *Streptococcus* sp. TISTR 1030, *B. coagu-*

lans JCM 2257, *B. coagulans* TISTR 1447 and *B. campeatris* NBRC 11547. The Gram-negative test strains included *P. fluorescens* TISTR 358, *P. fluorescens* JCM 5963 and A. *hydrophila* TISTR 1321. Bacteriocin activity was tested by spotting 10 μL of previously prepared cell-free supernatant (in different dilutions) of the isolate *L. plantarum* KL-1. The inhibition zone was observed after overnight incubation at the proper temperature for each indicator microorganisms and the spectrum was expressed at arbitrary units (AU) [22]. The results show that the antimicrobial activity of the bacteriocin was strain specific. The bacteriocin was most effective against both strains of *L. sakei*. The bacteriocin was less effective against certain Gram-positive bacteria (both strains of *E. faecalis*, *L. plantarum* and both strains of *L. mesenteroides* subsp. *mesenteroides*). However, it was not effective against *S. aureus*, both strains of *B. coagulans* and any of the chosen Gram-negative bacteria.

Tharmaraj and Shah [16] used the spot-on-lawn technique with wells to test the inhibition of chosen pathogenic bacteria (*E. coli*, *S. typhimurium*, *S. aureus* and *B. cereus*) and spoilage bacteria (*B. stearothermophilus* and *P. aeruginosa*) by one strain of *L. casei* (Shirota YLC); two strains of *L. paracasei* subsp. *paracasei* (LCS1, LC01), *L. acidophilus* (LA5, LAC1) and *B. animalis* (BB12, BLC1); three strains of *P. freudenreichii* subsp. *shermanii* (P, PS1, PB10360) and four strains of *L. rhamnosus* (LC705, LBA, LGG, LR1524). MRS agar was used for lactobacilli (*L. acidophilus*, *L. casei*, *L. paracasei* subsp. *paracasei* and *L. rhamnosus*), MRS agar + L-cysteine (0.05%) for *B. animalis*, NaLa agar for *P. freudenreichii* subsp. *shermanii* and nutrient agar was used for pathogenic bacteria. Suitable agar (25 mL) was poured into the plates and wells were cut with a sterile metal borer. The bottom of the wells was sealed with 0.8% agar. Active culture (50 μL) of producing probiotics was then filled into the wells and left at room temperature for 2 h, followed by incubating at 37°C for 3 h. The remaining depth of the well was sealed with 1% agar. Finally, the spotted plates were overlaid with 10 mL of 0.8% agar seeded with about 10^7 cfu/mL of pathogenic bacteria. The plates were incubated anaerobically for 72 h at 37°C for all chosen pathogenic and spoilage bacteria. Both chosen spoilage bacteria were additionally incubated aerobically for 24 h at 37°C. On average, among all the probiotic and spoilage bacterial interactions, the spore formers were inhibited by the probiotic microorganisms to a greater extent (average zone of inhibition, 19 mm) than the non-spore formers (average zone of inhibition, 14 mm). Also, the Gram-positive bacteria (average zone of inhibition, 18 mm) were inhibited more than the Gram-negative bacteria (average zone of inhibition, 14 mm). Strains of *P. freudenreichii* subsp. *shermanii* did not show notable inhibitory effect.

Soomro et al. [23] also used the spot-on lawn method to determine antimicrobial activity of various *Lactobacillus* species. They found that *L. acidophilus* J1 showed an inhibitory effect against *E. coli*. The plates were prepared by inoculating 100 μL of indicator strain *E. coli* grown in broth with 3.5 mL soft MRS agar and were overlaid over MRS agar. The plates were incubated for 2 h at 37°C after which 30 μL of cell-free supernatant of *L. acidophilus* J1 was spotted onto the overlaid surface. The pH of the cell-free supernatant was adjusted to 5.5 to eliminate the effect of organic acids and hydrogen peroxide. The plates were incubated at 37°C for 18 h and were subsequently examined for inhibition zones. It was found that the inhibitory effect against *E. coli* was due to the production of a bacteriocin.

Probiotic strains or strains with probiotic potential with efficient antimicrobial activity *in vitro*	**Indicator pathogenic microorganisms**	**Reference**
Lb:*L. casei* C1; *L. plantarum* C4	**G+:***L. monocytogenes* **G-:***S.* Typhimurium CECT 4157, *Y. enterocolitica* IP383	[35]
Lb:*Lactobacillus* MSMC64-1	**G+:** MRSA DMST 20651, 20654, **G-:** *S.* Typhi DMST 5784, *V. parahaemolyticus* DMST 5665, *S. dysenteriae* DMST 15111	[38]
Oth:*S.cerevisiae* JCM7255	**G+:***S. agalactiae*	[39]
Oth:*B. pumilus* B16, *B. mojavensis* J7	**G-:***V. parahaemolyticus*	[40]
Lb:*L. acidophilus* La-5, **Bb:** *B. longum* ATCC 15707	**G+:***S. aureus, L. monocytogenes;***G-:***E. coli* O157:H7	[41]
Lb:*L. acidophilus* JN188382, *L. fermentum* JN188383, *L. fermentum* JN188384, *L. buchneri* JN188385, *L. buchneri* JN188386, *L. buchneri* JN188387, *L. casei* JN188388, *L. casei* JN188389, *L. casei* JN188390	**G+:***E. faecium* ATCC 51558, *S. epidermidis ATCC 12228, P. acnes ATCC 6919, L. monocytogenes, S. aureus* S244; **G-:** *E. coli ATCC 29181, K. pneumoniae* K36, *E. cloacae, S. sonnei ATCC 25931, H. pylori ATCC 43579, V. parahaemolyticus,* **fng:** *C. albicans* ATCC 44831	[42]
Oth:*E. faecium* CV1, LPP29, *W. cibaria* P71, *L. lactis* subsp. *cremoris* SMF110, *Lc. mesenteroides* subsp. *cremoris* SMM69, *P. pentosaceus* SMM73, TPP3	**G-:***T. maritimum* NCIMB2154, LL01.8.3.8, *V. splendidus* CECT528, DMC-1	[43]
Lb:*L. plantarum* P6	**G+:***S. aureus ATCC 25923, B. cereus, L. ivanovii ATCC 19119;***G-:***E. coli ATCC 25921, S. enterica, P. aeruginosa*	[44]
Oth:*E. faecalis* AP-216, *E. faecalis* AP 45	**G+:***C. perfringens* KCTC 3269, KCTC 5100, *L. monocytogenes* KCTC 3569, 3586, 3710	[45]
Oth:*B. subtilis* DCU, *B. pumilus* BP, *B. cereus* HL7	**G-:***V. parahaemolyticus*	[46]
Lb: LAB 18, LAB 48	**G-:***S. enterica* serovar Enteritidis phage type 13A, *E. coli* O157:H7, *C. jejuni*	[47]
Lb:*L. plantarum* CK06, CK19, B01, B07, K09, K10, K21, LM11, ZS07, ZS11 and ZS15	**G+:***S. aureus SSV25, S. epidermidis SSV30, S. lentus CCM 3472, E. faecalis* V583, *L. monocytogenes* CCM *4699,* **G-:** *A. calcoaceticus* CCM *4503; S. paucimobilis* CCM *3293; S. enterica subsp. enterica* TA100 CCM 3812	[48]
Lb:*L. fermentum* PXN 44, *L. plantarum* PXN 47	**G+:***E. faecalis* NCTC 00775; **G-:** *E. coli* NCTC 9001	[49]
Lb:*L. paraplantarum* FT259	**G+:***L. monocytogenes* IAL 633, *L. innocua* ATCC 3309	[50]

Where probiotics are divided as follows: lb: lactobacilli; bb: Bifidobacterium; oth: other; and pathogens are divided as follows: G+: Gram positive; G−: Gram negative; fng: fungi.

Table 1. A selection of assays published since 2013 of successful antimicrobial activity of chosen probiotics using the spot-on lawn/agar spot assay on chosen pathogenic microorganisms.

Assays published since 2013 of antimicrobial activity of chosen probiotics using the spot-on lawn/agar spot assay on chosen pathogenic microorganisms are noted in **Table 1**.

As noted in **Table 1**, the most common investigated probiotic strains or strains with probiotic potential were from the genus *Lactobacillus* (*L. plantarum, L. acidophilus, L casei* and *L. fermentum*). Several studies included probiotic strains of the genus *Bacillus*. The most common pathogens included in the assays were *S. aureus, L. monocytogenes, E. coli, Vibrio* spp. and *Salmonella* spp. One study examined the antimycotic properties of probiotics against various strains of the genus *Aspergillus*. Different strains of *E. faecium* were on the one hand used as probiotics and on the other hand used as potential pathogen, thus proving the dualistic nature of this species.

4.2. Recent results of selected agar well diffusion assays/paper disc methods

The agar well diffusion assay was conducted in the research by Ali et al. [51], where 14 isolates with probiotic potential were screened for antimicrobial activity against *E. coli* and *S. aureus*. The probiotic isolates were identified as two *Lactobacillus* spp. (S2a3 and S4b1), eleven *Bifidobacterium* spp. (FCb1, Kb2, LZa7, LZb8, RC1b8, RC2b4, RC4a3, RC4b2, SCa4, SCb2 and Y2a5) and one *Streptococcus* spp. (RC2b3). A volume of 100 μL of cell-free supernatant of isolates with probiotic potential was filled in 7-mm wells cut in nutrient agar previously inoculated with *E. coli* or *S. aureus*. The diameter of inhibition zone was measured after 48 h of incubation. The supernatant obtained from all 14 isolates exhibited varying degrees of inhibitory activity against *S. aureus* and *E. coli*. The isolates LZb8, S4b1 and RC4a3 exhibited the superior antibacterial activity with inhibition zones ranged 8.3–8.4 mm. The least activity was recorded for the isolates SCa4 and RC4b2 (inhibition zone ranged 2.3–2.5 mm), whereas the isolates Kb2, LZa7, RC2b4, RC2b3, SCb2 and Y2a5 (inhibition zone ranged 3.5–4.8 mm) were moderately active against *S. aureus*. It is worth mentioning that the inhibitory activity of the tested isolates supernatants was slightly less against *E. coli* as compared to that obtained against *S. aureus*, indicating that *E. coli* could be less sensitive.

In the previously mentioned research by Soomro et al. [23], the paper disc method was also used. Sterile filter discs measuring 6-mm diameter with an absorbed aliquot of 20 μL of cell-free supernatant of *L. acidophilus* J1 were placed on MRS and nutrient agar plates containing the target strain *E. coli*. After incubation at 37°C, the inhibitory activity was evaluated. It was found that the paper disc assay yielded an inhibition zone of 10 mm and was more appropriate compared to the spot-on lawn assay.

Assays published since 2013 of antimicrobial activity of chosen probiotics using the agar well diffusion assay or the paper disc assay on chosen pathogenic microorganisms are noted in **Table 2**. The results show that the agar well diffusion assay or the paper disc assay is the most common method used for determining the antimicrobial or antagonistic effect. The most common investigated probiotic strains or strains with probiotic potential were again from the genus *Lactobacillus*. Some assays included bifidobacteria and bacteria from the genus *Pediococcus* and *Lactococcus*. The most common pathogens included in the assays were again *S. aureus, L. monocytogenes, E coli, Vibrio* spp., *Aeromonas* spp. *Salmonella* spp. and *Pseudomonas aeruginosa*. One study even assessed the antagonistic activity of probiotics against herpes simplex virus types 1 and 2 and one study investigated the antimicrobial activity of probiotics against the protozoa *Giardia lamblia*. However, using cell-free supernatants does not mimic real conditions. Therefore, further assays are necessary.

Probiotic strains or strains with probiotic potential with efficient antimicrobial activity *in vitro*	**Indicator pathogenic microorganisms**	**Reference**
Lb:*L. acidophilus* PBS066, *L. fermentum* PBS073, *L. plantarum* PBS067, *L. rhamnosus* PBS070, *L. reuteri* PBS072, **Bb:** *B. animalis* subsp. *lactis* PBS075, *B. longum* subsp. *longum* PBS108	**G+:***S. aureus* ATCC 6538, *E. faecalis* ATCC 29212, **G-:** *E. coli* ATCC 25922, *P. aeruginosa* ATCC 9027, **fng:** C. *albicans* ATCC 10231	[29]
Lb:*L. salivarius* JM41, JK21V, JM31, JS2A, JM14, JK22, JM2A1 and JM32, *L. plantarum PZ01* **Oth:** *P. acidilactici* JM241 and JH231, *P. pentosaceus* JS233, *E. faecium JS11*	**G+:***S. aureus* ATCC 29213, **G-:** *E. coli* K88, 25922 and 1569, *S. Enteritidis* ATCC 13076, *S.* Typhimurium ATCC 14082	[34]
Lb:*L. casei* C1, *L. plantarum* C4, *L. acidophilus*	**G+:***L. monocytogenes*,**G-:***E. coli* C17, *S. enterica* ser Typhimurium CECT4156, *Y. enterocolitica* IP383	[35]
Lb:*Lactobacillus* MSMC64-1	**G+:** MRSA DMST 20651, 20654, **G-:** *S.* Typhi DMST 5784, *V. parahaemolyticus* DMST 5665, *S. dysenteriae* DMST 15111	[38]
Lb:*L. acidophilus* La-5, **Bb:** *B. longum* ATCC15707	**G+:***S. aureus, L. monocytogenes*,**G-:***E. coli* O157:H7	[41]
Lb:*L. plantarum* WCFS1, *L. plantarum* NA7	**G+:***L. monocytogenes* CIP 81.3 ILSI NA 39, **G-:** *E. coli* O157:H7 ATCC 43888, *S. enterica* ser *Enteritidis* CIP 81.3	[52]
Lb:*L. casei* PTCC 1608, *L. rhamnosus* PTCC 1637	**G-:***P. aeruginosa* PTCC 1430	[53]
Oth:*B. amyloliqufaciens*	**G+:***C. difficile*	[54]
Oth:*P. pentosaceus* KID7	**G+:***S. aureus* KCCM1133515, MRSA CCM40510, *S. epidermidis* KCTC 191712, *L. monocytogenes* KACC1076420, *B. cereus* KACC11240 **G-:** *S.* Typhi KCTC2514, *S. choleraesuis* KCTC293215, *S. gallinarum* KCTC293126, *S. boydii* KACC10792 14, *Y. enterocolitica* KACC1532020, *E. coli* O138KCTC261511, O1KCTC2441, *P. aeruginosa* KCCM 1180218,	[55]
Lb:*L. rhamnosus* FM13, FM14, FM22, FS2, FS10, PS2, PS11, SF6, SP13, *L. paracasei* CM1, CM2, MF5, PM8	**G+:***S. aureus* ATCC 6538, *L. monocytogenes* DSM 12464, *E. faecalis*, **G-:** *E. coli* ATCC 25922	[56]
Lb: L. *casei* LC-01, *L. acidophilus* LA-5, *L. paracasei*	**fng:***A. niger* PTCC 5012, *A. flavus* PTCC 5004, *A. parasiticus* PTCC 5286, *P. chrysogenum* PTCC 5035	[57]

Probiotic strains or strains with probiotic potential with efficient antimicrobial activity *in vitro*	Indicator pathogenic microorganisms	Reference
Lb:*L. viridescens* NRRL B-1951	**G+:***L. monocytogenes* CWD 1002, CWD 1198	[58]
Lb:*L. plantarum* S2	**G+:***S. aureus* CMCC2607, **G-:** *E. coli* CMCC44825, *S.* Typhimurium CMCC50115, *S. flexneri* CMCC51061	[59]
Oth:*B. subtilis* JQ302302, *B. aerophilus* JQ312663	**G-:***A. hydrophila* ATCC 49140, MTCC 1739, *Aeromonas* sp. JX136697, JX136698, A. *enteropelogenes* JX136699, *P. rettgeri* JX 136696	[60]
Lb:*L. acidophilus* L-1, *L. bulgaricus* 6, *L. plantarum* 24-4B, *L. fermentum* 1, *L. brevis*, **Bb:** *B. animalis* subsp. *lactis* L-3	**G+:***S. aureus, B. cereus* **G-:***E. coli*	[61]
Lb:*L. plantarum* DK211, DK303; *L. paracasei* DK215, L. *sakei* DK301	**G+:***S. aureus* KCTC 3881, *E. faecalis* KCTC 2011, *B. cereus* KCTC 3624	[62]
Lb: L. *mesenteroides* subsp. *mesenteroides* SD1, SD23, SF2, SF3	**G+:***S. aureus* ATCC 25923, FRI 184, *L. monocytogenes* ATCC 19115, **G-:** *E. coli* ATCC43895, *S. enterica* ATCC 14028	[63]
Oth:*L. mesenteroides* MTCC 5442, *B. subtilis*	**G-:***V. cholerae*	[64]
Lb:*L. fermentum* M059, *L. fermentum* F-6, **Oth:** *W. cibaria* 4213	**G+:***S. aureus* ATCC 6538, *B. cereus* NCIM 245, *B. subtilis* ATCC 6633, **G-:** *E. coli* ATCC 25922, S. Typhi 25, *P. aeruginosa* ATCC 27853	[65]
Lb:*L. brevis* DT24	**G-:***E. coli* MTCC 729	[66]
Lb:*L. rhamnosus* (4 strains)	**G-:***Helicobacter pylori*	[67]
Lb:*L. plantarum, L. salivarius*	**G+:***S. aureus* ATCC 6538S, *C. perfringens* ATCC 13124, **G-:** *E. coli* ATCC 8734, *S. Enteritidis* ATCC 13311, *R. anatipestifer* ATCC 11845, *P. multocida* ATCC 43137	[68]
Lb:*L. acidophilus* P106, *L. plantarum* P164	**Prs:***Giardia lamblia*	[69]
Lb:*L. casei*	**G-:** S. *flexneri, S. sonnei*	[70]
Lb:*L. helveticus* PJ4, *L. plantarum* PJ7	**G+:***S. aureus* MTCC737, **G-:** *E. coli* MTCC443, *S.* Typhimurium MTCC733, *S. fleksneri* MTCC1457, *P. aeruginosa* MTCC1688	[71]
Lb:*L. salivarius* K35, K43	**G+:***S. mutans* ATCC 25175	[72]
Oth:*B. amyloliquefaciens* KATMIRA1933	**Vr:** Herpes simplex virus types 1 and 2	[73]
Oth:*B. amyloliquefaciens* FPTB16	**G-:***E. tarda, A. hydrophila, V. harveyi, V. parahaemolyticus*	[74]

Where probiotics are divided as follows: lb: lactobacilli; bb: Bifidobacterium; oth: other; and pathogens are divided as follows: G+: Gram positive; G–: Gram negative; fng: fungi; prs: parasite.

Table 2. A selection of assays published since 2013 of successful antimicrobial activity of chosen probiotics using the agar well diffusion assay or the paper disc assay on chosen pathogenic microorganisms.

4.3. Recent results of selected co-culturing assays

The influence of the potential pathogenic bacteria *P. aeruginosa* ATCC 27853 against various combinations of probiotic supplements and the kefir microbiota was investigated using the co-culturing method [6]. One multispecies, one oligospecies and one monospecies probiotic supplement as well as kefir microbiota from kefir grains originally from the Caucasian mountains were used. The multispecies supplement contained *L.* acidophilus (NIZO 3678; NIZO 3887), *L. paracasei* NIZO 3672, *L. plantarum* NIZO 3684, *L. rhamnosus* NIZO 3689, *L. salivarius* NIZO 3675, *B. bifidum* NIZO 3804, *B. lactis* NIZO 3680 and *E. faecium* NIZO 3886. The oligospecies supplement contained *L. acidophilus* LA-5, *B. infantis* BB-12 and *E. faecium.* The monospecies supplement contained *L. reuteri* DSM 17938. Co-culturing was conducted by adding 1 mL of probiotic samples and 1 mL of overnight *P. aeruginosa* suspension in 40 mL previously sterilized bovine milk. Samples were incubated for 4 days at 25°C with agitation (250/min). After incubation, serial 10-fold dilutions were prepared for all samples and the *P. aeruginosa* populations were enumerated on cetrimide agar with added glycerol. It was found that the *P. aeruginosa* population in milk without probiotics reached an average of 9.2 log/mL, whilst the *P. aeruginosa* population in milk reached 5.2, 8.3, 8.3 and 5.0 for the samples with the multispecies, oligospecies and monospecies probiotic supplement as well as the kefir microbiota respectively. This research thus found that the decrease of the potential pathogen *P. aeruginosa* was dependent on the type of probiotic microbiota and that both multispecies microbiota (multispecies probiotic supplement kefir microbiota) with a much more diverse population than the other two samples (oligospecies probiotic supplement and the monospecies supplement) exhibited an efficient synergistic effect [7]. Both samples also exhibited a higher increase in the total population of anaerobic microorganisms after fermentation with *P. aeruginosa* thus indicating that a more successful quorum-sensing regulatory network was established and yielded antagonistic effects against the potential pathogen *P. aeruginosa.*

Tharmaraj and Shah [16], as already mentioned in the previous section, also investigated the inhibition effect of various probiotics against chosen pathogenic and spoilage bacteria with the co-culturing method. Briefly, 9 mL of reconstituted skim milk was inoculated with 1 mL of overnight culture of probiotic bacteria and 0.1 mL of pathogenic or spoilage bacteria. The medium was mixed well and incubated at 37°C for 24 h. / were counted on nutrient agar and the log population calculated (**Table 6**). All four pathogenic bacteria were inhibited by all probiotic strains tested to varying degrees. On average, the probiotic bacteria reduced the population of pathogenic bacteria by 2.8 log units. *B. cereus* was inhibited to a greater degree by all probiotic bacteria and strains than other pathogenic bacteria. On average, the inhibitory effect of all probiotic bacteria and strains was the weakest against *E. coli. S. aureus* was inhibited to a greater degree by *B. animalis* and *L. rhamnosus* than the other probiotic bacteria.

Ratsep et al. [15] published their research of a microtitre plate assay on the antimicrobial effect of *L. plantarum* (five strains: N11, N27, N33, N44 and E) supernatant against various *C. difficile* strains (six clinical isolates from Norwegian patients, six clinical isolates from Estonian patients and two reference strains: VPI 10463 and M13042). Overnight *C. difficile* cultures were added to BHI broth with a density according to McFarland 3.0. Various reaction mixes were prepared (natural (acidic), neutral (pH 6.0) and neutral, heated for 20 min at 100°C) and incubated under anaerobic conditions for 48 h at 37°C. The optical density at 620 mm was measured at the beginning of incubation and after 48 h and the suppressive activity of *L. plantarum* strains calculated as a percentage of inhibition. The highest inhibitions of *C. difficile* growth were in the samples of heated neutralized supernatants and the lowest in cases of the neutralized samples. There was statistically higher inhibition in heated neutralized supernatants versus neutralized supernatants of N11 and E56 lactobacilli strains. When comparing antagonistic activity of *L. plantarum* strains, there was a relevant difference only between N11 and N33 strains in the samples of heated neutralized supernatants. The neutralization of supernatant did not reduce its inhibitory effect. Thus, lowering the pH of the environment is not the main mechanism in inhibition of *C. difficile* by lactobacilli. Also heating of supernatant did not reduce its activity; thus, some thermostable compounds may be involved in the inhibition. The above-mentioned authors [15] also performed the co-culturing assay with the *L. plantarum* strains and *C. difficile* strains by inoculating 50 mL of brain heart infusion broth with 50 μL of lactobacilli suspension and 50 μL of *C. difficile* suspension and incubating under anaerobic conditions for 48 h at 37°C. After incubation, serial 10-fold dilutions were prepared and the *C. difficile* populations were enumerated on fastidious anaerobe agar. It was found that the five *L. plantarum* strains (N11, N27, N33, N44 and E) were able to inhibit the growth of the 14 *C. difficile* strains (six clinical isolates from Norwegian patients and Estonian patients and two reference strains: VPI 10463, M13042) in the co-culture incubation as the average log cfu/mL after 48 h was 3.0, whereas the average log cfu/mL of the *C. difficile* strains alone was 7.0.

Another important co-culturing method is the use of cell lines as noted in the research by Abdel et al. [31] of 12 lactobacilli isolates interfering with the adherence and invasion of *S.* Typhi 66 using kidney epithelial cell line *Vero* (ATCC CCl-81). The same authors also investigated this interference with the co-culturing assay in MRS broth. It was found that nine lactobacilli isolates inhibited the growth of *S.* Typhi in the co-culturing assay. Nine lactobacilli isolates were also successful in achieving a >50% inhibition of adherence of *S.* Typhi isolate (SS6) to Vero cells.

Assays published since 2013 of antimicrobial activity of chosen probiotics using various co-culturing assays on chosen pathogenic microorganisms are noted in **Table 3**. The results were similar to the results of spot-on lawn and agar well diffuse assays.

Probiotic strains or strains with probiotic potential with efficient antimicrobial activity *in vitro*	**Indicator pathogenic microorganisms**	**Reference**
Lb:*L. plantarum* FH185	**G+:***S. aureus*,**G-:***S.* Typhimurium	[9]
Lb:*L. acidophilus* La-5, **Bb:** *B. longum* ATCC15707	**G+:***S. aureus, L. monocytogenes*,**G-:***E. coli* O157:H7	[41]
Lb:*L. acidophilus* P106, *L. plantarum* P164	**Prs:***Giardia lamblia*	[69]
Lb:*L. rhamnosus* GR-1, *L. reuteri* RC-14	**Fng:***C. glabrata*	[75]
Lb:*L. helveticus* KLDS 1.8701	**G+:***S. aureus* ATCC 25923, *L. monocytogenes* ATCC 19115, **G-:** *E. coli* O157:H7 ATCC 43889, *S.* Typhimurium ATCC 14028	[76]

Probiotic strains or strains with probiotic potential with efficient antimicrobial activity *in vitro*	Indicator pathogenic microorganisms	Reference
Lb:*L. reuteri***Oth:***B. subtilis* MA139	G-:*E. coli* K88	[77]
Lb:*L. plantarum* C014	G-:*A. hydrophila* TISTR 1321	[78]
Lb:*L. acidophilus*, **Oth:***Pediococcus*	G-:*S.* Enteritidis 13A	[79]
Lb:*L. paracasei* CNCM I-4034, *L. rhamnosus* CNCM I-4036, **Bb:** *B. breve* CNCM I-4035	G-:*E. coli* ETEC CECT 501, *S.* Typhimurium CECT 443 *S.* Typhi CECT 725, *S. sonnei* CECT 457	[80]
Lb:*L. fermentum* 907, **Bb:** *B. longum* 1011	G-:*E. coli* O157:H7, *E. coli* O86	[81]

Where probiotics are divided as follows: lb: lactobacilli; bb: Bifidobacterium; and pathogens are divided as follows: G+: Gram positive; G–: Gram negative; fng: fungi; prs: parasite.

Table 3. A selection of assays published since 2013 of successful antimicrobial activity of chosen probiotics using the co-culturing assay on chosen pathogenic microorganisms.

5. Recent results of *in vivo* antimicrobial/antagonistic assays for various probiotic strains

5.1. Recent results of determining the *in vivo* antimicrobial assays using animal models

In the research by Mazaya et al. [36], both *in vitro* and *in vivo* studies were conducted. The significant *in vitro* antimicrobial activity (no method specified) of two lactobacillus strains isolated from Egyptian dairy products (*L. plantarum* LA5 and *L. paracasei* LA7) was found against several potential pathogens: *S. aureus* ATCC 25923, *B. subtilis* ATCC 23857, *M. luteus* ATCC 21882, *P. aeruginosa* ATCC 27853 and *S.* Typhi. *In vivo* assays were also conducted on 5-week-old male mice, divided into six groups (10 mice/group). Animals within different treatment groups were treated daily for 8 days as follows: Group 1, untreated control; Group 2, animals challenged with single inoculation *S.* Typhi (200 μL aliquot of 1X 108/P.O); Group 3, animals treated orally with *L. plantarum* (LA5) (200 μL aliquot of 1X 108/P.O) for 7 days; Group 4, animals treated orally with *L. paracasei* (LA7) (200 μL aliquot of 1X 108/P.O) for 7 days; Group 5, animals challenged with single inoculation *S.* Typhi, then treated with LA5 for next 7 days; Group 6, animals challenged with single inoculation *S.* Typhi and treated with LA 7 for next 7 days. Administration of LA5 or LA7 counteracted the pathogenic effect resulting from Salmonella infection. The lactobacilli succeeded to get rid of salmonellosis based on its phagocytic and immunostimulant activity against typhoid antigen.

Lazarenko et al. [82] conducted an *in vitro* and *in vivo* assay to determine anti-staphylococcal actions of certain probiotic cultures (*L. casei* IMV B-7280, *L. acidophilus* IMV B-7279; *B. longum* VK1 and *B. bifidum* VK2). *In vitro* assay using perpendicular strokes yielded antagonistic activity against all three strains of *S. aureus* (209-P, 43, 8325-4). The *in vivo* study with *S. aureus* 8325-4 on mice showed that the combination of probiotics (*L. casei* IMV B-7280, *B. longum* VK1 and *B. bifidum* VK2) was most successful as after day 9 no colonies of *S. aureus* 8325-4 were found in the vagina of the mice.

http://dx.doi.org/10.5772/63141

In the study by Bujalance et al. [35], a lack of correlation between *in vitro* and *in vivo* methods of the antimicrobial activity of probiotic lactobacilli against enteropathogenic bacteria was determined. In this study, the *in vitro* assay using the agar spot test showed that 20 strains of probiotic lactobacilli successfully inhibited *Y. enterocolitica*, *S. enterica* ser Typhimurium and *L. monocytogenes*. However, in the *in vivo* study using mouse models the selected strains (*L. casei* C1 and *L. plantarum* C4) lacked protective effects against *S.* Typhimurium. Similar conclusions of finding no antagonism *in vivo* are noted in the study by Bratz et al. [83]. Another study [79] found that the tea Yerba mate exhibited antagonistic activity *in vitro* but as a feed additive did not reduce S. Enteritidis colonization *in vivo* in broiler chickens. These studies prove that successful *in vitro* assays do not necessarily mean that the chosen microorganism with probiotic properties will be successful in real conditions. On the other hand, *in vivo* animal studies do not automatically prove antagonism in humans or other species. Therefore, the justification of using vertebrate animal models is questionable [32]. Gupta et al. [84] used *Drosophila melanogaster* commonly known as the "fruit fly," instead of a vertebrate animal model. It is a eukaryotic organism and is considered an alternative in the drug discovery process, mainly because the key physiological processes are well conserved from fly to humans. Moreover, a short life cycle, distinct developmental stages, easy cultivation, numerous offspring and a strong cytogenetic/genetic background make *Drosophila* a model organism to study many biological processes including toxicity testing. Zhou et al. [30] used porcine neonatal jejunal epithelial cell lines (IPEC-J2) for *in vitro* assay and worms (*Caenorhabditis elegans*) for *in vivo* testing of lactobacilli isolates against enterotoxigenic *E. coli*

Probiotic strains or strains with probiotic potential with efficient antimicrobial activity *in vivo* using animal models	Indicator pathogenic microorganisms	Reference
Lb:*L. reuteri* CL9, K16, K67 and S33	G-:*E. coli* O149: K88 JG280	[30]
Lb:*L. salivarius* JM32, *L. plantarum* PZ01 **Oth:** *P. acidilactici* JH231	G-:*S. Enteritidis* ATCC 13076	[34]
Lb:*L. plantarum* LA5 and *L. paracasei* LA7	G-:*S.* Typhi	[36]
Oth:*B. amyloliqufaciens*	G+:*C. difficile*	[54]
Lb:*L. plantarum* C014	G-:*A. hydrophila* TISTR 1321	[78]
Lb:*L. casei* B–7280, **Bb:** *B. longum* VK1, *B. bifidum*VK2	G+: *S. aureus*8325–4	[82]
Lb:*L. plantarum* LR/14	**Ins:***Drosophila melanogaster*	[84]
Lb:*L. acidophilus* CH1	**Prs:***Enterocytozoon bieneusi*	[85]
Oth:*Pseudoalteromonas* sp.	G-:*V. harveryi* ATCC 14126	[86]

Where probiotics are divided as follows: lb: lactobacilli; bb: Bifidobacterium; oth: other; and pathogens are divided as follows: G+: Gram positive; G−: Gram negative; fng: fungi; prs: parasite; ins: insect.

Table 4. A selection of assays published since 2013 of successful antimicrobial activity of chosen probiotics using the *in vivo* animal models on chosen pathogenic microorganisms.

The most recent *in vivo* antagonistic assays using animal models are noted in **Table 4**. These results confirm the strain specific antagonistic activity of chosen probiotics.

5.2. Recent results of determining the *in vivo* antimicrobial assays using clinical trials

Most important research on the antagonistic effect of probiotics are clinical trials, however only a few well conducted clinical studies have been reported. Most clinical studies include the comparison of antibiotic therapy with adjuvant probiotic therapy. In the study by Dore et al. [87], in this prospective, single centre, open label pilot study, patients scheduled for upper endoscopy for any reason and found to be positive for *H. pylori* infection were invited to enter. The intervention consisted of *L. reuteri* (DSM 17938, Reuflor, BioGaia AB, Sweden) 10^8 cfu/tablet plus pantoprazole (proton pump inhibitor) 20 mg twice a day. A 76% decrease in urease activity was observed. The absence of a control group with pantoprazole without *L. reuteri* however prevents any definite conclusion.

In the study by Pendharkar et al. [88] the clinical outcome for women conventionally treated for bacterial vaginosis and yeast infection with probiotics bacilli was investigated. This study is an example of the antibiotic therapy with adjuvant probiotic therapy. In the clinical trial, women were recruited in three groups as follows: women with bacterial vaginosis receiving clindamycin and metronidazole treatment together with a prolonged administration of EcoVag® (containing *L. rhamnosus* DSM 14870 and *L. gasseri* DSM 14869) for 10 consecutive days after each antibiotic treatment followed by weekly administration of capsules for next four months, women with recurrent vulvovaginal candidiasis receiving extended fluconazole and EcoVag® treatment, and women receiving extended fluconazole treatments only. The 6- and 12-month cure rates for bacterial vaginosis were 67 %. The 6- and 12-month cure rates for vulvovaginal candidiasis were 100 and 89% in women receiving fluconazole and EcoVag®, and 100 and 70% in women receiving fluconazole only. The study suggests that the treatment with antibiotics or anti-fungal medication in combination with EcoVag® capsules provide long-term cure against bacterial vaginosis and R-VVC.

Some of the most recent *in vivo* antagonistic clinical trials are noted in **Table 5**. These results confirm that adjuvant therapy with antibiotics and chosen probiotics enhances the antagonistic activity.

Probiotic strains with efficient antimicrobial activity using *in vivo* clinical trials and other therapies	**Pathogenic microorganisms or treated disease**	**Basic therapy**	**Type of trial**	**Reference**
Lb:*L. reuteri* DSM 17938	**G+:***H. pylori*	Proton pump inhibitor: pantoprazole	CT	[87]
Lb:*L. rhamnosus* DSM 14870, *L. gasseri* DSM 14869	**Bc:** not specified, **Fng:** *Candida* spp.	Antibiotics: Clindamycin, metronidazole, fluconazole	CT	[88]
Lb:*L. rhamnosus* GG (LGG), **Bb:** *B. bacterium* BB-12	**G+:***H. pylori*	Standard triple *H. pylori* eradication therapy with	DBRCT	[89]

http://dx.doi.org/10.5772/63141

Probiotic strains with efficient antimicrobial activity using *in vivo* clinical trials and other therapies	Pathogenic microorganisms or treated disease	Basic therapy	Type of trial	Reference
		antibiotics: omeprazole, pantoprazole, clarithromycin, amoxicillin, or metronidazole		
Lb:*L. rhamnosus* GG (LGG), *L. acidophilus* La-5, **Bb:** *B. bacterium* BB-12	**Dis:** AAD	Antibiotics: broad spectrum oral antibiotics	DBRCT	[90]
Lb:*L. acidophilus, L. paracasei***Bb:***B. lactis* **At:** bismuth	**G+:***H. pylori*	Antibiotics: broad spectrum oral antibiotics: lansoprazole, amoxicillin, clarithromycin	BDRCT	[91]
Lb:*L. casei* DN-114001	**Dis:** AAD	Antibiotics: broad spectrum oral antibiotics	CT	[92]
Lb:*L. acidophilus, l. rhamnosus, L. acidophilus, L. bulgaricus,* **Bb:***B. bifidus***Oth:***S. Thermophilus*	**Dis:** bacterial vaginosis	Antibiotic: metronidazole	CT	[93]

Where probiotics are divided as follows: lb: lactobacilli; bb: Bifidobacterium; oth: other; pathogens are divided as follows: bc: bacteria; G+: Gram positive; G–: Gram negative; fng: fungi; and clinical trials are divided as follows: DBRCT: double-blinded randomized clinical trial; CT: clinical trial; AT: additional therapy; Dis: disease; AAD: antibiotic associated diarrhoea.

Table 5. A selection of published since 2013 of antimicrobial activity of chosen probiotics using *in vivo* clinical trials on chosen pathogenic microorganisms or treatment of diseases.

6. Discussion and conclusions

The antimicrobial ability of probiotics is a very important trait and includes the production of antimicrobial compounds, competitive exclusion of pathogens, enhancement of the intestinal barrier function and others. Usually, probiotic strains produce more than one antimicrobial substance that may act synergistically, increasing the spectrum of targeted microorganisms. This property may be desirable as long as this antimicrobial spectrum is restricted to pathogenic microorganisms but it cannot be excluded that it will not affect the normal microbiota of the gut or other microbiotas as well [94]. The results show that probiotic properties are strain dependent and that strain identification is imperative [3].

Probiotic candidates have been accessed from very diverse habitats including faeces of breast-fed human infants [65, 69, 80, 85, 95], faeces of healthy adults [9, 15, 65, 70], faeces of elderly [81], faeces of children [25, 96], breast milk [42], human saliva [52], vaginal isolates of healthy women [66, 75], various fermented foods or beverages including raw or fermented milk [23, 35, 44], kefir [97], cheese [51, 56, 98], whey [99], yogurt [16, 41], dahi [100, 101], other dairy products [25, 36, 61], sourdough [102], sausages [17], fermented meat [24], kimchi [10, 62], maize [25, 59], fermented olives [103], Yerba mate [79], ragi [64], soy sauce [86], soil [104], as well as animal origin including rat faeces [71], geese [68], calves [105], pigs [45], fish [39, 60, 63, 78] and other seafood [40, 43, 46] and many others.

By far, the most commonly investigated probiotic were bacteria of the genus *Lactobacillus* (*L. plantarum, L. acidophilus, L. fermentum, L. casei, L. paracasei* and *L. reuteri*). The genus *Bifidobacterium* and other probiotic microorganisms (*Lactococcus, Pediococcus, Enterococcus, Bacillus* and *Saccharomyces*) have been also been investigated, but to a somewhat lesser extent. Studies were also conducted on known probiotics from various tissue type collections. The most common pathogens used to test the antagonistic activity of probiotics were different strains of S. aureus, E. faecium, E. faecalis, L. monocytogenes, E. coli, various Salmonella, Vibrio and Yersinia spp., and P. aeruginosa.

The antimicrobial activity of probiotic microorganisms has a very wide area application including adjuvant therapy to antibiotic consumption or for correcting dysbiosis of the gastrointestinal tract microbiome due to diarrhoea [37, 38, 106], antagonistic activity in humans against urinary tract infections [26, 66, 75], eradicating *H. pylori* infections [87], nosocomial infections [15, 96], dental biofilm formation [72], lowering serum cholesterol [10, 55], treating fevers [31], as well as in the agro-food industry for manufacturing fermented products [44, 62, 107], preventing food spoilage [16, 23, 41], as food additives for functional foods [50, 56, 57, 59, 67, 97], as prophylactic agents, adjuvants or alternatives to antibiotic therapies to antibiotic therapy in poultry [34, 47, 68], cattle [105, 108], pigs [45], fish [74, 78] and other livestock industry [104], just to name a few.

The process of determining antimicrobial properties of probiotic is complex and includes *in vitro* assays, *in vivo* models or substitute models, clinical studies, metagenomic analyses and mathematical modelling. Only after all these steps are completed, a probiotic candidate can be identified as such [109]. *In vitro* studies are the most represented. Although, they are a crucial step in selecting probiotic candidates, they are only the first step as efficient antimicrobial activity via *in vitro* studies does not necessarily mean that the antimicrobial activity is present in *in vivo* assays. Therefore, further research methods (double-blinded randomized clinical trials) are necessary to prove the important antimicrobial trait of probiotic candidates. As noted in Section 5.2, there are only a few well-conducted published clinical studies. Most clinical studies include the comparison of antibiotic therapy with adjuvant probiotic therapy which is an important aim of probiotic consumption.

There is a clear need for more elaborate assays that would better represent the complex interactions between the probiotics and the host microbiome to understand the consequences of the *in situ* production of antimicrobials by the former [94]. Another important fact is that probiotics are often found to have higher antagonist activity as multispecies groups [6, 7, 26]. Quorum sensing among probiotics is also an important factor; however, quorum-sensing studies among probiotics are sparse. It is well known that microorganisms coordinate collective behaviour in response to environmental challenges using sophisticated intercellular communication networks and that they are not limited to communication within their own species but are capable of intercepting messages and coerce cohabitants into behavioural modifications [110], therefore probiotics are included. Although all these facts make research of the antimicrobial/antagonistic activity of probiotics even more complex, it also presents a great opportunity for future research.

Author details

Sabina Fijan

Address all correspondence to: sabina.fijan@um.si

Faculty of Health Sciences, University of Maribor, Maribor, Slovenia

References

[1] Peterson J, Garges S, Giovanni M, McInnes P. The NIH human microbiome project. Genome Res. 2009;19:2317–2323.

[2] Rijkers GT, De Vos WM, Brummer RJ, Morelli L, Corthier G, Marteau P. Health benefits and health claims of probiotics: bridging science and marketing. Br J Nutr. 2011;106:1291–1296.

[3] Fijan S. Microorganisms with claimed probiotic properties. Int J Environ Res Public Health. 2014;11:4745–4767.

[4] Food and Agriculture Organization of the United Nations/World Health Organization FAO/WHO. Health and Nutritional Properties of Probiotics in Food including Powder Milk with Live Lactic [Internet]; 2001. Available from: http://www.who.int/foodsafety/publications/fs_management/en/probiotics.pdf [Accessed: 11.1.2016]

[5] Working Group on Drafting Guidelines for the Evaluation of Probiotics in Food. Guidelines for the Evaluation of Probiotics in Food; Joint FAO/WHO. London, Ontario, Canada: Food and Agriculture Organization of the United Nations/World Health Organization FAO/WHO; 2002.

[6] Fijan S. Influence of the growth of Pseudomonas aeruginosa in milk fermented by multispecies probiotics and Kefir microbiota. J Probiotics Health. 2016;3:136. DOI: 10.4172/2329-8901.1000136.

[7] Koning CJ, Jonkers D, Smidt H, Rombouts F, Pennings HJ, Wouters E, Stobberingh E, Stockbrügger R. The effect of a multispecies probiotic on the composition of the faecal microbiota and bowel habits in chronic obstructive pulmonary disease patients treated with antibiotics. Br J Nutr. 2010;103:1452–1460.

[8] He F, Morita H, Ouwehand AC. Bifidobacteria and lactobacilli exhibited different mitogenic activity on murine splenocytes. Int J Probiotics Prebiotics. 2006;1:77–82.

[9] Park S-Y; Lim S-D. Probiotic characteristics of *Lactobacillus plantarum* FH185 isolated from human feces. Korean J Food Sci. 2015;35(5):615–621.

[10] Choi EA, Chang HC. Cholesterol-lowering effects of a putative probiotic strain *Lactobacillus plantarum* EM isolated from kimchi. LWT – Food Sci Technol. 2015;62(1): 210–217.

[11] Sanders ME. Probiotics: definition, sources, selection, and uses. Clin Infect Dis. 2008;46(2):S58–S61. DOI: 10.1086/523341.

[12] Sanders ME. Summary of probiotic activities of *Bifidobacterium lactis* HN019. J Clin Gastroenterol. 2006; 40:776–783.

[13] Saxelin M, Tynkkynen S, Mattila-Sandholm T, de Vos WM. Probiotic and other functional microbes: from markets to mechanisms. Curr Opin Biotechnol. 2005;16:204–211.

[14] Millette M, Luquet FM, Lacroix M. In vitro growth control of selected pathogens by *Lactobacillus acidophilus*—and *Lactobacillus casei*-fermented milk. Lett Appl Microbiol. 2007;44:314–319.

[15] Ratsep M, Naaber P, Koljalg S, Smidt I, Shkut E, Sepp E. Effect of *Lactobacillus plantarum* strains on clinical isolates of *Clostridium difficile* in vitro. J Probiotics Health. 2014;2:119.

[16] Tharmaraj N, Shah N P. Antimicrobial effects of probiotics against selected pathogenic and spoilage bacteria in cheese-based dips. Int Food Res J. 2009;16:261–276.

[17] Ammor S, Tauveron G, Dufour E, Chevallier I. Antibacterial activity of lactic acid bacteria against spoilage and pathogenic bacteria isolated from the same meat small-scale facility. Food Control. 2006;17:454–461.

[18] Arqués JL, Rodríguez E, Langa S, Landete JM, Medina M. Antimicrobial activity of lactic acid bacteria in dairy products and gut: effect on pathogens. BioMed Res Int. 2015;2015:9. DOI: 10.1155/2015/584183.

[19] Šušković J, Kos B, Beganovič J, Leboš Pavunc A, Habjanič K, Matošić S. Antimicrobial activity—the most important property of probiotic and starter lactic acid bacteria. Food Technol Biotechnol. 2010;48(3):296–307.

[20] Tagg JR, Dajani AS, Wannmaker LW. Bacteriocines of gram positive bacteria. Bacteriol Rev. 1976;40:722–756.

[21] Hoover DG, Harlander SK. Screening methods for detecting bacteriocin activity. In: Hoover DG, Steenson LR, editors. Bacteriocins of lactic acid bacteria. San Diego: Academic Press; 1993. p. 23–29.

[22] Parente E, Brienza C, Moles M, Ricciardi A. A comparison of methods for the measurement of bacteriocin activity. J Microbiol Methods. 1995;22:95–108.

[23] Soomro AH, Musad T, Sammiand S, Rathore HA. Comparison of different methods for detection of antimicrobial activity of *Lactobacillus* spp. Pakistan J Zool. 2007;39(4):265–268.

[24] Pilasombut K, Rumjuankiat K, Ngamyeesoon N, Duy le ND. In vitro characterization of bacteriocin produced by lactic acid bacteria isolated from Nem Chua, a traditional Vietnamese fermented pork. Korean J Food Sci Anim. 2015;35(4):473–478.

[25] Jacobsen CN, Rosenfeldt Nielsen V, Hayford AE, Møller PL, Michaelsen KF, Paerregaard A, Sandström B, Tvede M, Jakobsen M. Screening of probiotic activities of forty-seven strains of *Lactobacillus* spp. by in vitro techniques and evaluation of the colonization ability of five selected strains in humans. Appl Environ Microbiol. 1999;65:4949–4956.

[26] Chapman CM1, Gibson GR, Rowland I. In vitro evaluation of single- and multi-strain probiotics: inter-species inhibition between probiotic strains, and inhibition of pathogens. Anaerobe. 2012;18(4):405–413. DOI: 10.1016/j.anaerobe.2012.05.004.

[27] Fijan S, Šostar Turk, S. Influence of the microbial community in Kefir Grains on the survival and growth of *Staphylococcus aureus* in Milk. Abstracts from the meeting: 7th Probiotics, prebiotics & new foods, September 8-10 2013; Rome, Iniversità Urbaniana. J Clin Gastroenterol. 2014;48(1):S113–S114.

[28] Fijan S, Trunk M, Šostar Turk S. Influence of the microbial community in kefir grains on the survival and growth of *Candida albicans* in milk. In: International scientific conference on probiotics and prebiotics, Budapest, June 24–26, 2014. Kysucké Nové Mesto: Pamida; 2014. p. 89.

[29] Presti I, D'Orazio G, Labra M, La Ferla B, Mezzasalma V, Bizzaro G, Giardina S, Michelotti A, Tursi F, Vassallo M, Di Gennaro P. Evaluation of the probiotic properties of new *Lactobacillus* and *Bifidobacterium* strains and their in vitro effect. Appl Microbiol Biotechnol. 2015;99(13):5613–5626. DOI: 10.1007/s00253-015-6482-8.

[30] Zhou M, Zhu J, Yu H, Yin X, Sabour PM, Zhao L, Chen W, Gong J. Investigation into in vitro and in vivo models using intestinal epithelial IPEC-J2 cells and *Caenorhabditis elegans* for selecting probiotic candidates to control porcine enterotoxigenic *Escherichia coli.* J Appl Microbiol. 2014;117(1):217–226. DOI: 10.1111/jam.12505.

[31] Abdel-Daim A, Hassouna N, Hafez M, Ashor MS, Aboulwafa MM. Antagonistic activity of *Lactobacillus* isolates against *Salmonella typhi* in vitro. Biomed Res Int. 2013;2013:680605. DOI: 10.1155/2013/680605.

[32] Cencič A. Can functional cell models replace laboratory animals in biomedical research? J Bioanal Biomed. 2012;4:e105. DOI: 10.4172/1948-593X.1000e105.

[33] Cencič A, Langerholc T. Functional cell models of the gut and their applications in food microbiology—a review. Int J Food Microbial. 2010;141:S4–S14. DOI: 10.1016/j.ijfoodmicro.2010.03.026.

[34] Feng J, Wang L, Zhou L, Yang X, Zhao X. Using in vitro immunomodulatory properties of lactic acid bacteria for selection of probiotics against *Salmonella* infection in broiler chicks. PLoS One. 2016;11(1):e0147630. DOI: 10.1371/journal.pone.0147630.

[35] Bujalance C, Jiménez-Valera M, Moreno E, Ruiz-López MD, Lasserrot A, Ruiz-Bravo A. Lack of correlation between in vitro antibiosis and in vivo protection against enteropathogenic bacteria by probiotic lactobacilli. Res Microbiol. 2014;165(1):14–20. DOI: DOI: 10.1016/j.resmic.2013.10.006.

[36] Mazaya B, Hamzawy MA, Khalil MA, Tawkol WM, Sabit H. Immunomodulatory and antimicrobial efficacy of *Lactobacilli* against enteropathogenic infection of *Salmonella typhi*: In-vitro and in-vivo study. Int J Immunopathol Pharmacol. 2015;28(4):469–478. DOI: 10.1177/0394632015592099.

[37] Bendali F1, Madi N, Sadoun D. Beneficial effects of a strain of *Lactobacillus* paracasei subsp. paracasei in *Staphylococcus aureus*-induced intestinal and colonic injury. Int J Infect Dis. 2011;15(11):e787–e794. DOI: 10.1016/j.ijid.2011.07.003.

[38] Chimchang J, Theparee T, Ladda B, Tanasupawat S, Wongsatayanon BT, Taweechotipatr M. Antimicrobial properties of a potential probiotic *Lactobacillus* from Thai newborn feces. J Med Assoc Thai. 2015;98(9):S116–S122.

[39] Pinpimai K, Rodkhum C, Chansue N, Katagiri T, Maita M, Pirarat N. The study on the candidate probiotic properties of encapsulated yeast, *Saccharomyces cerevisiae* JCM 7255, in Nile Tilapia (*Oreochromis niloticus*). Res Vet Sci. 2015;102:103–111. DOI: 10.1016/j.rvsc.2015.07.021.

[40] Liu XF, Li Y, Li JR, Cai LY, Li XX, Chen JR, Lyu SX. Isolation and characterisation of *Bacillus* spp. antagonistic to *Vibrio parahaemolyticus* for use as probiotics in aquaculture. World J Microbiol Biotechnol. 2015;31(5):795–803. DOI: 10.1007/s11274-015-1833-2.

[41] El-Kholy AM, El-Shinawy SH, Meshref AMS, Korny AM. Screening of antagonistic activity of probiotic bacteria against some food-borne pathogens. J Appl Environ Microbiol. 2014;2(2):53–60.

[42] Shokryazdan P,Sieo CC, Kalavathy R, Liang JB, Alitheen NB, Jahromi MF, Ho YW. Probiotic potential of *Lactobacillus* strains with antimicrobial activity against some human pathogenic strains. BioMed Res Int. 2014;2014:16. DOI: http://dx.DOI.org/10.1155/2014/927268.

[43] Muñoz-Atienza E, Araújo C, Magadán S, Hernández PE, Herranz C, Santos Y, Cintas LM. In vitro and in vivo evaluation of lactic acid bacteria of aquatic origin as probiotics for turbot (Scophthalmus maximus L.) farming. Fish Shellfish Immunol. 2014;41(2): 570–580. DOI: 10.1016/j.fsi.2014.10.007.

[44] Mami A, Kerfouf A, Kihal M. Study of the antimicrobial and probiotic effect of *Lactobacillus Plantarum* isolated from raw goat's milk from the region of Western Algeria. Int J Sci Basic Appl Res. 2014;13(1):18–27.

[45] Han SK, Shin MS, Park HE, Kim SY, Lee WK. Screening of bacteriocin-producing Enterococcus faecalis strains for antagonistic activities against Clostridium perfringens. Korean J Food Sci Anim Resour. 2014;34(5):614–621.

[46] Wu HJ, Sun LB, Li CB, Li ZZ, Zhang Z, Wen XB, Hu Z, Zhang YL, Li SK. Enhancement of the immune response and protection against *Vibrio parahaemolyticus* by indigenous probiotic *Bacillus* strains in mud crab (*Scylla paramamosain*). Fish Shellfish Immunol. 2014;41(2):156–162. DOI: 10.1016/j.fsi.2014.08.027.

[47] Menconi A, Kallapura G, Latorre JD, Morgan MJ, Pumford NR, Hargis BM, Tellez G. Identification and characterization of lactic acid bacteria in a commercial probiotic culture. Biosci Microbiota Food Health. 2014;33(1):25–30. DOI: 10.12938/bmfh.33.25.

[48] Belicova A, Mikulašova M, Dušinsky R. Probiotic potential and safety properties of *Lactobacillus plantarum* from Slovak Bryndza cheese. Biomed Res Int. 2013;2013:760928. DOI: 10.1155/2013/760298.

[49] Chapman CM, Gibson GR, Todd S, Rowland I. Comparative in vitro inhibition of urinary tract pathogens by single- and multi-strain probiotics. Eur J Nutr. 2013;52(6): 1669–1677. DOI: 10.1007/s00394-013-0501-2.

[50] Tulini FL, Winkelströter LK, De Martinis EC. Identification and evaluation of the probiotic potential of *Lactobacillus paraplantarum* FT259, a bacteriocinogenic strain isolated from Brazilian semi-hard artisanal cheese. Anaerobe. 2013;22:57–63. DOI: 10.1016/j.anaerobe.2013.06.006.

[51] Ali F S, Saad O A O, Salwa AH. Antimicrobial activity of probiotic bacteria. Egypt Acad J Biol Sci. 2013;5(2):21–34.

[52] Aoudia N, Rieu A, Briandet R, Deschamps J, Chluba J, Jego G, Garrido C, Guzzo J. Biofilms of *Lactobacillus plantarum* and *Lactobacillus fermentum*: effect on stress responses, antagonistic effects on pathogen growth and immunomodulatory properties. Food Microbiol. 2016;53(Pt A):51–59. DOI: DOI: 10.1016/j.fm.2015.04.009.

[53] Aminnezhad S, Kermanshahi RK, Ranjbar R. Evaluation of synergistic interactions between cell-free supernatant of *Lactobacillus* Strains and Amikacin and genetamicin against *Pseudomonas aeruginosa*. Jundishapur J Microbiol. 2015;18(8):e16592. DOI: 10.5812/jjm.8(4)2015.16592.

[54] Geeraerts S, Ducatelle R, Haesebrouck F, Van Immerseel F. Bacillus amyloliquefaciens as prophylactic treatment for *Clostridium difficile*-associated disease in a mouse model. J Gastroenterol Hepatol. 2015;30(8):1275–1280. DOI: 10.1111/jgh.12957.

[55] Damodharan K, Lee YS, Palaniyandi SA, Yang SH, Suh JW. Preliminary probiotic and technological characterization of Pediococcus pentosaceus strain KID7 and in vivo

assessment of its cholesterol-lowering activity. Front Microbiol. 2015;6:768. DOI: 10.3389/fmicb.2015.00768.

[56] Caggia C, De Angelis M, Pitino I, Pino A, Randazzo CL. Probiotic features of *Lactobacillus* strains isolated from Ragusano and Pecorino Siciliano cheeses. Food Microbiol. 2015;50:109–117. DOI: 10.1016/j.fm.2015.03.010.

[57] Abbaszadeh S, Tavakoli R, Sharifzadeh A, Shokri H. Lactic acid bacteria as functional probiotic isolates for inhibiting the growth of *Aspergillus flavus, A. parasiticus, A. niger* and *Penicillium chrysogenum*. J Mycol Med. 2015;25(4):263–267. DOI: 10.1016/j.mycmed.2015.10.011.

[58] Ünlü G, Nielsen B, Ionita C. Production of Antilisterial Bacteriocins from lactic acid bacteria in dairy-based media: a comparative study. Probiotics Antimicrob Proteins. 2015;7(4):259–274. DOI: 10.1007/s12602-015-9200-z.

[59] Yu X, Yin J, Li L, Luan C, Zhang J, Zhao C, Li S. Prebiotic potential of xylooligosaccharides derived from corn cobs and their in vitro antioxidant activity when combined with *Lactobacillus*. J Microbiol Biotechnol. 2015;25(7):1084–1092. DOI 10.4014/jmb.1501.01022.

[60] Thankappan B1, Ramesh D, Ramkumar S, Natarajaseenivasan K, Anbarasu K. Characterization of Bacillus spp. from the gastrointestinal tract of *Labeo rohita*—towards to identify novel probiotics against fish pathogens. Appl Biochem Biotechnol. 2015;175(1):340–353. DOI: 10.1007/s12010-014-1270-y.

[61] Georgievaa R, Yochevab L, Tserovskab L, Zhelezovab G, Stefanovaa N, Atanasovaa A, Dangulevaa A, Ivanovaa G, Karapetkova N, Rumyana N, Karaivanovaa E. Antimicrobial activity and antibiotic susceptibility of Lactobacillus and Bifidobacterium spp. intended for use as starter and probiotic cultures. Biotechnol Biotech Equipm. 2015;29(1):84–91. DOI: 10.1080/13102818.2014.987450.

[62] Baick SC, Kim CH. Assessment of characteristics and functional properties of *Lactobacillus* species isolated from Kimchi for dairy use. Korean J Food Sci Anim Resour. 2015;35(3):339–349. DOI: 10.5851/kosfa.2015.35.3.339.

[63] Diana CR, Humberto HS, Jorge YF. Probiotic properties of *Leuconostoc mesenteroides* isolated from Aguamiel of *Agave salmiana*. Probiotics Antimicrob Proteins. 2015;7(2): 107–117. DOI: 10.1007/s12602-015-9187-5.

[64] VidyaLaxme B, Rovetto A, Grau R, Agrawal R. Synergistic effects of probiotic *Leuconostoc mesenteroides* and *Bacillus subtilis* in malted ragi (*Eleucine corocana*) food for antagonistic activity against *V. cholerae* and other beneficial properties. J Food Sci Technol. 2014;51(11):3072–3082. DOI: 10.1007/s13197-012-0834-5.

[65] Gomathi S, Sasikumar P, Anbazhagan K, Sasikumar S, Kavitha M, Selvi MS, Sadasivam Selvam G. Screening of indigenous oxalate degrading lactic acid bacteria from

human faeces and South Indian fermented foods: assessment of probiotic potential. Sci World J. 2014;2014:11. DOI: 10.1155/2014/648059.

[66] Trivedi D, Jena PK, Seshadri S. Colicin E2 Expression in *Lactobacillus brevis* DT24, a vaginal probiotic isolate, against uropathogenic *Escherichia coli*. ISRN Urol. 2014;2014:869610. DOI: 10.1155/2014/869610.

[67] Gotteland M, Cires MJ, Carvallo C, Vega N, Ramirez MA, Morales P, Rivas P, Astudillo F, Navarrete P, Dubos C, Figueroa A, Troncoso M, Ulloa C, Mizgier ML, Carrasco-Pozo C, Speisky H, Brunser O, Figueroa G. Probiotic screening and safety evaluation of Lactobacillus strains from plants, artisanal goat cheese, human stools, and breast milk. J Med Food. 2014;17(4):487–495. DOI: DOI: 10.1089/jmf.2013.0030.

[68] Dec M, Puchalski A, Urban-Chmiel R, Wernicki A. Screening of Lactobacillus strains of domestic goose origin against bacterial poultry pathogens for use as probiotics. Poult Sci. 2014;93(10):2464–2472. DOI: DOI: 10.3382/ps.2014-04025.

[69] Amer EI, Mossallam SF, Mahrous H. Therapeutic enhancement of newly derived bacteriocins against *Giardia lamblia*. Exp Parasitol. 2014;146:52–63. DOI: 10.1016/j.exppara.2014.09.005.

[70] Mirnejad R, Vahdati AR, Rashidiani J, Erfani M, Piranfar V. The antimicrobial effect of *Lactobacillus casei* culture supernatant against multiple drug resistant clinical isolates of *Shigella sonnei* and *Shigella flexneri* in vitro. Iran Red Crescent Med J. 2013;15(2):122–126. DOI: 10.5812/ircmj.7454.

[71] Jena PK, Trivedi D, Thakore K, Chaudhary H, Giri SS, Seshadri S. Isolation and characterization of probiotic properties of *Lactobacilli* isolated from rat fecal microbiota. Microbiol Immunol. 2013;57(6):407–416. DOI: 10.1111/1348-0421.12054.

[72] Wu CC, Lin CT, Wu CY, Peng WS, Lee MJ, Tsai YC. Inhibitory effect of *Lactobacillus salivarius* on *Streptococcus mutans* biofilm formation. Mol Oral Microbiol. 2015;30(1):16–26. DOI: 10.1111/omi.12063.

[73] Torres NI, Noll KS, Xu S, Li J, Huang Q, Sinko PJ, Wachsman MB, Chikindas ML. Safety, formulation, and in vitro antiviral activity of the antimicrobial peptide subtilosin against herpes simplex virus type 1. Probiotics Antimicrob Proteins. 2013;5(1):26–35. DOI: 10.1007/s12602-012-9123-x.

[74] Das A, Nakhro K, Chowdhury S, Kamilya D. Effects of potential probiotic Bacillus amyloliquefaciens [corrected] FPTB16 on systemic and cutaneous mucosal immune responses and disease resistance of catla (*Catla catla*). Fish Shellfish Immunol. 2013;35(5):1547-53. DOI: 10.1016/j.fsi.2013.08.022.

[75] Chew SY, Cheah YK, Seow HF, Sandai D, Than LT. Probiotic *Lactobacillus rhamnosus* GR-1 and *Lactobacillus reuteri* RC-14 exhibit strong antifungal effects against vulvovaginal candidiasis-causing *Candida glabrata* isolates. J Appl Microbiol. 2015;118(5):1180–1190. DOI: 10.1111/jam.12772.

[76] Bian X, Evivie SE, Muhammad Z, Luo GW, Liang HZ, Wang NN, Huo GC. In vitro assessment of the antimicrobial potentials of *Lactobacillus helveticus* strains isolated from traditional cheese in Sinkiang China against food-borne pathogens. Food Funct. 2016;7: 789-797. DOI: 10.1039/C5FO01041A.

[77] Yang JJ, Niu CC, Guo XH. Mixed culture models for predicting intestinal microbial interactions between *Escherichia coli* and *Lactobacillus* in the presence of probiotic *Bacillus subtilis*. Benef Microbes. 2015;6(6):871–877. DOI: 10.3920/BM2015.0033.

[78] Butprom S, Phumkhachorn P, Rattanachaikunsopon P. Effect of *Lactobacillus plantarum* C014 on innate immune response and disease resistance against *Aeromonas hydrophila* in hybrid catfish. ScientificWorldJournal. 2013;2013:392523. DOI: 10.1155/2013/392523.

[79] Gonzalez-Gil F, Diaz-Sanchez S, Pendleton S, Andino A, Zhang N, Yard C, Crilly N, Harte F, Hanning I. Yerba mate enhances probiotic bacteria growth in vitro but as a feed additive does not reduce Salmonella Enteritidis colonization in vivo. Poult Sci. 2014;93(2):434–440. DOI: 10.3382/ps.2013-03339.

[80] Muñoz-Quezada S, Bermudez-Brito M, Chenoll E, Genovés S, Gomez-Llorente C, Plaza-Diaz J, Matencio E, Bernal MJ, Romero F, Ramón D, Gil A. Competitive inhibition of three novel bacteria isolated from faeces of breast milk-fed infants against selected enteropathogens. Br J Nutr. 2013;109;(2):S63–S69. DOI: 10.1017/ S0007114512005600.

[81] Likotrafiti E, Tuohy KM, Gibson GR, Rastall RA. Development of antimicrobial synbiotics using potentially-probiotic faecal isolates of *Lactobacillus fermentum* and *Bifidobacterium longum*. Anaerobe. 2013;20:5–13. DOI: 10.1016/j.anaerobe.2013.01.002.

[82] Lazarenko L, Babenko L, Shynkarenko Sichel, Pidgorskyi V, Mokrozub V, Voronkova O, Spivak M. Antagonistic action of Lactobacilli and bifidobacteria in relation to *Staphylococcus aureus* and their influence on the immune response in cases of intravaginal Staphylococcosis in mice. Probiotics Antimicrob Proteins. 2012;4(2):78–89.

[83] Bratz K, Gölz G, Janczyk P, Nöckler K, Alter T. Analysis of in vitro and in vivo effects of probiotics against *Campylobacter* spp. Berl Munch Tierarztl Wochenschr. 2015;128(3–4):155–162.

[84] Gupta R, Sarkar S, Srivastava S. In vivo toxicity assessment of antimicrobial peptides (AMPs LR14) derived from *Lactobacillus plantarum* Strain LR/14 in *Drosophila melanogaster*. Probiotics Antimicrob Proteins. 2014;6(1):59–67. DOI: 10.1007/s12602-013-9154-y.

[85] Mossallam SF, Amer EI, Diab RG. Potentiated anti-microsporidial activity of *Lactobacillus acidophilus* CH1 bacteriocin using gold nanoparticles. Exp parasitol. 2014;144:14–21.

[86] Morya VK, Choi W, Kim EK. Isolation and characterization of *Pseudoalteromonas* sp. from fermented Korean food, as an antagonist to *Vibrio harveyi*. Appl Microbiol Biotechnol. 2014;98(3):1389–1395. DOI: 10.1007/s00253-013-4937-3.

[87] Dore MP, Cuccu M, Pes GM, Manca A, Graham DY. *Lactobacillus reuteri* in the treatment of *Helicobacter pylori* infection. Intern Emerg Med. 2014;9:649–654. DOI: 10.1007/s11739-013-1013-z

[88] Pendharkar S, Brandsborg E, Hammarström L, Marcotte H, Larsson PG. Vaginal colonisation by probiotic lactobacilli and clinical outcome in women conventionally treated for bacterial vaginosis and yeast infection. BMC Infect Dis. 2015;15:255. DOI: 10.1186/s12879-015-0971-3.

[89] Hauser G, Salkic N, Vukelic K, Jajac Knez A, Stimac D. Probiotics for standard triple *Helicobacter pylori* eradication: a randomized, double-blind, placebo-controlled trial. Medicine (Baltimore). 2015;94(17):e685, DOI: 10.1097/MD.0000000000000685.

[90] Fox MJ, Ahuja KD, Robertson IK, Ball MJ, Eri RD. Can probiotic yogurt prevent diarrhoea in children on antibiotics? A double-blind, randomised, placebo-controlled study. BMJ Open. 2015;5(1):e006474. DOI: 10.1136/bmjopen-2014-006474.

[91] Srinarong C, Siramolpiwat S, Wongcha-um A, Mahachai V, Vilaichone RK. Improved eradication rate of standard triple therapy by adding bismuth and probiotic supplement for *Helicobacter pylori* treatment in Thailand. Asian Pac J Cancer Prev. 2014;15(22): 9909–9913.

[92] Dietrich CG, Kottmann T, Alavi M. Commercially available probiotic drinks containing *Lactobacillus casei* DN-114001 reduce antibiotic-associated diarrhea. World J Gastroenterol. 2014;20(42):15837–15844. DOI: 10.3748/wjg.v20.i42.15837.

[93] Bodean O, Munteanu O, Cirstoiu C, Secara D, Cirstoiu M. Probiotics—a helpful additional therapy for bacterial vaginosis. J Med Life. 2013;6(4):434–436.

[94] Papadimitriou K, Zoumpopoulou G, Foligné B, Alexandraki V, Kazou M, Pot B, Tsakalidou E. Discovering probiotic microorganisms: in vitro, in vivo, genetic and omics approaches. Front Microbiol. 2015;6:58. DOI: 10.3389/fmicb.2015.00058.

[95] Basyigit Kilic G, Kuleasan H, Sömer VF, Akpinar D. Determining potential probiotic properties of human originated *Lactobacillus plantarum* Strains. Biotechnol Bioprocess Eng. 2013;18:479–485. DOI: 10.1007/s12257-012-0785-8.

[96] Jamalifar H, Rahimi HR, Samadi N, Shahverdi AR, Sharifian Z, Hosseini F, Eslahi H, Fazeli MR. Antimicrobial activity of different *Lactobacillus* species against multi-drug resistant clinical isolates of *Pseudomonas aeruginosa*. Iran J Microbiol. 2011;3(1):21–25.

[97] Carasi P, Díaz M, Racedo SM, De Antoni G, Urdaci MC, Serradell Mde L. Safety characterization and antimicrobial properties of kefir-isolated *Lactobacillus kefiri*. Biomed Res Int. 2014;2014:208974. DOI: 10.1155/2014/208974.

[98] Zavišić G, Ristić S, Petrièević S, Novaković Jovanović J, Janać Petković B, Strahinić I, Piperski V. Characterisation and preliminary lipid-lowering evaluation of *Lactobacillus* isolated from a traditional Serbian dairy product. Benef Microbes. 2015;6(1):119–128. DOI: 10.3920/BM2014.0018.

[99] Goyal N, Dixit K, Gandhi D. Antimicrobial activity of probiotic *Lactobacillus* strains towards *Salmonella enterica* ser enteritidis in whey. Internet J Microbiol. 2007;5(1):6.

[100] Shandilya UK, Sharma A, Kapila R, Kansal VK. Probiotic Dahi containing *Lactobacillus acidophilus* and *Bifidobacterium bifidum* modulates immunoglobulin levels and cytokines expression in whey proteins sensitized mice. J Sci Food Agric. 2015. DOI: 10.1002/jsfa.7497.

[101] Kaushal D, Kansal VK. Dahi containing *Lactobacillus acidophilus* and *Bifidobacterium bifidum* improves phagocytic potential of macrophages in aged mice. J Food Sci Technol. 2014;51(6):1147–1153. DOI 10.1007/s13197-012-0637-8.

[102] Tan Q1, Xu H, Aguilar ZP, Peng S, Dong S, Wang B, Li P, Chen T, Xu F, Wei H. Safety assessment and probiotic evaluation of *Enterococcus faecium* YF5 isolated from sourdough. J Food Sci. 2013;78(4):M587–M593. DOI: 10.1111/1750-3841.12079.

[103] Argyri AA, Zoumpopoulou G, Karatzas KA, Tsakalidou E, Nychas GJ, Panagou EZ, Tassou CC. Selection of potential probiotic lactic acid bacteria from fermented olives by in vitro tests. Food Microbiol. 2013;33(2):282–291. DOI: 10.1016/j.fm.2012.10.005.

[104] Isa K, Oka K, Beauchamp N, Sato M, Wada K, Ohtani K, Nakanishi S, McCartney E, Tanaka M, Shimizu T, Kamiya S, Kruger C, Takahashi M. Safety assessment of the *Clostridium butyricum* MIYAIRI 588® probiotic strain including evaluation of antimicrobial sensitivity and presence of Clostridium toxin genes in vitro and teratogenicity in vivo. Hum Exp Toxicol. 2015. DOI: 10.1177/0960327115607372.

[105] Eberhart LJ, Ochoa JN, Besser TE, Call DR. Microcin MccPDI reduces the prevalence of susceptible *Escherichia coli* in neonatal calves. J Appl Microbiol. 2014;117(2):340–346. DOI: 10.1111/jam.12535.

[106] Iordache F, Iordache C, Chifiriuc MC, Bleotu C, Smarandache D, Sasarman E, Laza V, Bucu M, Dracea D, Larion C, Cota A, Lixandru M. Antimicrobial and immunomodulatory activity of some probiotic fractions with potential clinical application. Arch Zootech. 2008;11(3): 41–51.

[107] Beganović J1, Kos B, Leboš Pavunc A, Uroić K, Džidara P, Šušković J. Proteolytic activity of probiotic strain *Lactobacillus helveticus* M92. Anaerobe. 2013;20:58–64. DOI: 10.1016/j.anaerobe.2013.02.004.

[108] Soleimani NA, Kermanshahi RK, Yakchali B, Sattari TN. Antagonistic activity of probiotic lactobacilli against *Staphylococcus aureus* isolated from bovine mastitis. Afr J Microbiol Res. 2010;4(20):2169–2173.

[109] Buffie CG, Bucci V, Stein RR, McKenney PT, Ling L, Gobourne A, No D, Liu H, Kinnebrew M, Viale A, Littmann E, van den Brink MR, Jenq RR, Taur Y, Sander C,

Cross JR, Toussaint NC, Xavier JB, Pamer EG. Precision microbiome reconstitution restores bile acid mediated resistance to *Clostridium difficile*. Nature. 2015;517(7533): 205–208. DOI: 10.1038/nature13828.

[110] Atkinson S, Williams PJ. Quorum sensing and social networking in the microbial world. R Soc Interface. 2009;6(40):959–978.

Chapter 11

Probiotics in Childhood Celiac Disease

Caterina Anania, Francesca Olivero,
Eugenia Olivero and Lucia Pacifico

Additional information is available at the end of the chapter

http://dx.doi.org/10.5772/63119

Abstract

Celiac disease (CD) is an autoimmune enteropathy induced by gluten ingestion in genetically susceptible individuals. Genetic predisposition plays an important role in the development of CD, but it is not sufficient by itself for the disease development. Although gluten proteins are the main environmental factor involved in CD pathogenesis and ingestion of gluten is necessary to manifest the disease, recent studies have suggested that alteration of the microbiota could be involved and, in particular, the interplay between gut microbiota and the mucosal immune system. Dysbiosis, the alteration of the microbiota, has been associated with a variety of intestinal pathologies including Crohn disease and CD. Most observational studies in children and adults with CD have shown alterations in the intestinal microbiota composition compared to control subjects, which is only partially recovered after treatment with a gluten-free diet (GFD). At this time, the only treatment for CD is lifelong adherence to a GFD, which involves the elimination of grains containing gluten, wheat, rye, and barley. However, it is difficult for many patients to follow a GFD. Abnormalities in the gut microbiome in CD patients have led to the use of probiotics as a promising alternative as a therapeutic or preventative approach.

Keywords: celiac disease, gluten free diet, intestinal microbiota, dysbiosis, probiotics

1. Introduction

Celiac disease (CD) is an autoimmune enteropathy induced by gluten ingestion in genetically susceptible individuals [1]. The major genetic risk factor for CD is represented by HLA-DQ genes. Ninety percent of affected individuals carry the HLA-DQ2 haplotype, 5% the DQ8 haplotype, and the remaining 5% carry at least one of the two DQ2 alleles [1, 2]. Genetic predisposition plays an important role in the development of CD but it is not sufficient by itself for the disease development [3]. Approximately, 30% of the general population carry the HLA-DQ2/8 CD susceptibility genes, however, only 2–5% of these individuals will develop CD, suggesting that additional environmental factors contribute to disease development [4]. Although gluten proteins are the main environmental factor involved in CD pathogenesis and ingestion of gluten is necessary to manifest the disease, recent studies have suggested that potential factors such as birth delivery, breast-feeding, infectious agents, and antibiotic intake could contribute to the development of CD [5–7]. The alteration of the microbiota could also be involved and, in particular, the interplay between gut microbiota and the mucosal immune system [8].

The microbiota, the set of microorganisms that colonize the human body, has a fundamental role for the host. It is important for both physiological and metabolic factors, ranging from the absorption of nutrients to the regulation and development of the immune system [9]. Dysbiosis, the alteration of the microbiota, has been associated with a variety of pathologies like Crohn disease and obesity [10, 11]. Most observational studies in children and adults with CD have shown alterations in the intestinal microbiota composition compared to control subjects, which is partially recovered after treatment with a gluten-free diet (GFD) [12–14]. It has been demonstrated that levels of *Bifidobacteria* and *Lactobacilli* are reduced in CD patients [14, 15]. Specific alterations in the microbiota could contribute to the etiopathogenesis of CD by providing proteolytic activities that influence the generation of toxic and immunogenic peptides from gluten, and compromise the intestinal barrier function [16]. Probiotics are nonpathogenic live microorganisms, which, when orally administered in adequate amounts, alter the microflora of the host and have beneficial health effect [17].

At this time, the only treatment for CD is lifelong adherence to a GFD, which involves the elimination of grains containing gluten, wheat, rye, and barley. However, it is difficult for many patients to follow a GFD. Some probiotics have been found to digest or alter gluten polypeptides [18]. Abnormalities in the gut microbiome in CD patients have led to the use of probiotics as a promising alternative as a therapeutic or preventative approach.

Here we focus on the role of microbiota in the pathogenesis of CD and on the chances for probiotics to be involved in an alternative treatment strategy.

2. Microbiota composition in celiac children

Several research papers have suggested that an important risk factor involved in the etiology of CD could be the gut microbiota. Multiple studies investigating the role of gut microbiota in CD have been performed on fecal samples and, later, on duodenal biopsies.

The studies that have addressed the relation between fecal microbiota and CD in the pediatric population are summarized in **Table 1** [13, 19–24]. In the earliest report involving a total of 49 children, 26 celiac patients aged 12–48 months and 23 age-matched controls, Collado et al. evaluated the composition of the fecal microbiota by both culture-dependent and culture-independent methods using fluorescent in situ hybridization (FISH) [13]. They showed a high level of *Bacteroides, Clostridium,* and *Staphylococcus* in fecal samples from CD children compared to healthy subjects when analyzed by culture methods. The numbers of *Bacteroides-Prevotella, Clostridium histolyticum, Eubacterium rectale-Clostridium coccoides, Atopobium,* and sulfate-reducing bacterial groups were also significantly higher in fecal samples from CD children analyzed by FISH [13]. Subsequently, Sanz et al. [19], using polymerase chain reaction (PCR) and denaturing gradient gel electrophoresis (DGGE) in 10 CD children aged 15–45 months and 10 age-matched healthy controls, demonstrated that the presence of species such as *Lactobacillus curvatus, Leuconostoc mesenteroides,* and *Leuconostoc carnosus* were characteristic of coeliac patients, while the *Lactobacillus casei* group was characteristic of healthy controls. Moreover, the authors found a reduction in *Bifidobacterium* population diversity in CD patients. Collado et al. [20], using real-time PCR, evaluated duodenal and fecal microbiota in three groups of children: (1) untreated CD patients on a gluten-containing diet (GCD); (2) treated CD patients who had been on a GFD for a minimum of two years; and (3) healthy controls. They found that feces and biopsies of CD patients had an increased presence of *Bifidobacterium, Bacteroides, and Clostridium leptum* groups with respect to the control group; *Escherichia coli and Staphylococcus* were otherwise predominant in CD subjects on GFD. GFD determined a complete normalization of gut microbiota [20]. De Palma et al. examined fecal microbiology and immunoglobulin-associated features in active and non-active stages of CD in children and in age-matched controls [21]. They found that in CD patients there was an alteration in the type of fecal immunoglobulin-coated bacteria along with a shift in the composition of the microbiota. In fact, they demonstrated a reduction of the percentages of the IgA-coated bacteria in CD patients on a GFD and in those not following a GFD compared to the control group. They also found a reduction of the percentages of IgG- and IgM-coated bacteria in treated CD patients with respect to untreated CD subjects and control group. Moreover, treated and untreated CD subjects showed a predominance of *Bacteroides-Prevotella* as well as an impaired mucosal barrier, as suggested by the reduction of IgA-coated bacteria with respect to the controls [21]. Sanchez et al., in an attempt to determine whether intestinal *Staphylococcus* spp. and their pathogenic features differed between CD patients and healthy controls, studied 40 CD children (20 active CD and 20 non-active CD) and 20 healthy controls [22]. *Staphylococci* were isolated from feces and identified by PCR and DNA sequencing. CD was associated with alterations in species diversity and composition of the fecal *Staphylococcus* population. *Staphylococcus epidermidis* isolates carrying the *mecA* gene and both the *mecA* and *atlE* genes were more abundant in CD patients than in controls, most likely reflecting increased exposure of these subjects to opportunistic staphylococcal pathogens and antimicrobials, which in turn affected the composition/features of their intestinal microbiota [22]. Di Cagno et al. in a study including seven CD patients on GFD, seven CD patients on a GCD, and seven healthy controls, utilizing DGGE analysis and gas chromatography-mass spectrometry-solid-phase microextraction analysis of fecal volatile organic compounds (VOCs), found that the fecal microbiota and VOCs of CD patients on GFD were more similar to those of healthy patients than to those of CD patients on GCD [23]. Consequently, the authors speculated that *Lactobacillus* and *Bifidobacterium* strains isolated from healthy children could be a potential probiotic treatment to restore the balance of intestinal microbiota in treated and untreated CD patients [23]. Similar conclusions have been reached by Lorenzo Pisarello et al. [24] in a very recent work. They found lower counts of *Lactobacillus* in the feces of CD compared to controls. Furthermore, the authors selected from feces of controls 5 *Lactobacillus* strains because of their high resistance percentages to gastrointestinal tract conditions. *Lactobacillus rhamnosus* (LC4) showed the highest percentage of autoaggregation and *Lactobacillus paracasei* showed high hydrophobicity suggesting a potential use of these strains as probiotics in CD [24].

Author/ References	Year	Country	Patients population and sample size	Methods	Main results
Collado et al. [13]	2007	Spain	26 untreated CD (mean age, 26 months) 23 controls (mean age, 23.1 months)	Culture+ FISH	In untreated CD: ↑ *Bacteroides* ↑ *Staphylococcus* ↑ *Clostridium* ↑ *Bacteroides-Prevotella,* ↑ *Clostridium hystoliticum,* ↑ *Eubacterium rectale-C. coccoides,* ↑ *Atopobium, Staphylococcus* ↓ *Bifidobacterium*
Sanz et al. [19]	2007	Spain	10 untreated CD (mean age, 28 months) 10 controls (mean age, 24 months)	Culture+qPCR +DGGE	In untreated CD: High diversity of fecal microbiota ↑ *Leuconostoc carnosum,* ↑ *Leuconostoc mesenteroides,* ↑ *Lactobacillus curvatus* ↓ *Lactobacillus casei,* ↓ *Bifidobacterium adolescentis*
Collado et al. [20]	2009	Spain	30 untreated CD (mean age, 38.5 months) 18 treated CD (mean age, 37.7 months) 30 controls (mean age, 33.5 months)	qPCR	In untreated and treated CD: ↑ Bacterial count ↑ *E. coli,* ↑ *Bacteroides,* ↑ *Clostridium leptum* *Staphylococcus* prevalence ↓ *Bifidobacterium* In treated CD: ↑ *Lactobacillus*
Di Cagno et al. [23]	2009	Italy	7 untreated CD (range, 6–12 years) 7 treated CD (range, 6–12 years) 7 (range, 6–12 years) controls	PCR+DGGE	In treated and untreated CD: ↓ Ratio of cultivable lactic acid bacteria and *Bifidobacterium* to *Bacteroides* and *Enterobacteria* In treated CD and in controls: *Lactobacillus brevis, Lactobacillus rossiae, Lactobacillus pentosus* Only in controls:

Author/ References	Year	Country	Patients population and sample size	Methods	Main results
					Lactobacillus fermentum, Lactobacillus delbrueckii subsp., *Lactobacillus bulgaricus, Lactobacillus gasseri*
De Palma et al. [21]	2010	Spain	24 untreated CD (mean age, 5.5 years) 18 treated CD (mean age, 5.5 years) 20 controls (mean age, 5.3 years)	FISH+ flow cytometry	In untreated CD: ↓ *Bifidobacterium,* ↓ *Clostridium histoliticum,* ↓ *Clostridium lituseburense,* ↓ *Fecalibacterium prausnitzii* ↑ *Bacteroides-Prevotella* In untreated CD and in controls: ↓ Levels of IgA coating the *Bacteroides-Prevotella*
Sanchez et al. [22]	2012	Spain	20 (mean age, 57.4 months) untreated CD 20 (mean age, 67.3 months) treated CD 20 (mean age, 54.0 months) controls	PCR+ DNA sequencing	In untreated CD: ↑ *Staphylococcus* spp. diversity ↑ *Staphylococcus haemolyticus* ↓ *Staphylococcus aureus* ↑ *mecA* and *atIE* genes in *S. epidermidis* clones
Lorenzo Pisarello et al. [24]	2015	Argentina	15 treated CD (mean age, 7.5 years) 15 controls (mean age, 6.5 years)	Culture (autoaggregation assay, hydrophobicity assay)	In treated CD ↓ *Lactobacilli* ↑ *Enterobacteria* *Lactobacillus rhamnosus and Lactobacillus paracasei* identified to improve sign and symptom in CD

CD celiac disease, *FISH* fluorescent in situ hybridization, *DGGE* denaturing gradient gel electrophoresis, *PCR* polymerase chain reaction, *qPCR* quantitative polymerase chain reaction.

Table 1. Fecal microbiota in celiac disease.

Duodenal microbial composition of pediatric CD patients was explored more extensively later on, with the main findings summarized in **Table 2** [20, 25–33]. Microbiota characterization from duodenal biopsy specimens was initially carried out on CD Spanish children by Nadal et al. [25] in 2007. The authors, in an attempt to identify the specific composition of the duodenal microbiota of celiac patients (with active and non-active disease), evaluated 20 CD patients on GCD, 10 CD patients on GFD for 1–2 years, and 8 healthy controls. Bacteriological analyses of duodenal biopsy specimens, carried out by fluorescent in situ hybridization coupled with flow cytometry, showed that the proportions of total and Gram-negative potentially pro-inflammatory bacteria were significantly higher in CD patients with active disease than in patients on GFD and controls. Although, the ratio of beneficial bacterial groups (*Lactobacillus*-

Bifidobacterium) to potentially harmful *Bacteroides-E. coli* was significantly reduced in CD patients on GFD, there was not a complete normalization of gut microbiota compared with controls [25]. Several subsequent Spanish studies confirmed these results [20, 26–28]. Particularly, these studies found that the *Bacteroides, E. coli, Bifidobacterium, Enterobacteriacae,* and *Staphylococcus* groups were significantly more abundant in GCD patients than in the controls with a greater diversity of these species [20, 26, 28], while, in contrast, members of the family Streptococcaceae were less abundant in CD patients [28]. Furthermore, the *Prevotella* genera were more frequent in healthy subjects than in celiac patients [27]. Ou et al. identified Clostridium, Prevotella and Actinomyces as predominant bacteria in the proximal small intestine biopsies from a cohort of 45 CD children and 18 healthy controls born during the so-called "Swedish CD epidemic" (2004-2007). This could explain the four-fold increase in the incidence of CD in children less than two years of age observed between 2004 and 2007 [29]. Schippa et al. [30] analyzed the mucosa-associated microbiota of CD children, before and after a GFD, and controls by temporal temperature gradient gel electrophoresis (TTGE). The most important findings of the study were: a demonstration of a presence of peculiar microbial TTGE profile and a significant higher biodiversity in CD pediatric patients' duodenal mucosa after 9 months of GFD compared to healthy controls. Di Cagno et al. [31], utilizing culture-dependent and culture-independent methods and metabolomics analyses, investigated the differences in the microbiota and metabolome of 19 treated CD patients and 15 controls. They confirmed the lower levels of *Lactobacillus* and increased levels of *Bacteroides* in CD patients. Moreover, the authors showed that a GFD lasting at least two years did not completely restore the microbiota and metabolome in CD patients [31]. A recent Spanish study demonstrated that the intestinal microbiota of patients with duodenal Marsh 3c lesions showed similarity of 98% and differed from that of CD patients with other type of histologic lesion as Marsh 3a, Marsh 3b, and Marsh 2 [32]. This indicated that the composition of duodenal microbiota differed depending on the grade of intestinal damage.

Authors/ references	**Years**	**Country**	**Patients population and sample size**	**Methods**	**Main results**
Nadal et al. [25]	2007	Spain	20 (untreated CD (mean age, 5.1 years) 10 treated CD (mean age, 5.6 years) 8 controls (mean age, 4.1 years)	FISH+ flow cytometry	In untreated CD: ↑ Total bacteria ↑ Gram-negative bacteria ↑ *Bacteroides* and *E. coli*, which normalized after GFD In treated and untreated CD: ↓ The ratio of *Lactobacillus-Bifidobacterium* to *Bacteroides*
Collado et al. [20]	2009	Spain	8 untreated CD (mean age, 56.4 months) 8 treated CD (mean age, 65.2 months)	qPCR	In untreated CD: ↑Bacterial counts ↑ *Lactobacillus* prevalence ↓ *C. coccoides* prevalence ↑ *Staphylococcus*

Authors/ references	Years	Country	Patients population and sample size	Methods	Main results
			8 controls (mean age, 45.0 months)		↑ *E. coli* ↓ *Bifidobacterium* In treated and untreated CD: ↑ *Bacteroides* ↑ *C. leptum*
Ou et al.[29]	2009	Sweden	33 untreated CD (median age, 5.9 years) 17 treated CD (median age, 7.5 years) 3 challenged CD (median age, 10.8 years) 18 controls (mean age, 3.2 years)	Culture +Scanning electron microscopy	In untreated CD ↑ *Streptococcus* ↑ *Neisseria*
Schippa et al. [30]	2010	Italy	20 CD (before and after GFD) (mean age, 8.3 years) 10 controls (mean age, 11.7 years)	TTGE	Differences in biodiversity between untreated CD and treated CD ↑*Bacteroides vulgatus* and *E. coli* in CD
Sanchez et al. [26]	2010	Spain	20 treated CD (mean age, 51.1 months) 12 untreated CD (mean age, 54.9 months) 8 controls (mean age, 50.1 months)	PCR-DDGE	In untreated and treated CD: ↓*Bacteroides* diversity In untreated CD: ↓ *Bacteroides dorei* ↑*Bifidobacterium* diversity ↑*Bifidobacterium adolescentis,* ↑ *Bifidobacterium animalis* ↓*Bacteroides diastonis,* ↓*Bacteroides fragilis* ↓ *Bacteroides thetaiotaomicron,* ↓ *Bacteroides uniformis* ↓ *Bacteroides Ovatus*
Di Cagno et al. [31]	2011	Italy	19 treated CD (mean age 9.7 years) 15 controls (mean age, 10.4 years)	PCR-DDGE	In treated CD: ↓ *Lactobacillus* ↓ *Enterococcus* ↓ *Bifidobacteria* ↑*Bacteroides,* ↑ *Staphylococcus,* ↑*Salmonella,* ↑ *Shigella, Klebsiella*
Sanchez et al. [28]	2013	Spain	32 untreated CD (mean age, 5.1 years) 17 treated CD (mean age, 5.9 years)	Culture +PCR	In untreated CD: ↑ *Proteobacteria, Enterobacteriaceae, Staphylococcaceae* (*Klebsiella oxytoca,*

Authors/ references	Years	Country	Patients population and sample size	Methods	Main results
			8 controls (mean age, 6.9 years)		*Staphylococcus epidermidis, Staphylococcus pausteri*) ↓ *Firmicutes* ↓ *Streptococcus anginosus,* ↓ *Streptococcus mutans*
Nistal et al. [27]	2012		8 untreated CD (mean age, 3.75 years) 5 controls (mean age, 7.2 years)	16SrRNA gene sequencing	↓ *Streptococcus* and *Prevotella*
De Meij et al. [32]	2013	Netherland	21 untreated CD (median age, 6.8 years) 21 controls (median age, 8.1 years)	IS-pro	In treated and untreated CD: ↑ *Streptococcus* ↑ *Lactobacillus* ↑ *Clostridium*
Cheng et al. [33]	2013	Finland	10 untreated CD (median age 9.5 years) 9 controls (median age, 8.5 years)	qRT-PCR+ HIPchip microarray	No significant differences in the abundance of bacterial phylum-like groups between CD and controls The bacterial diversity was comparable between CD and controls In treated and untreated CD: ↑ TLR2 expression ↑ IL-10, IFN-g, C-X-C chemokine receptor type 6 expression
Giron Fernandez-Crehuet et al. [34]	2015	Spain	11untreated CD (median age, 5.0 years) 6 controls (median age, 8.8 years)	DGGE	The intestinal microbiota of children with Marsh 3c lesion showed similarity of 98% and differs from other CD children with lesion as Marsh 3a, 3b and Marsh 2 In CD: ↓ Richness, diversity and abitability of *Lactobacillus* In untreated CD: ↓ *Streptococcus, Bacteroides, E. coli* In controls ↓ *Streptococcus, Bacteroides* ↑ *Bifidobacterium, Lactobacillus, Acinetobacter*

CD celiac disease, *FISH* fluorescent in situ hybridization, *DGGE* denaturing gradient gel electrophoresis, *GFD* gluten-free diet, *HIPchip* Human Intestinal Tract Chip, *IFN-g* interferon-gamma, *IL-10* interleukin-10, *IS-pro* 16S-23S interspacer, *PCR* polymerase chain reaction, *qPCR* quantitative polymerase chain reaction, *qRT-PCR* quantitative reverse-transcriptase-polymerase chain reaction, *TGGE* temporal temperature gradient gelelectrophoresis, *TLR2* toll-like receptor 2, C-X-C chemokine receptor type 6.

Table 2. Duodenal-associated microbiota in celiac disease.

In contrast, two recent studies reached different results. De Meij et al. [33], analyzing the total microbiome profile in small bowel biopsies of 21 untreated CD and 21 age-matched controls, found that mucosa-associated duodenal microbiome composition and diversity did not differ between children with untreated CD and controls. The same results were obtained by Cheng et al. using bacterial phylogenetic microarray to comprehensively profile the microbiota in duodenal biopsies of 10 CD and nine healthy children, suggesting that the duodenal mucosa-associated bacteria do not play an important role in the pathogenesis of CD [34].

In summary, although the majority of the studies available have confirmed the presence of intestinal dysbiosis in CD children characterized by low levels of *Lactobacilli* and *Bifidobacteria* and increase in Gram-negative bacteria (*Bacteroides*), which were not completely normalized after GFD, some of them have failed to find a distinct signature that defines celiac microbiota. The available articles regarding the relationship between the gut microbiota and GFD, demonstrated that a GFD only allows a partial recovery of the gut microbiota in CD patients [30, 34, 35].

3. Pathogenetic role of intestinal dysbiosis in CD

The intestinal microbiota composition and function play a fundamental role in the balance between the host's health and disease by different mechanisms: (1) regulation of epithelial cell proliferation and expression of tight junction proteins which act on intestinal permeability; (2) influence on mucin gene expression by goblet cells and their glycosylation pattern; 3) secretion of antimicrobial peptides (defensins, angiogenins, Reg3γ, etc.) by intestinal cells, which contribute to control gut bacterial adhesion. Certain components of the gut microbiota also affect the expression and activation of pattern recognition receptors (PRR), such as toll-like receptors (TLRs), which are expressed by epithelial cells and innate immune cells. The mammalian TLR recognizes specific patterns of microbial components, called pathogen-associated molecular patterns (PAMPs). After the PRR-PAMP interaction, activated innate immune cells start the adaptive immune response by presenting the antigen and by producing cytokines, which leads to antigen-specific, protective immune response. In inflammatory and autoimmune diseases this response causes damage to host's tissues [36]. The gut microbiota impacts on adaptive immunity. Recently, specific commensal bacteria have been shown to influence T lymphocyte production (Th1, Th17) or anti-inflammatory regulatory T cells (Tregs) [36].

To date, human microbiota and mucosal barrier function are the key players in etiology of many inflammatory and autoimmune diseases [37]. Changes in mechanisms regulating mucosal immunity and tolerance, can lead to impaired mucosal barrier function, increased penetration of microbial components from lumen into the mucosa and circulation, and consequently lead exaggeration of aberrant immune responses and inflammation.

The exact mechanisms through which the gut microbiota might influence CD onset or progression is unknown, but could include activation of innate immune system, modulation of the epithelial barrier, or exacerbation of the gliadin-specific immune response [38]. Moreover, the presence of microbiota can significantly influence the inflammatory effect of gluten. The microbiota may facilitate the access of gliadin peptides to the lamina propria and its interaction with infiltrated lymphocytes and antigen presenting cells (APCs) responsible for triggering the immune response via different mechanisms. In genetically predisposed individuals, gluten in association with microbial antigens can stimulate and modulate innate and adaptative immune response, sustaining a chronic mucosal inflammation, underlining this chronic disease [38].

4. Probiotics in the treatment of CD

Probiotics are nonpathogenic live microorganisms, which when orally administered in adequate amounts, alter the microflora of the host and have beneficial health effects. Probiotics have shown to preserve the intestinal barrier promoting its integrity both in vitro and in vivo [39, 40] as well as regulating the response of the innate and adaptative immune system. The association of CD with intestinal dysbiosis and the evidence supporting a role for the microbiota and specific bacteria in maintaining gut barrier function and regulating the response of the innate and adaptive immune system, have supported the potential use of probiotics in CD treatment [41, 42]. Although the data regarding the use of probiotics for CD are encouraging, most of these data come from in vitro experimental models of CD [43, 44]. Studies regarding probiotics and CD in humans are very scarce [45–47]. Smecuol et al. evaluated the effect of the *Bifidobacterium* infantis natren life start (NLS) on gut permeability, the occurrence of symptoms, and presence of inflammatory cytokines in adult CD patients on GCD. Results have shown that probiotics did not modify intestinal permeability probably due to an insufficient dose or a short time of administration. However, probiotic administration improved gastrointestinal symptoms, alleviating and reducing constipation [47].

In children, the clinical trials performed on the effect of probiotics on CD are summarized in **Table 3**. In the earliest study Olivares et al. [45] evaluated the influence of *Bifidobacterium longum* CECT 7347 in addition to a GFD in children newly diagnosed with CD. They showed a decrease in peripheral CD3+ T lymphocytes and a trend in the reduction of tumor necrosis factor (TNF)-α serum levels, and a reduction in the *Bacteroides fragilis* group(pro-inflammatory bacteria) and in the content of IgA in stools. Klemenak et al. [46] evaluated the effect of a combination of the strains *Bifidobacterium breve* BR03 and *B. breve* B632, as compared to placebo. They reported that *B. breve* strains decreased the production of the pro-inflammatory cytokine TNF-α in children CD on a GFD.

At this time, the only treatment for CD is lifelong GFD, which involves the elimination of grains containing gluten, wheat, rye, and barley in addition to food products and additives derived from them [48]. To date, adherence to a diet is difficult for many patients. Studies have shown that dietary transgression in patients with CD is common and can occur anywhere from 32% to 55% [49]. Moreover, a GFD may be rich in high glycemic index foods which can increase insulin resistance and, thus, the risk of obesity and cardiovascular disease. In the last decade, new therapies have been suggested to improve compliance to a GFD or to replace a GFD [50]. The use of probiotics appears to be able to reduce the damage caused by eating gluten-containing foods and may even accelerate mucosal healing after the initiation of GFD [50, 51]. A specific commercially available probiotic, VSL#3 (containing eight different bacteria), has been shown to reduce the toxicity of gluten when used in a fermentation process [52]. It is thought that the gut microbiota can be modified in its composition and function by probiotic administration. These may counteract or postpone the onset of CD, and it can be useful in patients on GFD, when the normal composition of the intestinal flora has not yet fully recovered.

Authors/ references	Years	Country	Study design	Patients population and sample size	Main results	Comments
Olivares et al. [45]	2013	Spain	DB, R, PC	18 CD (mean age, 6.8 years) received *B. longum* CECT 7347; 18 CD (mean age 8.5 years) received placebo for 3 months in parallel with the GFD	↓*B. fragilis* group ↓activated T-lymphocytes↓ TNF-α	*B. longum* CECT 7347 could improve the health status of CD patients
Klemenac et al. [46]	2015	Italy Slovenia	DB, R, PC	22 CD (age, 10.43) daily received *B. breve* 25 CD (age, 10.81) daily received placebo for 3 months 18 (age, 8.83) controls	↓TNF-α levels on CD group	Probiotic intervention with *B. breve* strains has shown a positive effect on decreasing the production of pro-inflammatory cytokine TNF-α in children with CD on GFD

CD celiac disease, DB double-blind, R randomized, PC placebo controlled.

Table 3. Clinical trials on the effect of probiotics for CD.

5. Conclusions

An alternative treatment that can improve CD patients' quality of life may lie in probiotics. In particular, probiotics such as *Lactobacilli* and *Bifidobacterium* could be useful to reset altered gut microbiota, as well as reduce gliadin toxicity and immune activation. Their use as a primary prophylactic treatment for children at high risk of CD is also a potential consideration. However, their use in routine clinical practice is hindered by limited data from human studies. The role of specific probiotics and their mechanism of action need to be identified in a larger experimental population to confirm their effectiveness.

Author details

Caterina Anania[1], Francesca Olivero[1], Eugenia Olivero[2] and Lucia Pacifico[1*]

*Address all correspondence to: lucia.pacifico@uniroma1.it

1 Policlinico Hospital Umberto I, Sapienza University of Rome, Rome, Italy

2 Ernst & Young Financial-Business Advisors, Rome, Italy

References

[1] Fasano A, Catassi C. Clinical practice. Celiac disease. N Engl J Med. 2012; 367:2419–2426. DOI: 10.1056/NEJMcp1113994.

[2] Track GJ, Verbeek WH, Schreurs MW, Mulder CJ. The spectrum of celiac disease: epidemiology, clinical aspects and treatment. Nat Rev Gastroenterol Hepatol. 2010;7:204–213. DOI: 10.1038/nrgastro.2010.23.

[3] Husby S, Koletzko S, Korponay-Szabo IR, Mearin ML, Phillips A, Shamir R, Troncone R, Giersiepen K, Branski D, Catassi C, Lelgeman M, Maki M, Ribes-Koninckx C, Ventura A, Zimmer KP. European Society for Pediatric Gastroenterology, Hepatology, and Nutrition guidelines for the diagnosis of coeliac disease. J Pediatr Gastroenterol Nutr. 2012;54:136–160. DOI: 10.1097/MPG.0b013e1821a23d0.

[4] Van Belzen MJ, Koeleman BPC, Crusius JBA, MeijervJWR, Bardoel AFJ, Pearson PL, Sandkuijl LA, Houwen RH, Wijmenga C. Defining the contribution of the HLA region to cis DQ2-positive coeliac disease patients. Gen Immun. 2004;5:215–220. http://dx.doi.org/10.1038/sj.gene.6364061.

[5] IavarsonA, Hernell O, Stenlud H, Persson LA. Breast-feeding protects against coeliac disease. Am J Clin Nutr. 2002;75:914–921. DOI

[6] Stene LC, Honeyman MC, Hoffenberg EJ, Haas JE, Sokol RJ, Emery L, Taki I, Norris JM, Erlich HA, Eisenbarth GS, Rewers M. Rotavirus infection frequency and risk of coeliac disease autoimmunity in early childhood: a longitudinal study. Am J Gastroenterol. 2006;101:2333–2340. DOI:10.1111/j.1572-0241.2006.00741.x.

[7] Akobeng AK, Ramanan AV, Buchan I, Heller R. Effect of breast feeding on risk of coeliac disease: a systematic review and meta-analysis of observational studies. Arch Dis Child. 2006;91:39–43. DOI: 10.1136/adc.2005.082016.

[8] Szebeni B, Veres G, Dezsofi A, Rusai K, Vannay A, Bokodi G, Vásárhelyi B, Korponay-Szabó IR, Tulassay T, Arató A. Increased mucosal expression of toll-like receptor

(TLR)2 and TLR4 in coeliac disease. J Pediatr Gastroenterol Nutr. 2007;45:187–193. DOI: 10.1097/MPG.0b013e318064514a.

[9] Vanderpool C, Yan F, Polk DB. Mechanisms of probiotic action: implications for therapeutic applications in inflammatory bowel diseases. Inflamm Bowel Dis. 2008;14:1585–1596. DOI: 10.1097/MPG.0b013e318064514a.

[10] Morgan XC, Tickle TL, Sokol H, Gevers D, Devaney KL, Ward DV, Reyes JA, Shah SA, LeLeiko N, Snapper SB, Bousvaros A, Korzenik J, Sands BE, Xavier RJ, Huttenhower C. Dysfunction of the intestinal microbiome in inflammatory bowel disease and treatment. Genome Biol. 2012;13:R79. DOI: 10.1186/gb-2012-13-9-r79.

[11] Miele L, Giorgio V, Alberelli MA, De Candia E, Gasbarrini A, Grieco A. Impact of gut microbiota on obesity, diabetes, and cardiovascular disease risk. Curr Cardiol Rep. 2015 17:120. DOI: 10.1007/s11886-015-0671-z.

[12] Forsberg G, Fahlgren A, Hörstedt P, Hammarström S, Hernell O, Hammarström ML. Presence of bacteria and innate immunity of intestinal epithelium in childhood celiac disease. Am J Gastroenterol 2004;99;894–904. DOI :10.1111/j.1572-0241.2004.04157.x.

[13] Collado MC, Calabuig M, Sanz Y. Differences between the fecal microbiota of coeliac infants and healthy controls. Curr Issues Intest Microbiol. 2007;8:9–14.

[14] Nadal I, Donat E, Ribes-Koninckx C, Calabuig M, Sanz Y. Imbalance in the composition of the duodenal microbiota of children with coeliac disease. J Med Microbiol. 2007;56:1669–1674. DOI: 10.1099/jmm.0.47410-0.

[15] Collado MC, Donat E, Ribes-Koninckx C, Calabuig M, Sanz Y. Imbalances in faecal and duodenal Bifidobacterium species composition in active and non-active coeliac disease. BMC Microbiol. 2008;8:232. DOI: 10.1186/1471-2180-8-232.

[16] Fernandez-Feo M, Wei G, Blumenkranz G, Dewhirst FE, Schuppan D, Oppenheim FG, Helmerhorst EJ. The cultivable human oral gluten-degrading microbiome and its potential implications in coeliac disease and gluten sensitivity. Clin Microbiol Infect. 2013;19:E386–394. DOI: 10.1111/1469-0691.12249.

[17] Food and Agriculture Organization of the United Nations, World Health Organization. Guidelines for the evaluation of probiotics in food: joint FAO/WHO Working Group report on drafting guidelines for the evaluation of probiotics in food. World Health Organization, Geneva, Switzerland. ftp://ftp.fao.org/es/esn/food/wgreport2.pdf. Accessed 27 April 2014.

[18] Lindfors K, Blomqvist T, Juuti-Uusitalo K, Stenman S, Venäläinen J, Mäki M, Kaukinen K. Live probiotic *Bifidobacterium lactis* bacteria inhibit the toxic effects induced by wheat gliadin in epithelial cell culture. Clin Exp Immunol. 2008;152:552–558. DOI: 10.1111/j.1365-2249.2008.03635.x.

[19] Sanz Y, Sánchez E, Marzotto M, Calabuig M, Torriani S, Dellaglio F. Differences in faecal bacterial communities in coeliac and healthy children as detected by PCR and dena-

turing gradient gel electrophoresis. FEMS Immunol Med Microbiol. 2007;51:562–568. DOI: http://dx.doi.org/10.1111/j.1574-695X.2007.00337.x.

[20] Collado MC, Donat E, Ribes-Koninckx C, Calabuig M, Sanz Y. Specific duodenal and faecal bacterial groups associated with paediatric coeliac disease. J Clin Pathol. 2009;62:264–269. DOI: 10.1136/jcp.2008.061366.

[21] De Palma G, Nadal I, Medina M, Donat E, Ribes-Koninckx C, Calabuig M, Sanz Y. Intestinal dysbiosis and reduced immunoglobulin-coated bacteria associated with coeliac disease in children. BMC Microbiol. 2010;10:63. DOI: 10.1186/1471-2180-10-63.

[22] Sánchez E, Ribes-Koninckx C, Calabuig M, Sanz Y. Intestinal Staphylococcus spp. and virulent features associated with coeliac disease. Clin Pathol. 2012;65:830–834. DOI: 10.1136/jclinpath-2012-200759.

[23] Di Cagno R, Rizzello CG, Gagliardi F, Ricciuti P, Ndagijimana M, Francavilla R, Guerzoni ME, Crecchio C, Gobbetti M, De Angelis M. Different fecal microbiotas and volatile organic compounds in treated and untreated children with celiac disease. Appl Environ Microbiol. 2009;75:3963–3971. DOI: 10.1128/AEM.02793-08.

[24] Lorenzo Pisarello MJ, Vintiñi EO, González SN, Pagani F, Medina MS. Decrease in lactobacilli in the intestinal microbiota of celiac children with a gluten-free diet, and selection of potentially probiotic strains. Can J Microbiol. 2015;61:32–37. DOI: 10.1139/cjm-2014-0472.

[25] Nadal I, Donat E, Ribes-Koninckx C, Calabuig M, Sanz Y. Imbalance in the composition of the duodenal microbiota of children with coeliac disease. J Med Microbiol. 2007;56:1669–1674. DOI: 10.1099/jmm.0.47410-0.

[26] Sánchez E, Donat E, Ribes-Koninckx C, Calabuig M, Sanz Y. Intestinal Bacteroides species associated with coeliac disease. J Clin Pathol. 2010;63:1105–1111. DOI: 10.1136/jcp.2010.07695.

[27] Nistal E, Caminero A, Herrán AR, Arias L, Vivas S, de Morales JM, Calleja S, de Miera LE, Arroyo P, Casqueiro J. Differences of small intestinal bacteria populations in adults and children with/without celiac disease: effect of age, gluten diet, and disease. Inflamm Bowel Dis. 2012;18:649–656. DOI: 10.1002/ibd.21830.

[28] Sánchez E, Donat E, Ribes-Koninckx C, Fernández-Murga ML, Sanz Y. Duodenal-mucosal bacteria associated with celiac disease in children. Appl Environ Microbiol. 2013;79:5472–5479. DOI: 10.1128/AEM.00869-13.

[29] Ou G, Hedberg M, Hörstedt P, Baranov V, Forsberg G, Drobni M, Sandström O, Wai SN, Johansson I, Hammarström ML, Hernell O, Hammarström S. Proximal small intestinal microbiota and identification of rod-shaped bacteria associated with childhood celiac disease. Am J Gastroenterol. 2009;104:3058–3067. DOI: 10.1038/ajg.2009.524.

[30] Schippa S, Iebba V, Barbato M, Di Nardo G, Totino V, Checchi MP, Longhi C, Maiella G, Cucchiara S, Conte MP. A distinctive 'microbial signature' in celiac pediatric patients. BMC Microbiol. 2010;10:175.DOI: 10.1186/1471-2180-10-175.

[31] Di Cagno R, De Angelis M, De Pasquale I, Ndagijimana M, Vernocchi P, Ricciuti P, Gagliardi F, Laghi L, Crecchio C, Guerzoni ME, Gobbetti M, Francavilla R. Duodenal and faecal microbiota of celiac children: molecular, phenotype and metabolome characterization. BMC Microbiol. 2011;11:219. DOI: 10.1186/1471-2180-11-219.

[32] Girón Fernández-Crehuet F, Tapia-Paniagua S, Moriñigo Gutiérrez MA, Navas-López VM, Juliana Serrano M, Blasco-Alonso J, Sierra Salinas C. The duodenal microbiota composition in children with active coeliac disease is influenced for the degree of enteropathy. An Pediatr (Barc). 2015; 18 pii: S1695–4033(15)00311-2. doi: 10.1016/j.anpedi.2015.06.014.

[33] de Meij TG, Budding AE, Grasman ME, Kneepkens CM, Savelkoul PH, Mearin ML. Composition and diversity of the duodenal mucosa-associated microbiome in children with untreated coeliac disease. Scand J Gastroenterol. 2013;48:530–536. DOI: 10.3109/00365521.2013.775666.

[34] Cheng J, Kalliomäki M, Heilig HG, Palva A, Lähteenoja H, de Vos WM, Salojärvi J, Satokari R. Duodenal microbiota composition and mucosal homeostasis in pediatric celiac disease. BMC Gastroenterol. 2013;13:113. DOI: 10.1186/1471-230X-13-113.

[35] Collado MC, Donat E, Ribes-Koninckx C, Calabuig M, Sanz Y. Imbalances in faecal and duodenal Bifidobacterium species composition in active and non-active coeliac disease. BMC Microbiol. 2008;8:232. DOI: 10.1186/1471-2180-8-232.

[36] Tlaskalová-Hogenová H, Stěpánková R, Kozáková H, Hudcovic T, Vannucci L, Tučková L, Rossmann P, Hrnčíř T, Kverka M, Zákostelská Z, Klimešová K, Přibylová J, Bártová J, Sanchez D, Fundová P, Borovská D, Srutková D, Zídek Z, Schwarzer M, Drastich P, Funda DP. The role of gut microbiota (commensal bacteria) and the mucosal barrier in the pathogenesis of inflammatory and autoimmune diseases and cancer: contribution of germ-free and gnotobiotic animal models of human diseases. Cell Mol Immunol. 2011;8:110–120. DOI: 10.1038/cmi.2010.67.

[37] Verdu EF, Galipeau HJ, Jabri B. Novel players in coeliac disease pathogenesis: role of the gut microbiota. Nat Rev Gastroenterol Hepatol. 2015;12:497–506. DOI: 10.1038/nrgastro.2015.90.

[38] Pagliari D, Urgesi R, Frosali S, Riccioni ME, Newton EE, Landolfi R, Pandolfi F, Cianci R. The interaction among microbiota, immunity, and genetic and dietary factors is the condicio sine qua non celiac disease can develop. J Immunol Res. 2015;2015:123653. DOI: 10.1155/2015/123653.

[39] Madsen K, Cornish A, Soper P, McKaigney C, Jijon H, Yachimec C, Doyle J, Jewell L, De Simone C. Probiotic bacteria enhance murine and human intestinal epithelial barrier

function. Gastroenterology 2001;121:580–591. DOI: http://dx.doi.org/10.1053/gast.2001.27224.

[40] Gupta P, Andrew H, Kirschner BS, Guandalini S. Is lactobacillus GG helpful in children with Crohn's disease? Results of a preliminary, open-label study. J Pediatr Gastroenterol Nutr. 2000;31:453–457.

[41] Sanz Y, De Pama G, Laparra M. Unraveling the ties between celiac disease and intestinal microbiota. Int Rev Immunol. 2011;30:207–218. DOI: 10.3109/08830185.2011.599084.

[42] Cenit MC, Olivares M, Codoñer-Franch P, Sanz Y. Intestinal microbiota and celiac disease: cause, consequence or co-evolution? Nutrients. 2015;7:6900–6923. DOI: 10.3390/nu7085314.

[43] Aloisio I, Santini C, Biavati B, Dinelli G, Cencič A, Chingwaru W, Mogna L, Di Gioia D. Characterization of Bifidobacterium spp. strains for the treatment of enteric disorders in newborns. Appl Microbiol Biotechnol. 2012;96:1561–1576. DOI: 10.1007/s00253-012-4138-5.

[44] Mogna L, Del Piano M, Mogna G. Capability of the two microorganisms *Bifidobacterium breve* B632 and *Bifidobacterium breve* BR03 to colonize the intestinal microbiota of children. J Clin Gastroenterol. 2014;48 Suppl 1:S37–9. DOI: 10.1097/MCG.0000000000000234.

[45] Olivares M, Castillejo G, Varea V, Sanz Y. Double-blind, randomised, placebo-controlled intervention trial to evaluate the effects of Bifidobacterium longum CECT 7347 in children with newly diagnosed coeliac disease. Br J Nutr. 2014;112:30–40. DOI: 10.1017/S0007114514000609.

[46] Klemenak M, Dolinšek J, Langerholc T, Di Gioia D, Mičetić-Turk D. Administration of Bifidobacterium breve decreases the production of TNF-α in children with celiac disease. Dig Dis Sci. 2015;60:3386–3392. DOI: 10.1007/s10620-015-3769-7.

[47] Smecuol E, Hwang HJ, Sugai E, Corso L, Cherñavsky AC, Bellavite FP, González A, Vodánovich F, Moreno ML, Vázquez H, Lozano G, Niveloni S, Mazure R, Meddings J, Mauriño E, Bai JC. Exploratory, randomized, double-blind, placebo-controlled study on the effects of Bifidobacteriuminfantis natren life start strain super strain in active celiac disease. J Clin Gastroenterol. 2013;47:139–147. DOI: 10.1097/MCG.0b013e31827759ac.

[48] Green PH, Jabri B. Coeliac disease. Lancet. 2003; 362:383–391. DOI: http// dx.doi.org/0.1016/s0140-6736(03)14027-5.

[49] Silvester JA, Rashid M. Long-term follow-up of individuals with celiac disease: an evaluation of current practiceguidelines. Can J Gastroenterol. 2007;21:557–564.

[50] Kaukinen K, Lindfors K, Mäki M. Advances in the treatment of coeliac disease: an immunopathogenic perspective. Nat Rev Gastroenterol Hepatol. 2014;11:36–44.DOI: 10.1038/nrgastro.2013.141.

[51] Lindfors K, Blomqvist T, Juuti-Uusitalo K, Stenman S, Venäläinen J, Mäki M, Kaukinen K. Live probiotic Bifidobacterium lactis bacteria inhibit the toxic effects induced by wheat gliadin in epithelial cell culture. Clin Exp Immunol. 2008;152:552–558. DOI: 10.1111/j.1365-2249.2008.03635.x.

[52] De Angelis M, Rizzello CG, Fasano A, Clemente MG, De Simone C, Silano M, De Vincenzi M, Losito I, Gobbetti M. VSL#3 probiotic preparation has the capacity to hydrolyze gliadin polypeptides responsible for Celiac Sprue. Biochim Biophys Acta. 2006;1762:80–93.

Chapter 12

Probiotics for Prevention and Treatment of Candidiasis and Other Infectious Diseases: *Lactobacillus* spp. and Other Potential Bacterial Species

Michelle Peneluppi Silva, Rodnei Dennis Rossoni,
Juliana Campos Junqueira and
Antonio Olavo Cardoso Jorge

Additional information is available at the end of the chapter

http://dx.doi.org/10.5772/64093

Abstract

The resident microbiota in the human body, such as the oral cavity, gastrointestinal tract and genitourinary tract, is able to provide resistance to disease. However, imbalances in the microbial components can promote the growth of opportunistic microorganisms, such as yeasts of genus *Candida*. Fungal infections present as a major cause of infectious diseases and the microorganisms of genus *Candida* are the most frequently isolated pathogenic fungi in human fungal infections. *Bacillus* spp. and *Lactobacillus* spp. are bacteria that have probiotic effects used in commercially available products and in studies that aim for the development of probiotics able to inhibit the microbial pathogenicity and restore the balance of resident microbiota. Thus, with increasing fungus resistance to the use of antifungal agents, which are capable of causing serious side effects to the host organism unable to destroy the target microorganism, it becomes important to develop therapeutic and/or prophylactic alternatives that have a different and an effective mechanism of action with capacity to combat fungal infections without harming the patient. Probiotic bacteria provide an alternative strategy for the prevention and treatment of candidiasis and other infectious diseases.

Keywords: probiotic, *Candida* spp., *Bacillus* spp., *Lactobacillus* spp., prevention and treatment

1. Introduction

The incidence of fungal infections has increased significantly in the past 25 years [1]. Human beings are colonized by a diverse and complex collection of microorganisms, contributing all of them to host nutrition, development of the immune system, response to pathogens and mucosal cell differentiation and proliferation [2].

Probiotic bacteria are also used in human and animal nutrition to influence beneficially the balance of intestinal microbiota of the host. Probiotics have several beneficial effects related to increasing digestion, strengthening the immune system and stimulating the production of vitamin. The use of probiotics is aimed to reduce the use of antibiotics and improve animal growth, as well as feed conversion [3].

Infectious diseases along with multidrug resistance are the major public health problem in developing countries with increased mortality and morbidity [4, 5]. Apart from the threat of multidrug resistance, several studies have confirmed that the continuous use of antibiotics can damage human commensal microbiota [5, 6]. Thus, an alternative and effective research focus is necessary to combat these pathogens with no effect on normal microbiota. In this regard, the use of probiotics and their natural metabolic compounds can be a substitute in various food and pharmaceutical industries [5].

There are around 600 pathogenic fungal species for humans and this group includes the fungi that cause infection of skin (e.g., *Malassezia* species) and fungi that have the potential to cause systemic infections (e.g., *Cryptococcus neoformans* and *Candida albicans*) [7]. The yeasts of the genus *Candida* are the fourth most common cause of systemic infections acquired in hospitals in the United States with 50% mortality rates. The most pathogenic species is *C. albicans* and can cause two major types of human infections: superficial infections, such as oral candidiasis, and systemic infections [8, 9].

The genus *Candida* is commonly found in the oral cavity of healthy individuals, isolated from approximately 75% of the population with a higher prevalence of *C. albicans*, followed by *C. tropicalis* and *C. glabrata* [10]. *Candida* species are a frequent cause of recurrent infections in the mucosa when favored by risk factors such as the use of antibiotics of broad spectrum and corticosteroids for long time, human immunodeficiency virus (HIV) infection, radiotherapy in the area of head and neck, the use of orthodontic appliances, deficient oral hygiene, among other factors affecting immunocompromised patients that may result in transition of commensal phase of *C. albicans* to pathogenic [11, 12].

Under certain conditions of immunosuppression, such as individuals with acquired immunodeficiency syndrome (AIDS), oral manifestations are the most important and earliest indicators of infection. The oral candidiasis is accepted internationally as a cardinal sign of HIV infection and is present in 50% of patients with HIV infection and in 80% of patients with AIDS [13, 14].

In Brazil during the period among 1996–2006, candidiasis was the second cause of deaths in HIV-positive patients due to fungal infections, being responsible for an average of 39 annual deaths [15]. Moreover, oral candidiasis remains clinically relevant in these individuals, where treatment is difficult and recurrent episodes are frequent, requiring multiple antifungal treatments, which may lead to resistance selection [16, 17]. Due to this, *C. albicans* can develop resistance to antifungals used to treat oral candidiasis, such as fluconazole and miconazole [18, 19].

Due to the high recurrence of *Candida* lesions, and the increased resistance of conventional antifungal drugs in clinical practice, the continuous use of probiotics to prevent fungal infections may be an interesting strategy. In this chapter, we discuss how probiotics can help in the prevention and/or adjuvant treatment of candidiasis.

2. Probiotic

The history of probiotics began with the history of man; cheese and fermented milk were well known to the Greeks and Romans who recommended their consumption, especially for children and convalescents. The first association of probiotics and health benefits was made at the turn of the century when the Russian scientist, Elie Metchnikoff, systematically studied the composition of the microbiota and suggested that the ingestion of fermented milk would improve this so-called autointoxication [20].

Probiotics play an important role in human health. There is general agreement on the important role of the gastrointestinal microbiota in the health and well-being status of humans and animals [21]. Probiotics are defined as live microorganisms, which when administered in adequate amounts confer a health benefit on the host. This term is defined by a United Nations and World Health Organization Expert Panel [22].

There was an increase in the number of searches, both in vivo and in vitro, related to the benefits of probiotics on health and described in the literature for the treatment of infectious diseases caused by fungi, viruses, and bacteria or diarrhea associated with the use of antibiotics, alleviation of inflammatory chronic bowel disease, decreased risk of colon cancer, reduced allergies, effect on intestinal microbiota [21], and anticancer therapies [23].

Other beneficial effects of probiotics include lowering serum cholesterol level [24–27], improving lactose intolerance, increasing the utilization of nutrients, decreasing the use of antibiotics [24, 27], and antidiabetic treatments [26, 28, 29]. In the context linking food and health, probiotics have been the subject of numerous scientific studies and publications demonstrating their therapeutic effectiveness on both systemic and gastrointestinal tract [21] (Figure 1).

Microorganisms commonly used as probiotics belong to the heterogeneous group including *Bacillus, Lactobacillus, Bifidobacterium, Saccharomyces cerevisiae,* and *Escherichia coli* [30, 31] (**Figure 1**).

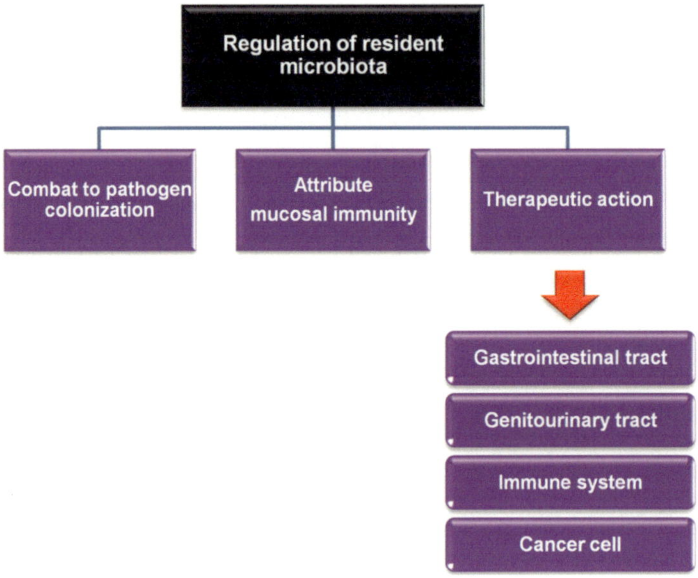

Figure 1. Some properties of probiotics.

3. *Lactobacillus* spp.

3.1. General characteristics

Lactobacillus spp. are Gram-positive bacteria, facultative anaerobic bacilli found in the normal microbiota of the gastrointestinal tract of birds and mammals, and genitourinary tract and oral cavity in the humans [31, 32]. This genre is heterogeneous and the number of species is constantly being modified due to the description of new species and reclassification of others [33]. Some members of the genus *Lactobacillus* were reclassified into *Carnobacterium* [34], *Atopobium* [35], *Weissella* [36], and *Paralactobacillus* [37]. In early 2007, 120 species composing the genus *Lactobacillus* [33] and in 2008 over 145 new species have already been identified [38, 39].

Different *Lactobacillus* species found in the gastrointestinal tract are concerned with the balance of microbiota and it has been widely studied due to their health-promoting properties [40]. Their effects on intestinal microbiota in terms of protection include competition for adhesion sites with pathogenic microorganisms and antimicrobial substance production, such as organic acids, lactic acid, carbon dioxide, and bacteriocins [41]. In addition, the regular use of probiotic appears to prevent certain gastrointestinal disorders such as lactose intolerance [42].

In 1907, Elie Metchnikoff won the Nobel Medicine Prize because he noticed that the daily consumption of Bulgarian yogurt (known for its rich composition in lactic acid bacteria) is beneficial to health. Metchnikoff worked at the Pasteur Institute in Paris and he discovered *L.*

bulgaricus and this strain was introduced into the commercial production of dairy products across Europe. He dedicated the last decade of his life to the study of bacteria that produce lactic acid as a means to increase human longevity. After the studies of Metchnikoff, the concept of probiotics was established and a new microbiology area started to develop [43].

3.2. *Lactobacillus* as probiotics and its mechanism of action

The main characteristics that a *Lactobacillus* strain needs to have to exercise an effective probiotic action against pathogenic microorganisms are related to three factors: the ability to inhibit the adhesion and colonization of pathogenic microorganisms in the host tissues, biosurfactant production, and hydrogen peroxide (H_2O_2). There is a collagen-binding protein called 29 kD present on the surface of some lactobacilli, which causes it to be capable of binding to collagen vaginal epithelial cells and to inhibit binding of pathogenic microorganisms to host tissues in significant numbers [44]. Some strains of lactobacilli produce biosurfactants generically known as surlactin, which are responsible for reducing the surface tension of liquid and thereby inhibiting the adherence of microorganisms. Surlactin studies are very important to help in the understanding of the urogenital tract microbiota and their maintenance for a balanced microbiota [45]. Other lactobacilli strains have the ability to produce hydrogen peroxide, which can be toxic to microorganisms that do not produce catalase [46, 47].

According to Reid and Bruce [46], not all probiotic strains have the same mechanisms of action and each has characteristics suitable for your application. For example, *L. casei* Shirota is ingested daily for about 24 million people who do not have the 29-kDa protein and do not produce H_2O_2. In the case of strain Shirota, its main action seems to be through the modulation of the host immune response.

In a recent study, Abedin-Do et al. [48] showed that some *Lactobacillus* strains exert innate and adaptive immune responses via their binding to pattern recognition receptors expressed on immune cells and many other tissues such as the intestinal epithelium. Furthermore, *Lactobacillus* can modulate the expression of genes involved in the regulation of immune system [49–53].

Members of our group evaluated the capacity of *L. rhamnosus* and its products to induce the synthesis of cytokines (tumor necrosis factor (TNF)-α, interleukin (IL)-1β, IL-4, IL-6, IL-10, and IL-12) by mouse macrophages. Jorjão et al. [54] used three microorganism preparations: live *L. rhamnosus* (LLR) suspension, heat-killed *L. rhamnosus* (HKLR) suspension, and the supernatant of a heat-killed *L. rhamnosus* (SHKLR) suspension. LLR and HKLR groups were able to significantly increase the production of TNF-α, IL-6, and IL-10. SHKLR also significantly increased the production of TNF-α and IL-10 but not IL-6. All the *L. rhamnosus* suspensions were not able to produce detectable levels of IL-1β or significant levels of IL-4 and IL-12. The authors concluded that live and heat-killed *L. rhamnosus* suspensions are able to induce the synthesis of different cytokines with pro-inflammatory (TNF-α and IL-6) or regulatory (IL-10) functions, suggesting the role of strain *L. rhamnosus* ATCC 7469 in the modulation or in the stimulation of immune responses.

In order for probiotic strains to have a satisfactory action, they must remain alive against stress challenges along the entire gastrointestinal tract, including the presence of bile in the small intestine. Bile is highly toxic to microorganisms not adapted to intestinal conditions. Moreover, some lactobacilli developed specific mechanisms to resist the deleterious effects caused by these compounds [55]. Among these mechanisms, we can cite the efflux pump that actively removes the acids and accumulated bile salts within the cytoplasm and the enzymatic activity of hydrolases, which are capable of neutralizing deleterious effect of bile [56–58].

According to FAO WHO [22], the ideal characteristics of a probiotic strain of *Lactobacillus* considered are as follows:

- Not pathogenic;
- Stable in acid and in the presence of bile;
- Adhesion ability in human mucosa;
- Colonize the intestine;
- Remain viable during storage and use;
- Have beneficial physiological effects and safe.

3.3. *Lactobacillus* in prevention and treatment of *Candida* infection

In vitro assays are important to evaluate the antifungal activity of each strain and characterization of the mechanisms of action, performing as a screening to in vivo tests with experimental models.

Sookkhee et al. [59] isolated and identified different species of lactic acid bacteria from the oral cavity of 130 volunteers in Thailand and they studied probiotic action against *C. albicans* in vitro. The authors found 3790 different samples of lactic acid bacteria including the genera *Lactococcus, Lactobacillus, Streptococcus, Leuconostoc,* and *Pediococcus,* and it was concluded that *L. paracasei* and *L. rhamnosus* strains were two species that had the greatest number of clinical isolates able to inhibit *C. albicans.*

Noverr and Huffnagle [60] examined the effect of living cultures, heat-killed cultures, and supernatants of probiotic bacteria (*L. casei, L. paracasei,* and *L. rhamnosus*) on the morphogenesis of *C. albicans* and observed an inhibition in the formation of germ tube when *C. albicans* interacted with living cells or supernatant of *Lactobacillus*. It was also found that supernatants obtained from cultures of 2 h inhibited germ tube formation of *C. albicans*. However, the addition of 24-h growth cultures took complete inhibition, suggesting that the accumulation of a soluble compound of the supernatant is responsible for this inhibition.

Coman et al. [61] evaluated the antifungal activities of two probiotic strains, *L. rhamnosus* IMC 501® and *L. paracasei* IMC 502®, and their 1:1 combination, named SYNBIO®, using agar well-diffusion method and liquid coculture assay. They tested probiotic strains in eight strains of *Candida*, including *C. albicans, C. krusei, C. glabrata, C. parapsilosis,* and *C. tropicalis*. All the *Candida* strains are strongly inhibited, except *C. glabrata* and *C. tropicalis,* and during the coculture assay, the inhibitory activity of probiotic bacteria against *Candida* strains was approximately 40% in some cases and absent in other cases, in particular against some strains of *C. albicans* and *C. tropicalis*. The authors concluded that in vitro screening of *Lactobacillus* strains according to their activity in various environmental conditions might be a valuable method that could precede clinical efficacy studies for adjunct treatment with probiotics in cure of different infections.

Parolin et al. [62] identified 17 clinical strains of *Lactobacillus* from the vaginal cavity of healthy premenopausal women, including the following species: *L. crispatus, L. gasseri*, and *L. vaginalis*, and evaluated their in vitro activity against *Candida* spp. (nine strains) and characterized their antifungal mechanisms of action. In general, the strains tested were more active toward *C. albicans*. No *Lactobacillus* strains showed activity against *C. krusei* and *C. parapsilosis*. All strains produced hydrogen peroxide and lactate, and in particular, *L. crispatus* BC2, *L. gasseri* BC10, and *L. gasseri* BC11 appeared to be the most active strains in reducing pathogen adhesion. It was concluded that these in vitro assays are prerequisites for the development of new therapeutic agents based on probiotics for prophylaxis and adjuvant therapy of *Candida* infection.

Some in vivo studies also show the effectiveness of probiotics in *Candida* infection. Wagner et al. [63] demonstrated that the inoculation of probiotics (*L. acidophilus, L. reuteri, L. casei* GG, and *B. animalis*) in immunodeficient mice reduced the density of *C. albicans* in gastrointestinal tract, incidence of systemic candidiasis, and prolonged the survival of adult and neonatal mice. Probiotic bacteria also modulated antibody and cell-mediated immune responses to *C. albicans*. The authors demonstrated that probiotic bacteria can protect immunodeficient mice from candidiasis; however, none of the probiotic bacteria we studied completely eliminated *C. albicans* from the alimentary tract.

Matsubara et al. [64] evaluated the oral colonization by *C. albicans* in experimental murine immunosuppressed and treatment with *L. acidophilus* and *L. rhamnosus*. The colonization by *C. albicans* on the oral mucosa, started on day 1 after inoculation, remained highest from day 3 until day 7 and then decreased significantly. Probiotic bacteria reduced *Candida* colonization on the oral mucosa significantly compared to the untreated group of animals (negative-control group). The reduction of yeast colonization in the group treated with *L. rhamnosus* was significantly higher compared to the group receiving nystatin (positive-control group). The authors concluded that the treatment with probiotics in this model may be an effective alternative to prevent it.

Deng et al. [65] evaluated the probiotic action in vitro and the anticolonization capacity of *L. paracasei* FJ861111.1 in vivo in mice infected with other selected pathogenic microorganisms. In vitro results showed that *Shigella dysenteriae, Staphylococcus aureus, Cronobacter sakazakii, E. coli*, and *C. albicans* were inhibited by *L. paracasei* FJ861111.1 that presented elevated survival at pH 2.5 and bile salt concentration at 0.3%. In vivo results demonstrated that the fermented milk with *L. paracasei* improved significantly the total population of bacteria, and the presence of *Lactobacillus* in the feces of mice. The colonization by *C. albicans* was significantly inhibited in the intestine of mice after infection and demonstrated the potential of this strain used as a probiotic organism for the production of functional fermented milk.

Although mice and rats are the gold standard for *Candida* studies, economic and ethical issues limit the use of mammals in these experiments, especially when a large number of strains need to be analyzed [66]. Invertebrate models have been used to study the microbial pathogenicity and pathogen-host interactions, which provided considerable insight into different aspects of microbial infection [67]. In this respect, *Galleria mellonella* has been found to be an interesting invertebrate model for the study of the pathogenicity of *C. albicans* [68–71]. Recently, our laboratory developed pioneering in vivo study to evaluate the probiotic action of *L. acidophilus* in the experimental candidiasis in *G. mellonella.* Vilela et al. [31] demonstrated that the inoculation of *L. acidophilus* into *G. mellonella* infected with *C. albicans* reduced the number of yeast cells in the larval hemolymph and increased the survival of these animals. However, *L. acidophilus* exerted no inhibitory effect on *C. albicans* filamentation in *G. mellonella* tissues. In this study, we verified that *G. mellonella* is an adequate model for the study of the probiotics.

4. *Bacillus* spp.

Bacillus spp. were classified a long time as only soil microorganisms, but they are also commensal microorganisms of the gut of humans and animals due to the great adaptability to the intestinal environment, representing part of your natural life cycle [72–74]. Some *Bacillus* species have been used as probiotics for at least 50 years, but scientific interest for these microorganisms has occurred mainly in the last 15 years [30, 75].

Among the large number of probiotic products in use today are bacterial spore formers, mostly of the genus *Bacillus. Bacillus* bacteria have been used widely as putative probiotics because they secrete many exoenzymes [76–78]. The species that have been most extensively examined include *B. subtilis, B. clausii, B. coagulans, B. licheniformis,* and *B. polyfermenticus* [26, 30, 79]. Although it requires an evaluation in each case, many species of *Bacillus* are considered as nonpathogenic and safe for animal and human consumption [79–81].

Used primarily in their spore form, these products have been shown to prevent gastrointestinal disorders and the diversity of species used and their applications are astonishing [30], then, demonstrating that exert immune stimulation, antimicrobial activity, and competitive exclusion. Studies have shown that these bacteria are able to grow inside the intestinal tract and could be considered temporary residents. This is important because it indicates that they are not exogenous microorganisms but may have unique symbiotic relationship with the host [74].

4.1. General characteristics

The members of genus *Bacillus* are Gram-positive, aerobic or facultative anaerobic, catalase-positive, and spore-forming bacteria [82, 83]. These microorganisms are saprophytic common in soil, water, dust, and air [84] and also involved in food spoilage [85]. These bacteria are considered allochthonous and enter the gut by association with food [30] or in an endosymbiotic relationship with their host, being able to survive temporarily and proliferate within the gastrointestinal tract [30, 86].

B. subtilis is a model microorganism for studies involving the genus *Bacillus* [87]. This species is a widely used oral vaccine delivery system since it has been classified as a novel food probiotic for both human and animal consumption [88, 89]. The beneficial effects of *B. subtilis* on the balance of the gastrointestinal microbiota justify its use as probiotic in pharmaceutical preparations, for the prevention and treatment of intestinal disorders and the reduction of inflammation [90–92].

4.2. Spores as probiotics

Sporulation of *Bacillus* spp. represents a protection process, which is usually induced by low levels of nutrients and conditions unfavorable to the survival of the bacteria in vegetative form [93]. The spores are extremely resistant cell structures that when exposed to appropriate abiotic factors, through the germination, they can return to vegetative form [94].

Bacterial spore formers are being used as probiotic supplements for use in animal feeds, for human dietary supplements, as well as in registered medicines [74]. The use of spore-based products raises a number of questions. Since the bacterial species being used are not considered resident members of the gastrointestinal microbiota, how do they exert a beneficial effect? According to Cutting [74], while often considered soil organisms this conception is misplaced and Bacilli should be considered as gut commensals. Therefore, in fact, the question to be answered is what produces the probiotic effect: the vegetative cells (spores germinated) or the spores themselves? The natural life cycle of spore-forming microorganisms involves spore germination, sporulation, and re-proliferation when nutrients are scarce [30]. According to these authors, although it is unlikely that they are true commensals, a unique dual life cycle of spore formers in the environment and within the gut of animals could represent a mechanism that may be responsible for probiotic action.

Bacillus spp. forms thermostable spores and shows advantages over other microorganisms non-spore-forming, but also have probiotic activity. Thus, the product can be stored at room temperature in the dried form without any deleterious effect on the viability. Furthermore, since spores are extremely stable and resistant, they are able to survive low pH of gastric barrier [95, 96]. Therefore, a particular dose of ingested spores can be stored indefinitely without refrigeration and the desired dose of vegetative bacteria will reach the small intestine intact [74].

The research efforts and the search for new perspectives for clinical and nutritional applications with probiotic preparations that last comparatively more than other pharmaceutical drugs are justified because the spores are more resistant than the vegetative cells. This allows for greater reliability in the treatment method with probiotics and reduces the cost of production [79].

4.3. Mechanism of action of *Bacillus* probiotic

Before a bacterial strain can be considered probiotic, some criteria must be assessed as inhibition capacity in the growth of harmful microorganisms, not toxic, not pathogenic, and be tolerant to acid, bile salt conditions, and pancreatic secretions in order to reach the small and large intestines, its ability to adhere to intestinal epithelial cells [82, 97–99], remain viable during transport and storage, exert beneficial effects on the host, stabilize the intestinal microbiota, adhere to the intestinal epithelial cell lining, and produce antimicrobial substances toward pathogen [82, 98].

Many authors have proposed that the properties of adhesion are a decisive factor for the selection of new probiotic strains. The mechanisms of action of probiotics against gastrointestinal pathogens consist principally on the following:

- Competition for nutrients and sites of accession;
- Production of antimicrobial metabolites [21, 100];
- Changes in environmental conditions;
- Modulation of the immune response of the host [21, 101].

The principal mechanism by probiotics is the production of antimicrobials that inhibit pathogenic microorganisms. *Bacillus* species produce a large number of antimicrobials and include bacteriocins and bacteriocin-like inhibitory substances, subtilin and coagulin, as well as antibiotics, surfactin, iturins A, C, D, E, and bacilysin [30, 102]. In 1979, Ozawa et al. [103] demonstrated that *B. subtilis* var. *natto* inhibited the growth of *C. albicans* in the intestinal tract and [104] showed that a surfactin had activity against yeast.

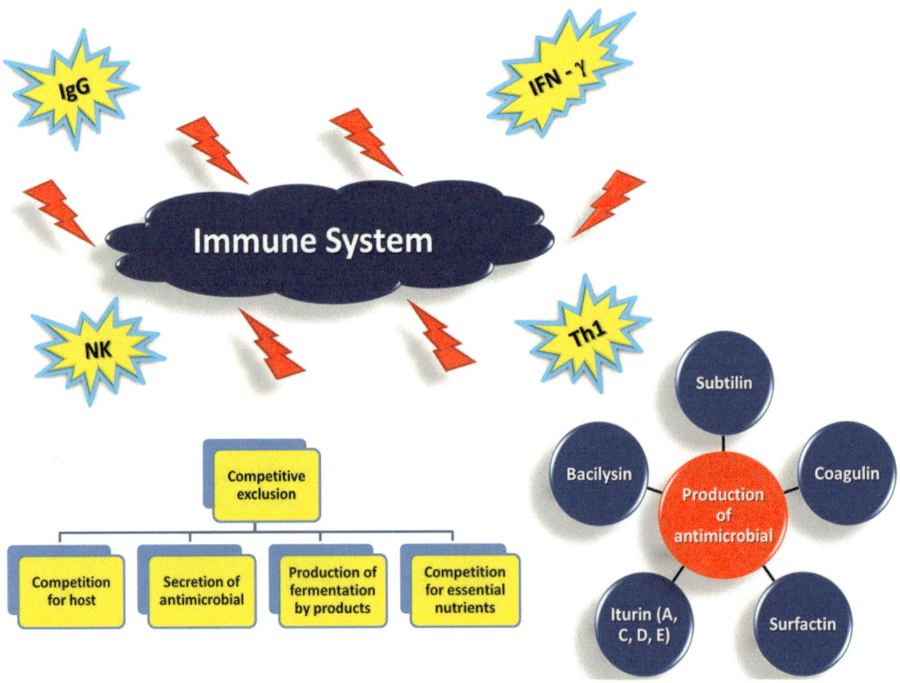

Figure 2. Mechanism of action of *Bacillus* probiotic.

Stimulation of the immune system or immunomodulation is considered an important mechanism to probiotics. Studies in humans and animal models have provided that the oral administration of spores stimulates the immune system, and this confirms that spores are neither innocuous gut passengers nor treated as a food. Helper lymphocyte (Th1) responses are important for IgG synthesis but more importantly for cytotoxic T-lymphocyte recruitment, and for the destruction of intracellular microorganisms, and involve presentation of antigens on the surface of the host cell by a class I major histocompatibility complex (MHC)-processing pathway [30].

Studies have shown that small amount of inoculum of *B. subtilis* spores can germinate in the small intestine, grow, proliferate, and then again sporulate [105, 106]. Thus, the spores of *Bacillus* spp. can germinate in significant numbers in the jejunum and ileum [107], and stimulate and regulate the synthesis of immunoglobulin A, the pro-inflammatory cytokines such as tumor necrosis factor and interferon γ, and the helper T lymphocytes [108]. Therefore, through colonization, immune stimulation, and antimicrobial activity developed by these bacteria it is possible to prove that they have the potential probiotic effect [109].

Different mechanisms have been proposed for competitive exclusion agents including competition for host-mucosal receptor sites, secretion of antimicrobials, production of fermentation by-products, such as volatile fatty acids, competition for essential nutrients, and stimulation of host immune functions [30] (**Figure 2**).

4.4. Studies with *Bacillus* spp. as probiotics

In literature, there are in vivo and in vitro studies of *Bacillus* spp. about the benefits of their probiotic action in humans and animals. However, despite its recognized probiotic action and its benefits to human and animal health, to date, there are no studies on the effect of *Bacillus* spp. in the genus *Candida*. Subsequent text describes some studies with the genus *Bacillus* as probiotic.

Lee et al. [26] studied the potential probiotic characteristics of *B. polyfermenticus* KU3 isolated from *kimchi*, a Korean dish made from fermented vegetables. The spore cell of *B. polyfermenticus* KU3 was highly resistant to artificial gastric juice and survived for 24 h in artificial bile acid. *B. polyfermenticus* KU3 did not generate the carcinogenic enzymes, β-glucosidase, N-acetyl-β-glucosaminidase, and β-glucuronidase, and adhered strongly to HT-29 human intestinal epithelial cell lines. The authors found that *B. polyfermenticus* KU3 strongly inhibited the proliferation of cancer cells such as HeLa, LoVo, HT-29, AGS, and MCF-7 cells. The supernatant of *B. polyfermenticus* KU3 had an anticancer effect against HeLa and LoVo cells. Conversely, the proliferation of normal MRC-5 cells was not inhibited. They also demonstrated the anti-inflammatory activity of *B. polyfermenticus* KU3 under inflammatory conditions, as shown by the reduction in nitric oxide and pro-inflammatory cytokines (TNF-α, IL-10, TGF-β2, and COX-2). This study demonstrated the probiotic characteristics of *B. polyfermenticus* KU3 and provided evidence for the effect of this bacterium against various cancer cells.

Studies performed by Thirabunyanon and Thongwittaya [99] investigated the activity of isolates of *Bacillus* spp. for possible use as potential probiotics, and their protective inhibition activity against *Salmonella enteritidis* infection. The gastrointestinal tracts of native chickens were evaluated for use as a potential probiotic. *Bacillus* demonstrated higher growth inhibition of seven food-borne pathogens, including *S. enteritidis, S. typhimurium, E. coli, B. cereus, S. aureus, Listeria monocytogenes*, and *Vibrio cholerae*. The authors concluded that *B. subtilis* NC11 has a protective activity against *S. enteritidis* infection, and is able to competitively exclude it from its original site in the gastrointestinal tract, which is the beginning of the route of food-pathogenic contamination.

Rhee et al. [110] studied the effect of bacteria administered orally on the development of the gut-associated lymphoid tissue (GALT) in infant rabbits and *B. subtilis* showed greater importance in GALT development. Besides, *B. subtilis* secretes antimicrobial agents, as coagulin, amicoumacin, and subtilisin, which may have probiotic effect by suppressing the growth of competing microorganisms, such as enteric pathogens.

Pinchuk and colleagues [90] demonstrated that a probiotic strain *B. subtilis* 3, originally isolated from animal feed, has inhibitory effect against *Helicobacter pylori* due to the production of antibiotics, including amicoumacin A. The group of isocoumarin antibiotics (which the amicoumacin A belongs) can exert, among other properties, anti-inflammatory and anti-tumor actions, and present potential for use in the treatment of *H. pylori* infection.

In the human and animal consumption, the spores of *B. subtilis* were used as probiotics and competitive exclusion agents [107, 111], and, in some countries, *B. subtilis* was applied in oral bacteriotherapy of gastrointestinal disorders [107].

Bacillus probiotics were developed for topical and oral treatment of uremia [30]. *B. coagulans* had the ability to secrete a bacteriocin, coagulin, that has activity against a broad spectrum of enteric microbes [112] and since 1983 [113] showed the beneficial effects of *Bacillus* probiotics on urinary tract infections.

Ghelardi and colleagues [114] aimed to investigate the survival and persistence of *B. clausii* in the human gastrointestinal tract following oral administration as spore-based probiotic formulation. The authors concluded that *B. clausii* strains can have different ability to survive in the intestinal environment. *B. clausii* spores administered as a liquid suspension or a lyophilized form behave similarly in vivo and *B. clausii* spores survive transit through the human gastrointestinal tract, and they can germinate, outgrowth, and multiply as vegetative forms.

The use of *Bacillus* species as probiotic is expanding rapidly with increasing number of studies demonstrating immune stimulation, antimicrobial activities, and competitive exclusion by these microorganisms. Most research with *Bacillus* has been performed in animals and some clinical studies also in humans. Thus, the question is: Are the findings relevant to probiotic research in humans?

Therefore, if the results are promising and not only the bacteria are becoming superbacteria, but also other microorganisms such as fungi, why not apply the probiotic properties of *Bacillus* spp. in the genus *Candida*?

5. Conclusion and future perspective

This chapter sought to provide the reader knowledge about the probiotic action of bacteria *Bacillus* spp. and *Lactobacillus* spp., describing the characteristics of microorganisms, the probiotic mechanism of action, and the studies described in the literature.

The high prevalence of *Candida* spp. associated with the increased resistance of microorganisms to conventional antifungal treatments boosts the development of research for new treatments to infections caused by *Candida*, such as probiotics. The treatment with probiotics promotes the reestablishment of the natural condition of microbiota with advantages over conventional antifungal because they do not induce microbial resistance, are nontoxic when administered in adequate amount, and therefore do not produce undesirable side effects, and also stimulate the immune system.

Infectious diseases along with the resistance of microorganisms to drugs represent serious problem in health. The knowledge of microorganisms that have characteristics capable of influencing the pathogenicity of *Candida*, and that characterize possible methods of prevention and treatment for candidiasis, is important, mainly, to provide alternative for microbial resistance without causing harmful side effects to the human organism and do not cause resistance to the fungus.

Author details

Michelle Peneluppi Silva*, Rodnei Dennis Rossoni, Juliana Campos Junqueira and Antonio Olavo Cardoso Jorge

*Address all correspondence to: michellepeneluppi@gmail.com

Department of Biosciences and Oral Diagnosis - Institute of Science and Technology, São Paulo State University/UNESP - São Jos dos Campos, São Paulo, Brazil

References

[1] Soni JN, Soman SS. Synthesis and antimicrobial evaluation of amide derivatives of benzodifuran-2-carboxylic acid. Eur J Med Chem. 2014;75:77–81.

[2] Nader-Macías ME, Juárez Tomás MS. Profiles and technological requirements of urogenital probiotics. Adv Drug Deliv Rev. 2015;92:84–104.

[3] De Baets L, Van Iwaarden P, Meeus N, Schimmel H, Philipp W, Emons H. First certified reference materials for molecular fingerprinting of two approved probiotic *Bacillus* strains. Int J Food Microbiol. 2009;129(1):16–20.

[4] World Health Organization (WHO). Antimicrobial Resistance: No Action Today, No Cure Tomorrow. Geneva, Switzerland: WHO Press, 2011.

[5] Abdhul K, Ganesh M, Shanmughapriya S, Vanithamani S, Kanagavel M, Anbarasu K, Natarajaseenivasan K. Bacteriocinogenic potential of a probiotic strain *Bacillus coagulans* [BDU3] from Ngari. Int J Biol Macromol. 2015;79:800–6.

[6] Blaser M. Antibiotic overuse: stop the killing of beneficial bacteria. Nature. 2011;476(7361):393–4.

[7] Brown GD, Denning DW, Levitz SM. Tackling human fungal infections. Science. 2012;336(6082):647.

[8] Pfaller MA, Diekema DJ. Epidemiology of invasive candidiasis: a persistent public health problem. Clin Microbiol Rev. 2007;20(1):133–63.

[9] Mayer FL, Wilson D, Hube B. *Candida albicans* pathogenicity mechanisms. Virulence. 2013;4(2):119–28.

[10] Ruhnke M. Skin and mucous membrane infections. In: Calderone RA, editor. *Candida* and Candidiasis. Washington, DC: ASM Press; 2002. pp. 307–25.

[11] Pappas PG, Kauffman CA, Andes D, Benjamin DK Jr, Calandra TF, Edwards JE Jr, Filler SG, Fisher JF, Kullberg BJ, Ostrosky-Zeichner L, Reboli AC, Rex JH, Walsh TJ, Sobel JD; Infectious Diseases Society of America. Clinical practice guidelines for the management of candidiasis: 2009 update by the Infectious Diseases Society of America. Clin Infect Dis. 2009;48(5):503–35.

[12] Salvatori O, Puri S, Tati S, Edgerton M. Innate immunity and saliva in *Candida albicans*-mediated oral diseases. J Dent Res. 2016 Jan 8. pii: 0022034515625222.

[13] Coogan MM, Greenspan J, Challacombe SJ. Oral lesions in infection with human immunodeficiency virus. Bull World Health Organ. 2005;83(9):700–6.

[14] Warrier SA, Sathasivasubramanian S. Human immunodeficiency virus induced oral candidiasis. J Pharm Bioallied Sci. 2015;7(Suppl 2):S812–4.

[15] Prado M, Silva MB, Laurenti R, Travassos LR, Taborda CP. Mortality due to systemic mycoses as a primary cause of death or in association with AIDS in Brazil: a review from 1996 to 2006. Mem Inst Oswaldo Cruz. 2009;104(3):513–21.

[16] Cassone A, Cauda R. *Candida* and candidiasis in HIV-infected patients: where commensalism, opportunistic behavior and frank pathogenicity lose their borders. AIDS. 2012;26(12):1457–72.

[17] De Paula SB, Morey AT, Santos JP, Dos Santos PM, Gameiro DG, Kerbauy G, Sena EM, Ueda LT, Carneiro M, Pinge-Filho P, Yamauchi LM, Yamada-Ogatta SF. Oral *Candida* colonization in HIV-infected patients in Londrina-PR, Brazil: antifungal susceptibility and virulence factors. J Infect Dev Ctries. 2015;9(12):1350–9.

[18] Sánchez-Vargas LO, Ortiz-López NG, Villar M, Moragues MD, Aguirre JM, Cashat-Cruz M, Lopez-Ribot JL, Gaitán-Cepeda LA, Quindós G. Point prevalence, microbiology and antifungal susceptibility patterns of oral *Candida* isolates colonizing or infecting Mexican HIV/AIDS patients and healthy persons. Rev Iberoam Micol. 2005;22(2):83–92.

[19] Delgado AC, de Jesus Pedro R, Aoki FH, Resende MR, Trabasso P, Colombo AL, de Oliveira MS, Mikami Y, Moretti ML. Clinical and microbiological assessment of patients with a long-term diagnosis of human immunodeficiency virus infection and *Candida* oral colonization. Clin Microbiol Infect. 2009;15(4):364–71.

[20] Gismondo MR, Drago L, Lombardi A. Review of probiotics available to modify gastrointestinal flora. Int J Antimicrob Agents. 1999;12(4):287–92.

[21] Saad N, Delattre C, Urdaci M, Schmitter JM, Bressollier P. An overview of the last advances in probiotic and prebiotic field. LWT – Food Sci Technol. 2013;50(1):1–16.

[22] FAO/WHO. Guidelines for the Evaluation of Probiotics in Food. London, Ontario: Food and Agriculture Organization of the United Nations and World Health Organization Working Group Report; 2002. pp. 1–11.

[23] Chen C, Khismatullin DB. Lipopolysaccharide induces the interactions of breast cancer and endothelial cells via activated monocytes. Cancer Lett. 2014;345(1):75–84.

[24] Guo XH, Kim JM, Nam HM, Park SY, Kim JM. Screening lactic acid bacteria from swine origins for multistrain probiotics based on in vitro functional properties. Anaerobe. 2010;16(4):321–6.

[25] Guo CF, Zhang S, Yuan YH, Yue TL, Li JY. Comparison of lactobacilli isolated from Chinese susan-tsai and koumiss for their probiotic and functional properties. J Funct Foods. 2015;12:294–302.

[26] Lee NK, Son SH, Jeon EB, Jung GH, Lee JY, Paik HD. The prophylactic effect of probiotic *Bacillus polyfermenticus* KU3 against cancer cells. J Funct Foods. 2015;14:513–18.

[27] Angmo K, Kumari A, Savitri, Bhalla TC. Probiotic characterization of lactic acid bacteria isolated from fermented foods and beverage of Ladakh. LWT – Food Sci Technol. 2016;66:428–35.

[28] Giraffa G. Selection and design of lactic acid bacteria probiotic culture. Eng Life Sci. 2012;12(4):391–8.

[29] Chen P, Zhang Q, Dang H, Liu X, Tian F, Zhao J, Chen Y, Zhang H, Chen W. Screening for potential new probiotic based on probiotic properties and α-glucosidase inhibitory activity. Food Control. 2014;35(1):65–72.

[30] Hong HA, Duc le H, Cutting SM. The use of bacterial spore formers as probiotics. FEMS Microbiol Rev. 2005;29(4):813–35.

[31] Vilela SF, Barbosa JO, Rossoni RD, Santos JD, Prata MC, Anbinder AL, Jorge AO, Junqueira JC. *Lactobacillus acidophilus* ATCC 4356 inhibits biofilm formation by *C.*

albicans and attenuates the experimental candidiasis in *Galleria mellonella*. Virulence. 2015;6(1):29–39.

[32] Caufield PW, Schön CN, Saraithong P, Li Y, Argimón S. Oral lactobacilli and dental caries: a model for niche adaptation in humans. J Dent Res. 2015 Sep;94(9 Suppl):110S–8S.

[33] Delfederico L, Hollmann A, Martínez M, Iglesias NG, De Antoni G, Semorile L. Molecular identification and typing of lactobacilli isolated from kefir grains. J Dairy Res. 2006 ;73(1):20–7.

[34] Huch Née Kostinek M, Hanak A, Specht I, Dortu CM, Thonart P, Mbugua S, Holzapfel WH, Hertel C, Franz CM. Use of *Lactobacillus* strains to start cassava fermentations for Gari production. Int J Food Microbiol. 2008;128(2):258–67.

[35] McLeod A, Nyquist OL, Snipen L, Naterstad K, Axelsson L. Diversity of *Lactobacillus sakei* strains investigated by phenotypic and genotypic methods. Syst Appl Microbiol. 2008;31(5):393–403.

[36] Molenaar D, Bringel F, Schuren FH, de Vos WM, Siezen RJ, Kleerebezem M. Exploring *Lactobacillus plantarum* genome diversity by using microarrays. J Bacteriol. 2005;187(17):6119–27.

[37] Tamang JP, Tamang B, Schillinger U, Franz CM, Gores M, Holzapfel WH. Identification of predominant lactic acid bacteria isolated from traditionally fermented vegetable products of the Eastern Himalayas. Int J Food Microbiol. 2005;105(3):347–56.

[38] Claesson MJ, van Sinderen D, O'Toole PW. *Lactobacillus* phylogenomics – towards a reclassification of the genus. Int J Syst Evol Microbiol. 2008;58(Pt 12):2945–54.

[39] Parolo CC, Do T, Henssge U, Alves LS, de Santana Giongo FC, Corção G, Maltz M, Beighton D. Genetic diversity of *Lactobacillus paracasei* isolated from *in situ* human oral biofilms. J Appl Microbiol. 2011;111(1):105–13.

[40] Veljovic K, Terzic-Vidojevic A, Vukasinovic M, Strahinic I, Begovic J, Lozo J, Ostojic M, Topisirovic L. Preliminary characterization of lactic acid bacteria isolated from Zlatar cheese. J Appl Microbiol. 2007;103(6):2142–52.

[41] Al-Allaf MAH, Al-Rawi AMM, Al-Mola AT. Antimicrobial activity of lactic acid bacteria isolated from minced beef meat against some pathogenic bacteria. Iraqi J Vet Sci. 2009;23:115–7.

[42] Zavisic G, Petricevic S, Radulovic Z, Begovic J, Golic N, Topisirovic L, Strahinic I. Probiotic features of two oral *Lactobacillus* isolates. Braz J Microbiol. 2012;43(1):418–28.

[43] Meurman JH. Probiotics: do they have a role in oral medicine and dentistry? Eur J Oral Sci. 2005;113(3):188–96.

[44] Heinemann C, van Hylckama Vlieg JE, Janssen DB, Busscher HJ, van der Mei HC, Reid G. Purification and characterization of a surface-binding protein from *Lactobacillus*

fermentum RC-14 that inhibits adhesion of *Enterococcus faecalis* 1131. FEMS Microbiol Lett. 2000;190(1):177–80.

[45] Reid G, Heinemann C, Velraeds M, van der Mei HC, Busscher HJ. Biosurfactants produced by *Lactobacillus*. Methods Enzymol. 1999;310:426–33.

[46] Reid G, Bruce AW. Selection of *Lactobacillus* strains for urogenital probiotic applications. J Infect Dis. 2001;183 Suppl 1:S77–80.

[47] Balkus JE, Mitchell C, Agnew K, Liu C, Fiedler T, Cohn SE, Luque A, Coombs R, Fredricks DN, Hitti J. Detection of hydrogen peroxide-producing *Lactobacillus* species in the vagina: a comparison of culture and quantitative PCR among HIV-1 seropositive women. BMC Infect Dis. 2012;12:188.

[48] Abedin-Do A, Taherian-Esfahani Z, Ghafouri-Fard S, Ghafouri-Fard S, Motevaseli E. Immunomodulatory effects of *Lactobacillus* strains: emphasis on their effects on cancer cells. Immunotherapy. 2015;7(12):1307–29.

[49] Galdeano CM, Perdigón G. The probiotic bacterium *Lactobacillus casei* induces activation of the gut mucosal immune system through innate immunity. Clin Vaccine Immunol. 2006;13(2):219–26.

[50] Chon H, Choi B, Lee E, Lee S, Jeong G. Immunomodulatory effects of specific bacterial components of *Lactobacillus plantarum* KFCC11389P on the murine macrophage cell line RAW 264.7. J Appl Microbiol. 2009;107(5):1588–97.

[51] Chon H, Choi B, Jeong G, Lee E, Lee S. Suppression of proinflammatory cytokine production by specific metabolites of *Lactobacillus plantarum* 10hk2 via inhibiting NF-kB and p38 MAPK expressions. Comp Immunol Microbiol Infect Dis. 2010;33(6):e41–9.

[52] Kim YG, Ohta T, Takahashi T, Kushiro A, Nomoto K, Yokokura T, Okada N, Danbara H. Probiotic *Lactobacillus casei* activates innate immunity via NF-kappaB and p38 MAP kinase signaling pathways. Microbes Infect. 2006;8(4):994–1005.

[53] Wagner RD, Johnson SJ. Probiotic *lactobacillus* and estrogen effects on vaginal epithelial gene expression responses to *Candida albicans*. J Biomed Sci. 2012;19:58.

[54] Jorjão AL, de Oliveira FE, Leão MV, Carvalho CA, Jorge AO, de Oliveira LD. Live and heat-killed *Lactobacillus rhamnosus* ATCC 7469 may induce modulatory cytokines profiles on macrophages RAW 264.7. Sci World J. 2015;2015:716749.

[55] Sánchez B, Ruiz L, Gueimonde M, Ruas-Madiedo P, Margolles A. Adaptation of bifidobacteria to the gastrointestinal tract and functional consequences. Pharmacol Res. 2013;69(1):127–36.

[56] Piddock LJ. Multidrug-resistance efflux pumps – not just for resistance. Nat Rev Microbiol. 2006;4(8):629–36.

[57] Duary RK, Batish VK, Grover S. Relative gene expression of bile salt hydrolase and surface proteins in two putative indigenous *Lactobacillus plantarum* strains under in vitro gut conditions. Mol Biol Rep. 2012;39(3):2541–52.

[58] Ruiz L, Margolles A, Sánchez B. Bile resistance mechanisms in *Lactobacillus* and *Bifidobacterium*. Front Microbiol. 2013;4:396.

[59] Sookkhee S, Chulasiri M, Prachyabrued W. Lactic acid bacteria from healthy oral cavity of Thai volunteers: inhibition of oral pathogens. J Appl Microbiol. 2001;90(2):172–9.

[60] Noverr MC, Huffnagle GB. Regulation of *Candida albicans* morphogenesis by fatty acid metabolites. Infect Immun. 2004;72(11):6206–10.

[61] Coman MM, Verdenelli MC, Cecchini C, Silvi S, Orpianesi C, Boyko N, Cresci A. *In vitro* evaluation of antimicrobial activity of *Lactobacillus rhamnosus* IMC 501(®), *Lactobacillus paracasei* IMC 502(®) and SYNBIO(®) against pathogens. J Appl Microbiol. 2014;117(2):518–27.

[62] Parolin C, Marangoni A, Laghi L, Foschi C, Ñahui Palomino RA, Calonghi N, Cevenini R, Vitali B. Isolation of vaginal lactobacilli and characterization of anti-*candida* activity. PLoS One. 2015;10(6):e0131220.

[63] Wagner RD, Pierson C, Warner T, Dohnalek M, Farmer J, Roberts L, Hilty M, Balish E. Biotherapeutic effects of probiotic bacteria on candidiasis in immunodeficient mice. Infect Immun. 1997;65(10):4165–72.

[64] Matsubara VH, Silva EG, Paula CR, Ishikawa KH, Nakamae AE. Treatment with probiotics in experimental oral colonization by *Candida albicans* in murine model (DBA/2). Oral Dis. 2012;18(3):260–4.

[65] Deng K, Chen T, Wu Q, Xin H, Wei Q, Hu P, Wang X, Wang X, Wei H, Shah NP. *In vitro* and *in vivo* examination of anticolonization of pathogens by *Lactobacillus paracasei* FJ861111.1. J Dairy Sci. 2015;98(10):6759–66.

[66] Jacobsen ID. *Galleria mellonella* as a model host to study virulence of *Candida*. Virulence. 2014;5(2):237–9.

[67] Fedhila S, Buisson C, Dussurget O, Serror P, Glomski IJ, Liehl P, Lereclus D, Nielsen-LeRoux C. Comparative analysis of the virulence of invertebrate and mammalian pathogenic bacteria in the oral insect infection model *Galleria mellonella*. J Invertebr Pathol. 2010;103(1):24–9.

[68] Cotter G, Doyle S, Kavanagh K. Development of an insect model for the *in vivo* pathogenicity testing of yeasts. FEMS Immunol Med Microbiol. 2000;27(2):163–9.

[69] Fuchs BB, O'Brien E, Khoury JB, Mylonakis E. Methods for using *Galleria mellonella* as a model host to study fungal pathogenesis. Virulence. 2010;1(6):475–82.

[70] Junqueira JC, Fuchs BB, Muhammed M, Coleman JJ, Suleiman JM, Vilela SF, Costa AC, Rasteiro VM, Jorge AO, Mylonakis E. Oral *Candida albicans* isolates from HIV-posi-

tive individuals have similar *in vitro* biofilm-forming ability and pathogenicity as invasive *Candida* isolates. BMC Microbiol. 2011;11:247.

[71] Rossoni RD, Barbosa JO, Vilela SF, dos Santos JD, de Barros PP, Prata MC, Anbinder AL, Fuchs BB, Jorge AO, Mylonakis E, Junqueira JC. Competitive interactions between *C. albicans, C. glabrata* and *C. krusei* during biofilm formation and development of experimental candidiasis. PLoS One. 2015;10(7):e0131700.

[72] Fakhry S, Sorrentini I, Ricca E, De Felice M, Baccigalupi L. Characterization of spore forming Bacilli isolated from the human gastrointestinal tract. J Appl Microbiol. 2008;105(6):2178–86.

[73] Hong HA, Huang JM, Khaneja R, Hiep LV, Urdaci MC, Cutting SM. The safety of *Bacillus subtilis* and *Bacillus indicus* as food probiotics. J Appl Microbiol. 2008;105(2): 510–20.

[74] Cutting SM. *Bacillus* probiotics. Food Microbiol. 2011;28(2):214–20.

[75] Sanders ME, Morelli L, Tompkins TA. Spore formers as human probiotics: *Bacillus, Sporolactobacillus,* and *Brevibacillus*. Compr Rev Food Sci Food Saf. 2003;2(3):101–10.

[76] Moriarty, DJ. Microbial biotechnology: a key ingredient for sustainable aquaculture. Infofish Int. 1996;4:29–33.

[77] Moriarty DJ. Control of luminous Vibrio species in penaeid aquaculture ponds. Aquaculture. 1998;164:351–8.

[78] Ziaei-Nejad S, Rezaei MH, Takami GA, Lovett DL, Mirvaghefi AR, Shakouri M. The effect of *Bacillus* spp. bacteria used as probiotics on digestive enzyme activity, survival and growth in the Indian white shrimp *Fenneropenaeus indicus*. Aquaculture. 2006;252(2–4):516–24.

[79] Foligné B, Peys E, Vandenkerckhove J, Van Hemel J, Dewulf J, Breton J, Pot B. Spores from two distinct colony types of the strain *Bacillus subtilis* PB6 substantiate anti-inflammatory probiotic effects in mice. Clin Nutr. 2012;31(6):987–94.

[80] Sorokulova I. Preclinical testing in the development of probiotics: a regulatory perspective with *Bacillus* strains as an example. Clin Infect Dis. 2008;46(Suppl.2):S92e5.

[81] Endres JR, Qureshi I, Farber T, Hauswirth J, Hirka G, Pasics I, Schauss AG. One-year chronic oral toxicity with combined reproduction toxicity study of a novel probiotic, *Bacillus coagulans,* as a food ingredient. Food Chem Toxicol. 2011;49(5):1174–82.

[82] Patel AK, Deshattiwar MK, Chaudhari BL, Chincholkar SB. Production, purification and chemical characterization of the catecholate siderophore from potent probiotic strains of *Bacillus* spp. Bioresour Technol. 2009;100(1):368–73.

[83] Selim KM, Reda RM. Improvement of immunity and disease resistance in the Nile tilapia, *Oreochromis niloticus,* by dietary supplementation with *Bacillus amyloliquefaciens*. Fish Shellfish Immunol. 2015;44(2):496–503.

[84] Nicholson WL. Roles of *Bacillus* endospores in the environment. Cell Mol Life Sci. 2002;59(3):410–6.

[85] Granum PE. *Bacillus cereus* and food poisoning In: Berkeley R, Heyndrickx M, Logan NA, De Vos P, editors. Applications and Systematics of *Bacillus* and Relatives. Oxford: Blackwell Science; 2002. pp. 37–46.

[86] Jensen GB, Hansen BM, Eilenberg J, Mahillon J. The hidden lifestyles of *Bacillus cereus* and relatives. Environ Microbiol. 2003;5(8):631–40.

[87] Earl AM, Losick R, Kolter R. Ecology and genomics of *Bacillus subtilis*. Trends Microbiol. 2008;16(6):269–75.

[88] Huang JM, Hong HA, Van Tong H, Hoang TH, Brisson A, Cutting SM. Mucosal delivery of antigens using adsorption to bacterial spores. Vaccine. 2010;28(4):1021–30.

[89] Wang X, Chen W, Tian Y, Mao Q, Lv X, Shang M, Li X, Yu X, Huang Y. Surface display of Clonorchis sinensis enolase on *Bacillus subtilis* spores potentializes an oral vaccine candidate. Vaccine. 2014;32(12):1338–45.

[90] Pinchuk IV, Bressollier P, Verneuil B, Fenet B, Sorokulova IB, Mégraud F, Urdaci MC. In vitro anti-Helicobacter pylori activity of the probiotic strain *Bacillus subtilis* 3 is due to secretion of antibiotics. Antimicrob Agents Chemother. 2001;45(11):3156–61.

[91] Taillade P, Urdaci MC. Strain for the treatment and/or prevention of chronic inflammatory diseases. Patent WO/2014/207360. 2014.

[92] Dudonné S, Varin TV, Anhê FF, Dubé P, Roy D, Pilon G, Marette A, Levy E, Jacquot C, Urdaci M, Desjardins Y. Modulatory effects of a cranberry extract co-supplementation with *Bacillus subtilis* CU1 probiotic on phenolic compounds bioavailability and gut microbiota composition in high-fat diet-fed mice. PharmaNutrition. 2015;3(3):89–100.

[93] Setlow P. Spores of *Bacillus subtilis*: their resistance to and killing by radiation, heat and chemicals. J Appl Microbiol. 2006;101(3):514–25.

[94] Moir A. How do spores germinate? J Appl Microbiol. 2006;101(3):526–30.

[95] Spinosa MR, Braccini T, Ricca E, De Felice M, Morelli L, Pozzi G, Oggioni MR. On the fate of ingested *Bacillus* spores. Res Microbiol. 2000;151(5):361–8.

[96] Barbosa TM, Serra CR, La Ragione RM, Woodward MJ, Henriques AO. Screening for *Bacillus* isolates in the broiler gastrointestinal tract. Appl Environ Microbiol. 2005;71(2): 968–78.

[97] Salminen S, von Wright A, Morelli L, Marteau P, Brassart D, de Vos WM, Fondén R, Saxelin M, Collins K, Mogensen G, Birkeland SE, Mattila-Sandholm T. Demonstration of safety of probiotics – a review. Int J Food Microbiol. 1998;44(1–2):93–106.

[98] Tomasik PJ, Tomasik P. Probiotics and prebiotics. Cereal Chem. 2003;80(2):113–7.

[99] Thirabunyanon M, Thongwittaya N. Protection activity of a novel probiotic strain of *Bacillus subtilis* against *Salmonella enteritidis* infection. Res Vet Sci. 2012;93(1):74–81.

[100] Alvarez-Olmos MI, Oberhelman RA. Probiotic agents and infectious diseases: a modern perspective on a traditional therapy. Clin Infect Dis. 2001;32(11):1567–76.

[101] Tien MT, Girardin SE, Regnault B, Le Bourhis L, Dillies MA, Coppée JY, Bourdet-Sicard R, Sansonetti PJ, Pédron T. Anti-inflammatory effect of *Lactobacillus casei* on *Shigella*-infected human intestinal epithelial cells. J Immunol. 2006;176(2):1228–37.

[102] Urdaci MC, Pinchuk I. Antimicrobial activity of *Bacillus* probiotics In: Ricca E, Henriques AO, Cutting SM, editors. Bacterial Spore Formers: Probiotics and Emerging Applications. Norfolk, UK: Horizon Bioscience; 2004. pp. 171–82.

[103] Ozawa K, Yagu-Uchi K, Yamanaka K, Yamashita Y, Ueba K, Miwatani T. Antagonistic effects of *Bacillus natto* and *Streptococcus faecalis* on growth of *Candida albicans*. Microbiol Immunol. 1979;23(12):1147–56.

[104] Nagal S, Okimura K, Kaizawa N, Ohki K, Kanatomo S. Study on surfactin, a cyclic depsipeptide. II. Synthesis of surfactin B2 produced by *Bacillus natto* KMD 2311. Chem Pharm Bull (Tokyo). 1996;44(1):5–10.

[105] Hoa TT, Duc LH, Isticato R, Baccigalupi L, Ricca E, Van PH, Cutting SM. Fate and dissemination of *Bacillus subtilis* spores in a murine model. Appl Environ Microbiol. 2001;67(9):3819–23.

[106] Tam NK, Uyen NQ, Hong HA, Duc le H, Hoa TT, Serra CR, Henriques AO, Cutting SM. The intestinal life cycle of *Bacillus subtilis* and close relatives. J Bacteriol. 2006;188(7):2692–700.

[107] Casula G, Cutting SM. *Bacillus* probiotics: spore germination in the gastrointestinal tract. Appl Environ Microbiol. 2002;68(5):2344–52.

[108] Duc le H, Hong HA, Barbosa TM, Henriques AO, Cutting SM. Characterization of *Bacillus* probiotics available for human use. Appl Environ Microbiol. 2004;70(4):2161–71.

[109] Deng J, Li Y, Zhang J, Yang Q. Co-administration of *Bacillus subtilis* RJGP16 and *Lactobacillus salivarius* B1 strongly enhances the intestinal mucosal immunity of piglets. Res Vet Sci. 2013;94(1):62–8.

[110] Rhee KJ, Sethupathi P, Driks A, Lanning DK, Knight KL. Role of commensal bacteria in development of gut-associated lymphoid tissues and preimmune antibody repertoire. J Immunol. 2004;172(2):1118–24.

[111] Mazza P. The use of *Bacillus subtilis* as an antidiarrhoeal microorganism. Boll Chim Farm. 1994;133(1):3–18.

[112] Hyronimus B, Le Marrec C, Urdaci MC. Coagulin, a bacteriocin-like inhibitory substance produced by *Bacillus coagulans* I4. J Appl Microbiol. 1998;85(1):42–50

[113] Meroni PL, Palmieri R, Barcellini W, De Bartolo G. Zanussi, C. Effect of long-term treatment with *B. subtilis* on the frequency of urinary tract infections in older patients. Chemioterapia 1983;2:142–4.

[114] Ghelardi E, Celandroni F, Salvetti S, Gueye SA, Lupetti A, Senesi S. Survival and persistence of *Bacillus clausii* in the human gastrointestinal tract following oral administration as spore-based probiotic formulation. J Appl Microbiol. 2015;119(2): 552–9.

Chapter 13

Phosphorus Nutrition and Health: Utilization of Phytase-producing Bifidobacteria in Food Industry

Long Chen, Fengshou Tian and Zhongke Sun

Additional information is available at the end of the chapter

http://dx.doi.org/10.5772/63644

Abstract

Phosphorus plays vital roles in human health and nutrition. In nature, phosphorus exists as phosphate, either inorganic or organic. The major form of phosphate in plant-derived diets is phytate that cannot be degraded by monogastric animal, as well as humans. Initially, this chapter reviews current research of phosphorus in human nutrition and health. Subsequently, problems of phytate degradation and phosphorus utilization in plant-derived diet are outlined. Next, as the main part, the enzymes of phytase, which catalyze the release of inorganic phosphorus from phytate, are compared, especially those produced by gut microbiota. Meanwhile, how probiotic bifidobacteria can be used for producing phytase and therefore enhance their beneficial effects are discussed. Phytase-producing bifidobacteria can be either isolated rarely in nature or constructed by genetic cloning of phytase genes from other well-characterized enzymes. The combination of bifidobacteria and highly active phytase may improve human health and nutrition especially as supplementary probiotic foods. Therefore, potential application is prospected. Finally, other considerations related to industrial production and usage of phosphorus-enriched additives are remarked. In conclusion, improving and maintaining the phosphorus balance in food by bifidobacteria may be promising for a healthier life.

Keywords: bifidobacteria, phytate, phytase, phosphorus, nutrition

1. Introduction

Phosphorus is an essential nutrient for the body and is routinely consumed through food. After consumption, phosphorus is usually bound with oxygen and exists as phosphate in the body. Both organic and inorganic forms of phosphate are present in regularly consumed foods. The amount of total phosphate ingestion can be significantly influenced by processed food. Following a meal, inorganic phosphate can be rapidly absorbed across the small intestine and enter the bloodstream causing an elevation in serum phosphate levels. An increase in serum levels of inorganic phosphate usually reduces serum levels of ionic calcium by forming a calcium phosphate complex. High ratio of phosphate to calcium usually leads to hypophosphatemia. In contrast, dietary phosphate deficiency, mostly due to malnutrition, can also impair the bone mineralization process and eventually lead to the development of rickets [1]. Nevertheless, phosphorus homeostasis is important for versatile functions, especially skeletal growth, development, and maintenance [2].

Despite the essential role of phosphate in living cells and wide application of phosphate additives in kinds of food, humans cannot efficiently digest plant-derived phosphate, namely, phytate that is the main form in both cereals and vegetables [3]. Degradation of phytate is catalyzed by phytases, which are predominately presented on bacteria and fungi. Bifidobacteria are the most frequently used microbial supplements in functional foods and probiotic formulations [4]. Probiotics have many beneficial effects in human intestine [5]. Phytase activity was detected in a few species of bifidobacteria [6,7]. Furthermore, heterologous secretion of phytases cloned from other bacteria was reported in bifidobacteria as well [8]. These strains can be used in fermented foods for conversion of poorly digestible phytate enriched in plant materials, which serves an alternative approach for dietary phosphorus supplementation in humans, especially those health-compromised individuals.

2. Role of phosphorus in human nutrition and health

2.1. General biochemistry and distribution of phosphorus

In biological systems, phosphorus involves in many important reactions, including forming cell membrane and nucleic acids, generation of ATP, cell signaling through protein phosphorylation or dephosphorylation, urinary buffering, and bone mineralization. In addition, phosphorus widely takes part in biochemical reactions, e.g., glucose and triacylglycerol (triglyceride) utilize phosphate to synthesize glucose 6-phosphate and glycerol 3-phosphate respectively. Phosphorus is the sixth abundant element in the human body and comprises approximately 1% of total body weight [9]. In mammals, phosphorus is presented as phosphate, which is a predominantly intracellular anion. There is 85% phosphate in bone and teeth, 14% in other tissues, and 1% in extracellular fluid.

Under steady state, a regular Western diet provides approximately 20 mg/kg/day of phosphorus [10]. Around 16 mg/kg/day is absorbed in the proximal intestine, mainly in the jejunum. The normal range of serum phosphate concentration is 4.5–8.3 mg/dl and higher in infants who require more of the mineral for bone growth and soft tissue buildup [11]. At zero metabolic balance, about 13 mg/kg/day phosphorus is excreted in the urine in adults. Thus, under phosphate equilibrium state and normal renal function, the amount of urine phosphorus can be an indicator of the amount absorbed in the intestine [12]. Reasonably, phosphate absorption and reabsorption decline along human aging, respectively, in both the intestinal tract and kidney. Meanwhile, expression of sodium-phosphate co-transporters decreases [13].

2.2. Phosphorus for nutrition and health

Phosphorus can be supplied in two forms, namely, organic phosphate and inorganic phosphate. Inorganic phosphate additives have greater bioavailability than organic sources of phosphorus that are the main form of phosphate in plant-derived foods. Phosphorus serves vital roles in the human body and is essential component of nutrient. It is crucial for bone growth and mineralization. Both bench and clinical researches show that phosphate is one of the major factors in the maintenance of bone health, and its deficiency results in bone pathology and clinical illness, such as rickets and osteomalacia [14]. Inorganic phosphorus is one of the two main ionic components required for hydroxyapatite formation during the mineralization of the extracellular matrix [15].

Roughly, 80–90% of the mineral content of bone is calcium and phosphorus, and 85% of the phosphorus is in the skeleton. Adequate phosphorus intake is essential for skeletal mineralization. Although calcium plays an important role in regulating chondrocyte maturation, apoptosis of hypertrophic chondrocytes is dependent upon circulating phosphate at normal levels [16]. Diets high in phosphorus often lead to diminished intestinal calcium absorption, reducing serum calcium concentration, and stimulating parathyroid hormone (PTH) secretion [17]. Phosphorus also directly regulates the production of 1,25(OH)2D by kidney cells. Furthermore, phosphorus is considered to be a major dietary source of acid [18].

2.3. Phosphate homeostasis and health

As more than 2000 chemical reactions in living cells use phosphate, optimal phosphate balance is essential for effective regulation. Generally, phosphate homeostasis is determined by both intestinal absorption from consumed food and renal excretion of the serum phosphate. Sodium-dependent phosphate (NaPi) transporters actively regulate the intestinal phosphate absorption and partially mediate renal phosphate excretion and reabsorption as well. Parathyroid hormone (PTH) facilitates urinary phosphate excretion because of strong inhibition of NaPi transporters function [10]. Dietary phosphate restriction induces an adaptive increase of intestinal phosphate uptake, and prolonged restriction increases NaPi-2a activity, thereby attempting to restore the balance by increasing kidney phosphate reabsorption [19].

The maintenance of optimal phosphate balance is managed by complex interactions between the gut, kidney, and bone, as well as "phosphatonins" involving multiple regulators. More precisely, the duodenum and jejunum are responsible for phosphorus absorption in the diet via both passive diffusion and active sodium-dependent transportation [20]. The kidney is the major organ involved in the regulation of phosphate homeostasis. A variety of factors along the proximal convoluted and straight tubule of the kidney, including serum PTH, calcium, 1,25(OH)2D3, and bicarbonate concentrations, take part in the regulation of phosphate. In animals with intact parathyroid glands, the phosphate concentration in the proximal tubules is 70% of the plasma level. There is little phosphate reabsorption in the proximal straight tubule in the presence of PTH. However, in the absence of PTH, phosphate is avidly reabsorbed along the proximal straight tubule. As previously reported, phosphate renal losses were enhanced by increasing fibroblast growth factor 23 (FGF-23).

2.4. Phosphate toxicity

Excessive retention of phosphate in the body is toxic to humans and can cause a wide range of cellular and tissue injuries; partial toxicities are shown in **Figure 1** [21]. Common toxicity of phosphate in humans includes impaired renal function, rhabdomyolysis, and tumor lysis syndrome [22]. Occasionally, exogenous phosphate toxicity is also documented in patients when exposed to hypertonic phosphate enemas [23]. Horribly, excessive exogenous phosphate administration can be fatal though the lethal dose in humans is unknown [24]. Overall, it is convincingly demonstrated that phosphate accelerates various pathologies. Acute toxicity can provoke hypocalcemia and associated symptoms including tetany, hypotension, and tachycardia. Moderate toxicity leads to deposition of calcium phosphate crystals, including often fatal cardiovascular calcification that usually irreversible. For instance, phosphate toxicity has been implicated as independent risk factor for high mortality in chronic kidney disease patients [25]. In an animal study, a 7–20-fold higher commercial phosphate-containing enema induced 100% mortality [26]. In another study, the *NaPi2a/klotho* double-knockout mice lost their fertility when fed with a high-phosphate diet [27]. Phosphate toxicity can induce an increased rate of apoptosis in various tissues. It has been found that phosphate toxicity accelerates the mammalian aging process by inflicting tissue damage and reducing survival as well [28]. Meanwhile, several studies reported links between high dietary inorganic phosphate intake and cancer development [17,29], as well as bone health problems [10, 30].

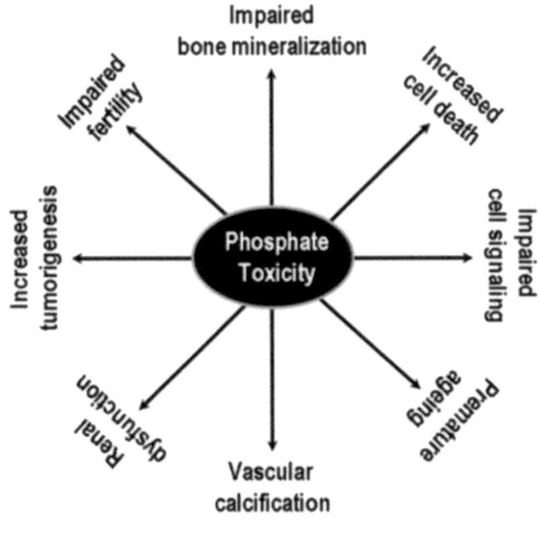

Figure 1. Partial list of pathological events related to phosphate toxicity composed by Razzaque [21] from related literatures in both human and animal studies.

3. Phytate in plant-derived diets

Phytate, the salt form of phytic acid, represents 60–80% of total phosphorus in plant seeds that can be hydrolyzed by phytase. Even milk and its related products are the richest phosphate sources in human diet; the major sources of phosphate in all natural foods are protein-rich foods and cereal grains. However, humans do not encode genes for phytase and hence can poorly digest phytate in plant-derived diets. Lacking of phytase causes three major problems in simple-stomached animals as well as humans: (1) environmental pollution from manure phosphorus, (2) dietary addition of inorganic phosphorus, and (3) depletion of rock phosphorus deposits. For instance, in a crossover trial with chronic kidney disease-suffering patients, the fasting serum phosphorus concentration was lower after the vegetarian diet than after the meat diet that contained identical phosphorus. More notably, secretion of plasma FGF-23 was about 40% lower in subjects treated with vegetarian diet after one week [31].

Phosphate interacts with several dietary minerals, such as calcium, sodium, and magnesium. Therefore, deficiency of these minerals is more common than deficiency of phosphate when its bioavailability is low. It was noted that the phosphorus bioavailability of natural foods is variable. Particularly, the bioavailability of phosphorus in phosphate-rich plant foods such as whole grains, legumes, peas, nuts, and seeds is relatively low, because a high proportion of it is tied up in poorly absorbed phytates. Considering many studies link high phosphorus intakes that are mainly supplied by inorganic phosphate additives to increased morbidity and mortality, natural plant foods may favorite health outcomes as their relatively low bioavailability of phosphorus.

4. Phytases and gut microbiota

Phytases (myoinositol hexakisphosphate phosphohydrolase) are enzymes that catalyze the stepwise removal of phosphates from phytic acid (myoinositol hexakisphosphate) or its salt phytate. Until now, a plenty of phytases were discovered and they show different catalytic mechanisms. The first and most extensively studied group of phytases, such as *Escherichia coli* AppA, belongs to the class of histidine acid phosphatases (HAPs) [32]. The other three groups of phytase are classified as b-propeller phosphatase (BPP; also referred to as alkaline phytase, exampled by *Bacillus amyloliquefaciens* phytase) [33], protein tyrosine phosphatase (PTP; also referred to as dual-specificity phosphatase) [34], and purple acid phosphatase (PAP; metalloenzymes) [35]. Corresponding three-dimensional structures and catalytic sites of these phytases are created using protein sequences. As shown in **Figure 2**, they have different secondary structures together with different active sites [36]. The currently known distribution of different types of phytases had been summarized in a previous review [3]. Among them, the majority are encoded by bacteria and fungi even a few species of animal and plant possess phytase activity as well.

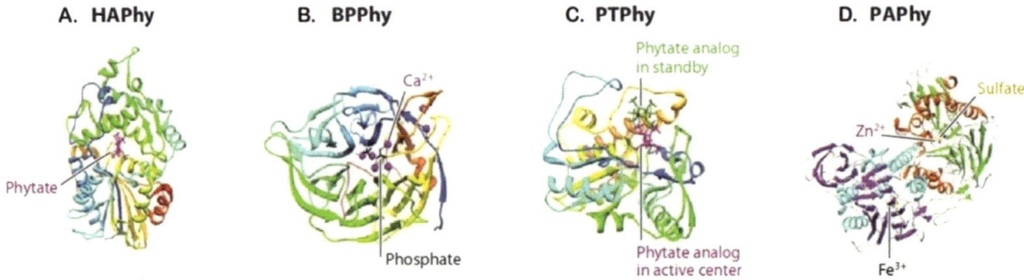

Figure 2. Secondary structure structures of representatives of each of the four structural classes of phytases. (A) Histidine acid phytase (HAPhy), (B) b-propeller phytase (BPPhy), (C) protein tyrosine phytase (PTPhy), and (D) purple acid phytase (PAPhy). Pictures are adapted from the work done by Lei et al. [3].

Phylum	Number	Class
Proteobacteria	124	a-Proteobacteria (57)
		b-Proteobacteria (4)
		g-Proteobacteria (61)
Actinobacteria	39	Streptomycetales (20)
		Micromonosporales (11)
		Corynebacteriales (4)
		Pseudonocardiales (3)
		Bifidobacteriales (1)
Firmicutes	18	Bacillales (9)
		Clostridiales (8)
		Lactobacillales (1)
CFB group bacteria	7	Flavobacteriales (5)
Cyanobacteria	6	Gloeobacterales (4)
GNS bacteria	2	
Dictyoglomales	2	

BBPR_1292, which is annotated as lipoprotein in *Bifidobacterium bifidum* PRL2010, has two conserved domains that are phytase-like or esterase-like (pfam13449) and NHL repeat unit of beta-propeller proteins (cl18310).

Table 1. Existence of phytase genes in bacteria.

The gut, especially the jejunum, is the most active site, responsible for the absorption of two thirds of phosphate intake in humans. However, as mentioned above, gut cannot absorb organic phosphorus presented as phytate in plant-derived diets. We know that human gut consists of a complex community of microorganisms, namely, gut microbiota. One main role of gut microorganisms is they benefit the host by fermentation of human readily undigested substrates to absorbable nutrients. Some gut microorganisms produce kinds of enzymes and many of these enzymes are deficient in host, thereby symbiotic relationship is developed. Such a case is phytase producing microbe, like Escherichia coli, Streptomyces coelicolor, Clostridium spp., and so on. Search of "phytase" in the NCBI gene database yielded 198 genes annotated as bacterial phytase. A detailed presence of phytase genes in bacteria is demonstrated in **Table 1**. Among them, Proteobacteria and Actinobacteria are the most predominating groups that are also natural habitants of human gut.

5. Phytate degradation by bifidobacteria

5.1. Phytase-encoding genes

As shown in **Table 1**, there is only one gene in *B. bifidum* PRL2010 that was annotated as possible phytase-encoding gene. Meanwhile, two enzymes in bifidobacteria, exactly *B. pseudocatenulatum* ATCC 27919 and *B. longum* subsp. *infantis* ATCC 15697 with phytase activity, have been characterized [37]. Therefore, protein sequences of these three enzymes (BBPR_1292, BIFPSEUDO_03792, and BLON_0263) were used for searching homologues in *Bifidobacterium* (taxid: 1678).

Organism	Protein name	Accession	Locus_tag	Length (aa)
B. dentium ATCC 27678	Histidine acid phosphatase	WP_003838654	BIFDEN_01159	637
B. dentium ATCC 27679	Histidine acid phosphatase	WP_003843340	HMPREF0168_2166	631
B. dentium Bd1	Histidine acid phosphatase	WP_012902513	BDP_1985	643
B. longum DJO10A	Histidine acid phosphatase	WP_010081042	Blon03000750	617
B. longum DJO10A	Histidine acid phosphatase	WP_012472023	BLD_1202	622
B. longum NCC2705	Histidine acid phosphatase	WP_011068470	BL0400	606
B. longum subsp. *infantis* 157F	Histidine acid phosphatase	WP_015713264	BLIF_0216	622
B. longum subsp. *infantis* ATCC 15697=JCM 1222	Histidine acid phosphatase	WP_012576702	Blon_0263	623

Organism	Protein name	Accession	Locus_tag	Length (aa)
B. longum subsp. *infantis* ATCC 15697=JCM 1222	Histidine acid phosphatase	WP_014484530	BLIJ_0267	618
B. longum subsp. *infantis* CCUG 52486	Histidine acid phosphatase	WP_007051528	BLIG_00414	617
B. longum subsp. *longum* 35B	Histidine acid phosphatase	WP_007057720	HMPREF1314_0451	572
B. longum subsp. *longum* 44B	Histidine acid phosphatase	WP_007056476	HMPREF1312_1349	617
B. longum subsp. *longum* BBMN68	Histidine acid phosphatase	WP_013410389	BBMN68_1139	622
B. longum subsp. *longum* F8	Histidine acid phosphatase	WP_015512490	BIL_17170	617
B. long um subsp. *longum* JCM 1217	Histidine acid phosphatase	WP_007054753	BLLJ_0234	617
B. longum subsp. *longum* KACC 91563	Histidine acid phosphatase	WP_014485906	BLNIAS_02473	617
B. pseudocatenulatum DSM 20438=JCM 1200	Histidine acid phosphatase	WP_004222312	BIFPSEUDO_03792	639
B. sp. 12_1_47BFAA	Histidine acid phosphatase	WP_008783259	HMPREF0177_01170	561

Table 2. Protein list of histidine acid phosphatase in *Bifidobacterium* sp.*.

Available from http://www.ncbi.nlm.nih.gov/proteinclusters/?term=BIFPSEUDO_03792.

BLAST searches revealed that (1) BBPR_1292-like proteins are exclusively presented on the genomes of all *B. bifidum* strains with at least 99% identity and (2) BIFPSEUDO_03792 and BLON_0263 are presented in a few strains of *Bifidobacterium*. Though there is the presence of BBPR_1292-like proteins, there is no specific phytase activity that had been detected in *B. bifidum*. Based on sequence comparisons, these two characterized enzymes are more close to the phytases of plants, fungi, and vertebrates. However, in the protein clusters database of histidine acid phosphatase (PCLA_3557679), there are 18 proteins that belong to 16 *bifidobacteria* strains as listed in **Table 2**. Notably, all these predicted phytases belong to *B. dentium*, *B. longum*, and *B. pseudocatenulatum*. Nevertheless, phytase activity has been detected in some *Bifidobacterium* sp. even it is not a common metabolic feature.

5.2. Phytase enzyme activities

Initially, it was believed that bifidobacteria are phytase negative, as very low level activity may be because of unspecific release by phosphatase, except *B. pseudocatenulatum* ATCC 27919 [6].

To further evaluate the enzyme activities, five strains of different bifidobacterial species, i.e., *B. animalis, B. bifidum, B. infantis, B. longum,* and *B. pseudolongum,* were inoculated to degrade myoinositol hexaphosphate (InsP(6)). In a complex medium in which phytic acid was the only source of phosphorus, *B. infantis* ATCC 15697 showed the highest level of phytate-degrading activity. The optimal condition is at slight acid pH (6.0–6.5) and higher temperature (50°C). Maximum activity appears at the stationary phase of growth and when 1% lactose was used as carbon source [7]. The same research team compared phosphatase and phytase activities of 23 bifidobacterial strains (13 from infants and 10 from adults) belonging to three different species (*B. longum, B. breve,* and *B. catenulatum*). The highest phytate-degrading activity is displayed in *B. longum* BIF307, similar to previous comparison in which is *B. infantis,* a subspecies of *B. longum* has the highest phytase activity.

Although two novel phytases from *B. pseudocatenulatum* and *B. longum* subsp. *infantis* had been characterized, parallel comparison of bifidobacterial phytase activities to *E. coli* AppA is difficult, as they were expressed as relative percentage activity. Nevertheless, the enzymes that belong to a new subclass are highly specific for the hydrolysis of phytate and render *myo*inositol triphosphate as the final hydrolysis product [37]. From our experience, native phytase activity in bifidobacteria is extremely lower than commercial enzymes. Therefore, we constructed a series of recombinant *B. bifidum* S17 that can secrete heterologous AppA within high specific activity to phytate; even our primary aim is using appA as a suitable secretion reporter [8]. Among these constructs, *B. bifidum* S17/pMgapS6P using the GAP promoter and BBIF_1761 signal direct the most efficient phytase secretion (**Figure 3**).

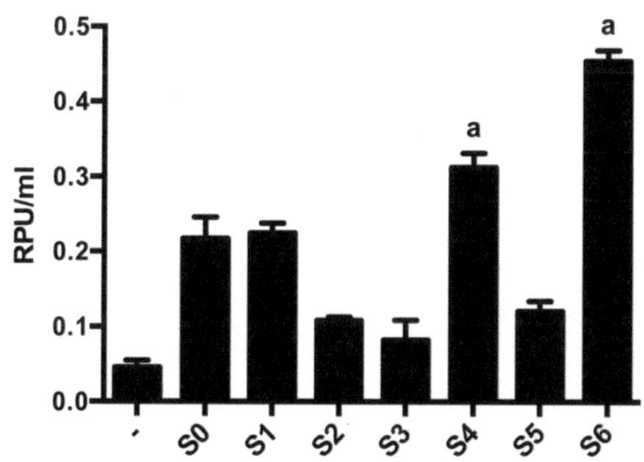

Figure 3. Phytase activity in spent cell-free medium of recombinant *B. bifidum* S17 strains. *B. bifidum* S17-harboring pMgapP-derived plasmids containing different SPs (S0–S6) were grown in 5 ml reinforced clostridia medium under anaerobic condition. The control plasmid pMgapP (–) contains no SP and serves as a background control for expression of a nonsecreted phytase. Values are relative phytase units (RPU) per ml supernatant and are mean ± standard deviation of three independent cultures measured in technical triplicates. The figure is adapted from Osswald et al. [8].

6. Potential application of phytase-producing bifidobacteria in foods

Despite phytase's main application in animal feeds, its applications in human foods can be equally important, if not exceed. To a large extent, using phytase in human foods is not primarily the target to improve phosphorus consumption, because depletion of phytate is more important as it chelates essential minerals, including iron, zinc, and calcium, contributing to deficiencies of these nutrients. It was estimated that there are approximately two to three billion people around the world suffering from mineral deficiency. The application of phytase in human health may be more exciting but need further in-depth study of potential adverse effects. Because certain inositol phosphates are beneficial to human health, phytase and phytase-producing cells can be immobilized as cost-effective bioreactors for large-scale production of these compounds [39]. There are many successful attempts to use phytase in brewing, baking, and dephytination of soy milk [25].

In fact, application of phytase or phytase-producing bacteria in food has already been illustrated. For example, *B. pseudocatenulatum* ATCC 27919 was tested as a starter in sourdough for the production of whole rye-wheat mixed bread [40]. In situ production of phytase during fermentation by probiotics results higher mineral availability in breads. The ability of *B. infantis* ATCC 15697 to degrade InsP(6) and accumulate InsP(3) could contribute to the reduction of the anti-nutritional properties of InsP(6) and generation of intermediate compounds with beneficial properties. *B. longum* BIF307, another phytase producer, was used in whole wheat bread making and decreased InsP(6) content. In another study, phytase-producing bifidobacterial strains significantly reduced the InsP(6) + InsP(5) concentrations compared to control samples during the bread-making process. Meanwhile, dialyzable Fe contents were increased from 2.3- to 5.6-folds. However, the effects appeared to be still insufficient to improve Fe bioavailability in Caco-2 cells [41]. Anyway, with similar technological and sensorial quality, levels of InsP(6) are significantly lower in bifidobacteria-fermented bread. Collectively, probiotic bifidobacteria are particularly suitable to reduce the content of InsP(6) in rich fiber products for human consumption [42].

7. Advantages of using phytase-producing bifidobacteria

One of the most important advantages of using phytase-producing bifidobacteria is safety. As widely known, several species of bifidobacteria are generally regarded as safe (GRAS) or qualified presumption of safety (QPS). The GRAS status made these strains particularly attractive for application in both food and pharmaceutical industries. Currently, probiotic bifidobacteria are widely used as micro-ecological reagent in many countries. These micro-ecological reagents had been added into both foods and pharmaceuticals without additional toxicity test.

Secondly, as important as the safety issue, many beneficial effects of bifidobacteria made them promising in industry especially ameliorating gastrointestinal disorders (both bacterial- and viral-induced gastroenteritis), allergic diseases, antibiotic-associated diarrhea, lactose intolerance, constipation, and irritable bowel disease. Let alone increasing iron accessibility, phytase-producing bifidobacteria has expanded nutrition profile [41,42]. In the gut of human eating plant-derived diets, phytase-producing bifidobacteria can degrade phytate-based components, therefore improving their adaptability or cross-feeding other symbiotic inhabitants in the same niche.

Thirdly, intake of phytase-producing bifidobacteria is superior to eating inorganic phosphate additives for human. In one aspect, phosphorus homeostasis can be easily disturbed after eating external inorganic phosphate additives. In another aspect, phytase-producing bifidobacteria can improve organic phytate-originated phosphorus. Thereby, supplementation of external inorganic phosphate additives becomes unnecessary. This is particularly significant for avoiding excessive phosphate, resulting in different kinds of toxicities that are largely caused by phosphate-containing additives in foods and drinks. For example, phosphorus-based food additives may pose high risk in people suffering chronic kidney disease, as this made dietary management of hyperphosphatemia practically difficult. In dialysis patients, managing hyperphosphatemia may require using phosphate binder other than restricting protein intake as this allows patients to eat more protein-rich foods [43]. In addition, a study evaluated 93 premature infants with a mean gestational age of 27.5 ± 2.0 weeks. The result demonstrated that elevated serum phosphorus was inversely correlated to the day of life of the infant after receiving human milk-derived fortifier though the incidence of hyperphosphatemia was mild and transient in this population [44]. For those health promised people, intake of phytase-producing bifidobacteria supplied a novel interventional approach.

Lastly but not least, bifidobacteria can produce phytase in human gut as microbial cell factories. They can be ingested as live cells and then colonized in the intestine to facilitate the degradation of plant-derived diets. The relatively constant replication of bifidobacteria in human intestine can either enlarge the bioavailability of organic phytate or downsize the toxicity of excessive phosphorus, hence maintaining the balance of phosphorus in a long term.

8. Final remarks

Phosphorus salts are added to foods as additives in many countries. Thus, dietary intake of phosphorus is higher than the recommended daily allowance in these countries and populations. For instance, phosphorus additives were particularly common in the categories of small goods, bakery goods, frozen meals, and biscuits in Australia [45]. In the United States, it has been estimated that phosphorus additives may add as much as 1 g of phosphorus to the diet [46]. However, high phosphorus intake has been shown to inhibit the increase in serum $1,25(OH)_2D$ concentration in response to low dietary calcium intake [30].

Collectively, although long-term and large amount consumption of phosphorus additives, little is known about risk associated with dietary phosphorus intake. A prospective cohort study of healthy adults reveals that high dosage of dietary phosphorus intake is associated with increased mortality [47]. Considering that the deleterious effects of chronic ingestion of unrestricted amounts of phosphate in individuals are not clear, consumption of high phosphate-containing processed foods and soft drinks should be alarming, particularly for health-compromised individuals [48,49]. Under those circumstances as mentioned above, using phytase-producing bifidobacteria may be a new way for increasing bioavailability of phosphorus from plant-derived diets, therefore avoiding supplementation of inorganic additives.

Author details

Long Chen[1], Fengshou Tian[2] and Zhongke Sun[1*]

*Address all correspondence to: Sunzh@daad-alumni.de

1 College of Life Sciences and Agronomy, Zhoukou Normal University, Chuanhui District, Zhoukou City, China

2 School of Chemistry and Chemical Engineering, Zhoukou Normal University, Chuanhui District, Zhoukou City, China

References

[1] Fukagawa M, Hamada Y, Nakanishi S, Tanaka M. The kidney and bone metabolism: nephrologists' point of view. J Bone Miner Metab. 2006; 24: 434–438.

[2] Huttunen MM, Pietila PE, Viljakainen HT, Lamberg-Allardt CJ. Prolonged increase in dietary phosphate intake alters bone mineralization in adult male rats. J Nutr Biochem. 2006; 17: 479–484.

[3] Lei XG, Weaver JD, Mullaney E, Ullah AH, Azain MJ. Phytase, a new life for an "old" enzyme. Annu Rev Anim Biosci. 2013; 1: 283–309.

[4] Kleerebezem M, Vaughan EE. Probiotic and gut lactobacilli and bifidobacteria: molecular approaches to study diversity and activity. Annu Rev Microbiol. 2009; 63: 269–290.

[5] Gareau MG, Sherman PM, Walker WA. Probiotics and the gut microbiota in intestinal health and disease. Nat Rev Gastroenterol Hepatol. 2010; 7: 503–514.

[6] Haros M, Bielecka M, Sanz Y. Phytase activity as a novel metabolic feature in *Bifidobacterium*. FEMS Microbiol Lett. 2005; 247: 231–239.

[7] Haros M, Bielecka M, Honke J, Sanz Y. Myo-inositol hexakisphosphate degradation by *Bifidobacterium infantis* ATCC 15697. Int J Food Microbiol. 2007; 117: 76–84.

[8] Osswald A, Westermann C, Sun Z, Riedel CU. A phytase-based reporter system for identification of functional secretion signals in bifidobacteria. PLoS ONE. 2015; 10(6): e0128802.

[9] Farrow EG, White KE. Recent advances in renal phosphate handling. Nat Rev Nephrol. 2010; 6: 207–217.

[10] Trautvetter U, Jahreis G, Kiehntopf M, Glei M. Consequences of a high phosphorus intake on mineral metabolism and bone remodeling in dependence of calcium intake in healthy subjects – a randomized placebo-controlled human intervention study. Nutr J. 2016; 15(1): 7.

[11] Bergwitz C, Huppner H. Regulation of phosphate homeostasis by PTH, vitamin D and FGF-23. Annu Rev Med. 2010; 61: 91–104.

[12] Berndt TJ, Schiavi S, Kumar R. "Phosphatonins" and the regulation of phosphorus homeostasis. Am J Physiol Renal Physiol. 2005; 289: F1170–F1182.

[13] Xu H, Bai L, Collins JF, Ghishan FK. Age-dependent regulation of rat intestinal type IIb sodium–phosphate cotransporter by 1,25-(OH)2 vitamin D3. Am J Physiol Cell Physiol. 2002; 282: C487–C493.

[14] Penido MG, Alon Uri S. Phosphate homeostasis and its role in bone health. Pediatr Nephrol. 2012; 27(11): 2039–2048.

[15] Magne D, Bluteau G, Faucheux C, Palmer G, Vignes-Colombeix C, Pilet P, Rouillon T, Caverzasio J, Weiss P, Daculsi G, Guicheux J. Phosphate is a specific signal for ATDC5 chondrocyte maturation and apoptosis-associated mineralization: possible implication of apoptosis in the regulation of endochondral ossification. J Bone Miner Res. 2003; 18: 1430–1442.

[16] Sabbagh Y, Carpenter TO, Demay MB. Hypophosphatemia leads to rickets by impairing caspase-mediated apoptosis of hypertrophic chondrocytes. Proc Natl Acad Sci U S A. 2005; 102: 9637–9642.

[17] Wilson KM, Shui IM, Mucci LA, Giovannucci E. Calcium and phosphorus intake and prostate cancer risk: a 24-y follow-up study. Am J Clin Nutr. 2015; 101(1): 173–183.

[18] Remer T, Manz F. Estimation of the renal net acid excretion by adults consuming diets containing variable amounts of protein. Am J Clin Nutr. 1994; 59: 1356–1361.

[19] Lotscher M, Kaissling B, Biber J, Murer H, Levi M. Role of microtubules in the rapid regulation of renal phosphate transport in response to acute alterations in dietary phosphate content. J Clin Invest. 1997; 99: 1302–1312.

[20] Amanzadeh J, Reilly RF Jr. Hypophosphatemia: an evidence-based approach to its clinical consequences and management. Nat Clin Pract Nephrol. 2006; 2: 136–148.

[21] Razzaque MS Phosphate toxicity: new insights into an old problem. Clin Sci (Lond). 2011; 120(3): 91–97.

[22] Berner YN, Shike M. Consequences of phosphate imbalance. Annu Rev Nutr. 1988; 8: 121–148.

[23] Ismail EA, Al-Mutairi G, Al-Anzy H. A fatal small dose of phosphate enema in a young child with no renal or gastrointestinal abnormality. J Pediatr Gastroenterol Nutr. 2000; 30: 220–221.

[24] Perlman JM. Fatal hyperphosphatemia after oral phosphate overdose in a premature infant. Am J Health Syst Pharm. 1997; 54: 2488–2490.

[25] Van-Etten RL, Davidson R, Stevis PE, MacArthur H, Moore DL. Covalent structure, disulfide bonding, and identification of reactive surface and active site residues of human prostatic acid phosphatase. J Biol Chem. 1991; 266: 2313–2319.

[26] Martin RR, Lisehora GR, Braxton M Jr, Barcia PJ. Fatal poisoning from sodium phosphate enema. Case report and experimental study. J Am Med Assoc. 1987; 257: 2190–2192.

[27] Ohnishi M, Razzaque MS. Dietary and genetic evidence for phosphate toxicity accelerating mammalian aging. FASEB J. 2010; 24(9): 3562–3571.

[28] Ohnishi M, Nakatani T, Lanske B, Razzaque MS. Reversal of mineral ion homeostasis and soft-tissue calcification of klotho knockout mice by deletion of vitamin D 1α-hydroxylase. Kidney Int. 2009; 75: 1166–1172.

[29] Lee YS, Ha YC, Chae CH, Beck GR Jr, Cho MH. High dietary inorganic phosphate increases lung tumorigenesis and alters Akt signaling. Am J Respir Crit Care Med. 2009; 179: 59–68.

[30] Takeda E, Yamamoto H, Yamanaka-Okumura H, Taketani Y. Increasing dietary phosphorus intake from food additives: potential for negative impact on bone health. Adv Nutr. 2014; 5(1): 92–97.

[31] Moe SM, Zidehsarai MP, Chambers MA, Jackman LA, Radcliffe JS, Trevino LL, Donahue SE, Asplin, JR. Vegetarian compared with meat dietary protein source and phosphorus homeostasis in chronic kidney disease. Clin J Am Soc Nephrol. 2011; 6(2): 257–264.

[32] Voormolen N, Noordzij M, Grootendorst DC, Beetz I, Sijpkens YW, van Manen JG, Boeschoten EW, Huisman RM, Krediet RT, Dekker FW. High plasma phosphate as a risk factor for decline in renal function and mortality in pre-dialysis patients. Nephrol Dial Transplant. 2007; 22: 2909–2916.

[33] Ha NC, Kim YO, Oh TK, Oh BH. Preliminary X-ray crystallographic analysis of a novel phytase from a *Bacillus amyloliquefaciens* strain. Acta Crystallogr D Biol Crystallogr. 1999; 55: 691–693.

[34] Chu HM, Guo RT, Lin TW, Chou CC, Shr HL, Lai HL, Tang TY, Cheng KJ, Selinger BL, Wang AH. Structures of *Selenomonas ruminantium* phytase in complex with persulfat-

ed phytate: DSP phytase fold and mechanism for sequential substrate hydrolysis. Structure. 2004; 12: 2015–2024.

[35] Hegeman CE, Grabau EA. A novel phytase with sequence similarity to purple acid phosphatases is expressed in cotyledons of germinating soybean seedlings. Plant Physiol. 2001; 126: 1598–1608.

[36] Mullaney EJ, Ullah AHJ. Phytases: attributes, catalytic mechanisms and applications. In Inositol Phosphates Linking Agriculture and the Environment, 2007. eds. BL Turner, AE Richardson, EJ Mullaney, pp. 97–110. Cambridge, MA: CABI

[37] Tenenhouse HS. Regulation of phosphorus homeostasis by the type IIa Na/phosphate cotransporter. Annu Rev Nutr. 2005; 25: 197–214.

[38] Palacios MC, Haros M, Rosell CM, Sanz Y. Selection of phytate-degrading human bifidobacteria and application in whole wheat dough fermentation. Food Microbiol. 2008; 25: 169–176.

[39] Meyer AS. Enzyme technology for precision functional food ingredient processes. Ann NY Acad Sci. 2010; 1190: 126–132.

[40] García-Mantrana I, Monedero V, Haros M. Myo-inositol hexakisphosphate degradation by *Bifidobacterium pseudocatenulatum* ATCC 27919 improves mineral availability of high fibre rye–wheat sour bread. Food Chem. 2015; 178: 267–275.

[41] Sanz-Penella JM, Laparra JM, Sanz Y, Haros M. Assessment of iron bioavailability in whole wheat bread by addition of phytase-producing bifidobacteria. J Agric Food Chem. 2012; 60(12): 3190–3195.

[42] Sanz-Penella JM, Tamayo-Ramos JA, Sanz Y, Haros M. Phytate reduction in bran-enriched bread by phytase-producing bifidobacteria. J Agric Food Chem. 2009; 57(21): 10239–10244.

[43] Fouque D, Horne R, Cozzolino M, Kalantar-Zadeh K. Balancing nutrition and serum phosphorus in maintenance dialysis. Am J Kidney Dis. 2014; 64(1): 143–150.

[44] Chetta KE, Hair AB, Hawthorne KM, Abrams SA. Serum phosphorus levels in premature infants receiving a donor human milk derived fortifier. Nutrients. 2015; 7(4): 2562–2573.

[45] McCutcheon J, Campbell K, Ferguson M, Day S, Rossi M. Prevalence of phosphorus-based additives in the Australian food supply: a challenge for dietary education? J Ren Nutr. 2015; 25(5): 440–444.

[46] Bell RR, Draper HH, Tzeng DY, Shin HK, Schmidt GR. Physiological responses of human adults to foods containing phosphate additives. J Nutr. 1977; 107: 42–50.

[47] Chang AR, Lazo M, Appel LJ, Gutiérrez OM, Grams ME. High dietary phosphorus intake is associated with all cause mortality: results from NHANES III. Am J Clin Nutr. 2014; 99(2): 320–327.

[48] Fernando GR, Martha RM, Evangelina R. Consumption of soft drinks with phosphoric acid as a risk factor for the development of hypocalcemia in postmenopausal women. J Clin Epidemiol. 1999; 52: 1007–1010.

[49] Jin H, Xu CX, Lim HT, Park SJ, Shin JY, Chung YS, Park SC, Chang SH, Youn HJ, Lee KH, Lee YS, Ha YC, Chae CH, Beck GR Jr, Cho MH. High dietary inorganic phosphate increases lung tumorigenesis and alters Akt signaling. Am J Respir Crit Care Med. 2009; 179(1): 59–68.

[50] Lee KJ, Kim KS, Kim HN, Seo JA, Song SW. Association between dietary calcium and phosphorus intakes, dietary calcium/phosphorus ratio and bone mass in the Korean population. Nutr J. 2014; 13(1): 114.

[51] Segawa H, Hanazaki A, Miyamoto K. Intracellular and extracellular functions of phosphorus compound in the body. Clin Calcium. 2016; 26(2): 187–191.

[52] Taal MW, Thurston V, McIntyre NJ, Fluck RJ, McIntyre CW. The impact of vitamin D status on the relative increase in fibroblast growth factor 23 and parathyroid hormone in chronic kidney disease. Kidney Int. 2014; 86(2): 407–413.

[53] Tamayo-Ramos JA, Sanz-Penella JM, Yebra MJ, Monedero V, Haros M. Novel phytases from *Bifidobacterium pseudocatenulatum* ATCC 27919 and *Bifidobacterium longum* subsp. *infantis* ATCC 15697. Appl Environ Microbiol. 2012; 78(14): 5013–5015.

[54] Ushasree MV, Gunasekaran P, Pandey A. Single-step purification and immobilization of MBP-phytase fusion on starch agar beads: application in dephytination of soy milk. Appl Biochem Biotechnol. 2012; 167: 1–10.

[55] Wesseling-Perry K. FGF-23 in bone biology. Pediatr Nephrol. 2010; 25: 603–608.

Chapter 14

Probiotic Microorganisms in Dry Fermented Meat Products

Katarzyna Neffe-Skocińska, Karolina Wójciak and Dorota Zielińska

Additional information is available at the end of the chapter

http://dx.doi.org/10.5772/64090

Abstract

In the modern lifestyle, food is supposed not only to feed the hunger but also to provide an appropriate amount and quality of nutrients necessary for proper functioning of the body. The interest of consumers in functional food, including fermented products with probiotic properties, has been growing for several years. Meat and meat products represent one of the most important components of contemporary human diet. Meat fermentation is one of the oldest methods of preserving food. This is a low-energy, biological acidulation which results in unique flavour and palatability, colour, microbiological safety and tenderness. Changes of muscle form into fermented meat product are caused by homo- or heterofermentative starter cultures or "wild" microorganisms which lower the pH. Fermented meat products are one of the most cherished and valuable food products. Fermentation and ageing process would deliver most aromatic and rich in flavour products, which is incomparable with other processes. A new solution is dry-aged meats with the use of new probiotic starter cultures with a high degree of health safety and long shelf life due to the inhibition of growth of the pathogenic microorganisms and therefore reduction of the formation of harmful compounds from protein transformation or lipid oxidation.

Keywords: dry-fermented meat, probiotic starter cultures, lipid oxidation, biogenic amine, bioactive peptides

1. Introduction

Meat and meat products are one of the most important components of human nutrition. Manufacturing raw cured sausages has a very long tradition and its origin is to be sought in the

Roman times in the Mediterranean area. In the past, raw cured sausages were manufactured only in the cool and cold time of the year and, therefore, it was possible to avoid the risk of spoilage. Nowadays, the preservation role of meat fermentation has become largely obsolete due to the introduction of the cold chain. Nevertheless, fermented meat products remain very popular and are still produced in large amounts, especially in Europe, probably because of their unique and specific sensory properties, their convenience and their alleged rootedness in culinary and cultural heritage [1].

One of the most promising areas of development in the human nutritional field over the last two decades has been the use of probiotics and recognition of their role in human health and disease. Lactic acid-producing bacteria are the most commonly used probiotics in foods and supplements. The means by which probiotic bacteria elicit their health effects are not understood fully, but may include competitive exclusion of enteric pathogens, neutralization of dietary carcinogens, production of antimicrobial metabolites and modulation of mucosal and systemic immune function [2]. According to the currently adopted definition by the Food and Agriculture Organization/World Health Organization [3], probiotics are defined as "live microorganisms which when administered in adequate amounts confer a health benefit on the host".

Although dairy products are the most commonly used food vehicles for the delivery of probiotics, several investigations dealing with the use of probiotics in cereal products [4, 5] vegetables and fruit juices [6, 7] and fermented meat products [8–13] to improve their nutritional value as functional foods have been reported.

The commercial application of probiotics in meat products is not yet popular, mainly because of technological issues. As fermented meat products are processed without heating, they could be suitable products for assessing probiotic LAB as starter cultures [14]. However, probiotics may be inactivated due to low pH or water activity value, as well as presence of native microorganisms or curing salt. The most important problem is to find compromise between technology, safety, quality and health-beneficial value of food [15].

2. Lactic acid bacteria in meat fermentation

2.1. Traditional starter cultures

Starter cultures are live, defined and specially selected microorganisms with the GRAS (generally recognized as safe) safety status, responsible for the proper course of meat ageing. Starter cultures may consist of selected bacteria, moulds or yeasts. Their use in the production of dry-aged cold meats is always intentional and aims at obtaining the specified sensory and microbiological characteristics in the end product [16–18].

The fermentation of food is known from centuries. First fermentation processes were driven by adventitious microbiota, represented by unknown microorganisms naturally present in the raw food ingredients and in the environment. A number of fermented foods, such as traditional cheeses, dry-fermented sausages and fermented beverages, are still produced without the addition of microbial inoculation [19]. Over time, with the aim to improve and standard-

http://dx.doi.org/10.5772/64090

ize the foods, the subsequent evolutionary step has been constantly associated with the back-slopping approaches, where higher counts of microorganisms are added to activate the fermentation. However, these natural starter cultures were often variable in load and composition, and if, on one hand, they can confer to the product peculiar characteristics of uniqueness and quality, on the other hand, they are continuously evolving according to seasonal and environmental variations and may result in variable qualities of the final product. For this reason, since the beginning of the past century, strains isolated from the best natural fermentations have been cultivated and studied under defined conditions by industrial companies and research institutions and used as selected starter cultures in food productions [20].

Group of microorganisms	Technological function and changes in meat>
Lactic acid bacteria	Natural preservative: lactic acid production, acidifying bacteria;
Lactobacillus sakei	inhibiting
Lactobacillus curvatus	the development of putrefactive and pathogenic microorganisms;
Lactobacillus plantarum	storage stabilization Good sensory quality, flavour and aroma
Lactobacillus pentosus	development
Lactobacillus casei	Proteolysis and lipolysis stabilization
Pediococcus acidilactici	
Pediococcus pentosaceus	
Gram-positive cocci	Bacteria redox flavouring: nitrates and nitrites reduction; using up
Staphylococcus carnosus	the oxygen; decomposition of peroxides; lipolysis stabilization (delaying
Staphylococcus xylosus	rancidity); colour stabilization; good sensory quality, flavour and aroma
Micrococcus varians	development
Yeasts	The surface microflora: using up the oxygen; decomposition of
Debaryomyces hansenii	peroxides;
Candida famata	delaying rancidity colour stabilization; good sensory quality, flavour
	and aroma development
Moulds	The surface microflora: using up the oxygen; decomposition of
Penicillium nalgiovense	peroxides;
Penicillium camemberti	proteolysis and lipolysis stabilization; good sensory quality, flavour and
Penicillium chrysogenum	aroma development
Mixed composition of yeasts and moulds	
Penicillium nalgiovense + Debaryomyces hansenii	
Penicillium candidum + Debaryomyces hansenii	

Table 1. The starter cultures composition for dry-fermented meat production [15].

Currently, the production of commercial starter preparations uses primarily lactic acid bacteria which show favourable technological effect. Typical starter cultures (**Table 1**) which are used to all types of fermented cold meats are composed of mildly acidifying bacteria cultures of the following species: *Lactobacillus sakei, L. curvatus, L. plantarum, Pediococcus acidilactici* and *Pediococcus pentosaceus.* In Europe, mainly cultures of *L. sakei* and *L. curvatus* are used to manufacture dry-aged cold meats [14, 16]. Strains of bacteria belonging to one species often differ in various physiological and metabolic properties among each other. Due to the fact that most strains of *L. curvatus* demonstrate the ability to produce biogenic amines, *L. sakei* bacteria are more often used in practice. These microorganisms are not capable of catalysing the decarboxylation of amino acids, thereby reducing or even inhibiting the formation of biogenic amines in dry-fermented meat products [14, 15, 21–23].

In spite of LAB, starter cultures may also contain micrococci, most frequently those of *Micrococcus varians* species and of *Staphylococcus xylosus*, *Staphylococcus carnosus* and *Streptomyces griseus* [15].

Apart from providing consistent quality and typical sensory features, the primary function of LAB bacteria included in such starter cultures is mainly to preserve the product through the production of lactic acid during metabolic changes and competition with microbiota naturally occurring in the meat product and pathogenic microorganisms. The composition of starter cultures impacts the duration of the ageing process and storage stability of such products but also on their flavour, odour and texture [16, 24].

2.2. Development of novel starter cultures

One of the major focuses of the current innovation in development of novel starter cultures to meat industry seems to be on improved food safety and health properties. The isolation and selection of lactic acid bacteria which can be used as starter cultures in meat fermentation present a considerable challenge to standardization and management of quality of dry-fermented sausage. The basic starter cultures used in meat industry are selected strains of homofermentative *Lactobacillus* (lactic acid bacteria (LAB)) and/or *Pediococcus* and Gram-positive catalase-positive cocci (GCC), nonpathogenic, coagulase-negative staphylococci and/or *Kocuria*. Lactic acid bacteria originating from fermented meats are specially adapted to the ecology of meat fermentation. The rapid production of lactic acid in those products is primarily responsible for the quality and safety of the product [16, 25].

First of all the addition of selected starter cultures usually induces a higher acidification, compared to the standard product, which was reported by several authors [13, 26–28]. Moreover, in Spanish raw-fermented sausage with addition of probiotic starter cultures, the reduction of fat and salt has been achieved [27]. Also flavour, texture and taste are very important components of the final quality of dry-fermented meat products, and most of these traits are related to the metabolic activities of microorganisms [20].

Selected LAB starter cultures could have positive influence on sensorial acceptation of dry-fermented meat products. For example, in [29], they have found that *Lb. sakei* and *Staphylococcus equorum* added to the Dacia sausage resulted in better smell intensity, overall quality and mastication attributes, as well as lower biogenic amines content in comparison to control samples. In Ref. [30], they studied the effect of selected LAB starter cultures in Italian dry-fermented sausage and found that the obtained products were saltier, juicier and more tasty as compared to the control.

It has been also found that probiotic starter cultures may have been successfully used in fermentation process of meat products. In Ref. [31], they found that probiotic bacteria did not change the characteristic flavour and aroma of raw sausages in comparison to product obtained from commercial starter cultures. Also in studies [12, 27], they have obtained the sausages with probiotic cultures addition and recorded a satisfactory overall sensory quality without any noticeable off-flavour.

The recent literature is also well consistent in indicating advantages of selected starter cultures in the control of pathogenic bacteria and other spoilage microflora. Fermented meat products are commonly considered safe for consumption, and the acidification by lactic acid starter bacteria is one of the main preserving factors. The most frequently isolated lactic acid bacteria from dry sausages processed with different technologies are *L. sakei, L. curvatus* and *L. plantarum* [32, 33].

The lactic acid bacteria (LAB) produce an array of antimicrobial substances (such as organic acids, diacetyl, acetoin, hydrogen peroxide, reuterin, reutericyclin, antifungal peptides and bacteriocins) [34, 35]. Therefore, there is an increasing interest in lactic acid bacteria (LAB) derived from meat that can be used as starter or adjunct cultures in dry sausage fermentation. Their ability to produce bacteriocins and nonproteinaceous low-molecular-mass antimicrobial compounds (mainly lactic acid and hydrogen peroxide) is of importance [36]. As there is no sufficient glucose in meat to reduce the pH, the addition of glucose is essential to develop the desired metabolic activity to produce lactic acid via glycolysis. Hydrogen peroxide is produced after glucose is consumed by cells [37].

Bacteriocins are the peptides produced by lactic acid bacteria with antibacterial properties. These peptides can reduce or inhibit the growth of other Gram-positive [38–40], and thus they can be used to control the growth of food-borne pathogens such as *L. monocytogenes* in food products [41]. In Ref. [38], they isolated *P. acidilactici* from Spanish dry-fermented sausages and found that they had a strong inhibitory effect against members of Gram-positive genera. It has been observed that starter cultures containing *L. sakei* reduced the growth of *Listeria* in fermented sausages [42, 43]. Also *L. curvatus* and *L. plantarum* in sausage starter cultures have shown antilisterial effect [44, 45]. In the other study [46], they reported antilisterial effect of a lactic acid bacterium isolated from Italian salami. In Ref. [47], they found that nine strains of *Lactobacillus casei* and three strains of *L. plantarum* isolated from dry-fermented sausages had an antagonistic activity against the indicator species tested. The bacteriocin produced by *L. casei* was named as Lactocin 705 and showed antibacterial effects against *L. plantarum, L. monocytogenes, S. aureus* and a wide range of Gram-negative bacteria. Bacteriocinogenic starter cultures are recommended as an additional hurdle to reduce the risk of *L. monocytogenes* in dry sausage [48]. In contrast sakacin P, synthesized by *L. sakei* subsp. *sakei* 2a isolated from pork sausage, inhibits the growth of *Listeria monocytogenes* [49]. The addition of the bacteriocinogenic *L. sakei* CTC494 in combination with some ingredients (i.e. pepper, salt and nitrite) in sausage batter has a dramatic effect on *L. monocytogenes* survival in fermented sausages [50]. Sakacins produced by *L. sakei* are mainly active against other LAB and *L. monocytogenes* as well as against the Gram-negative psychrotroph *Aeromonas hydrophila* [51, 52].

Besides prevention of microbiological hazards, also probiotic starter cultures have been developed. Many advantages and disadvantages are connected with application of probiotic bacteria to dry-fermented meat products.

2.3. Probiotic starter cultures: benefits and problems

Dynamic development of the functional food market has contributed to the attempt to use starter cultures consisting of probiotic LAB in meat processing. Two trends may be observed during development of new probiotic starter cultures. One of them is an attempt to apply already known probiotic cultures (from the gastrointestinal tract of healthy humans) used, e.g. in the production of fermented milk beverages. The second one consists in isolating of the strains of lactic acid bacteria from naturally fermented meat products and examining them in terms of probiotic qualities as well as of safety of use in an industrial scale [25, 53–55].

The number of benefits arising from the use of probiotic starter cultures is worth noticing (**Table 2**). The important aspect of using cultures of probiotic bacteria in the production of dry-fermented meat, in addition to the possibilities of growth and survival in meat environment and exercising favourable effect of these microorganisms on human body, is the ability to inhibit the growth of pathogenic microflora, which usually is capable of producing biogenic amines. Model studies with the use of probiotic bacteria as a starter culture to manufacture ripening meat products revealed that strains of *Lactobacillus acidophilus, L. lactis* subsp. *lactis, Lactococcus lactis* subsp. *lactis, L. plantarum, L. reuteri* and *L. fermentum* reduce or even inhibit the production of biogenic amines in the products discussed [56–58].

Advantages	Disadvantages
Meat, as a rich source of nutrition components, is a suitable medium for probiotic bacteria growth	Technological issues: • Presence of native microflora can inhibit growth of probiotic bacteria • Presence of other inhibitory factors: low water activity, low sugar contents, nitrates and salt additives • Difficulties with inoculation probiotic in appropriate number of bacteria • Stability of probiotic during storage
Beneficial effect on human health corresponding with applied probiotic strain	Difficulties with identification of probiotic strains in meat matrix
Inhibition of pathogen growth, production of bacteriocin and antimicrobial compounds	Non-sterile environment can affect the spontaneous fermentation or spoilage
Unique sensorial quality	No detailed procedure for production of probiotic meat products
Reduction of fat oxidation, proteolytic reactions	Possibilities of biogenic amine production

Table 2. Benefits and issues related to application of probiotic starter cultures.

As a result of their own metabolic changes, the probiotic starter cultures produce a number of bacteriostatic and bactericidal substances (e.g. lactic acid, acetic acid, formic acid, ethanol and bacteriocins), thereby inhibiting the growth of undesired and pathogenic microbiota, including Gram-negative strains from family *Enterobacteriaceae* (e.g. *Escherichia coli*) and *Pseudomonaceae* as well as species such as *Listeria monocytogenes* or *Staphylococcus aureus*, thus naturally preserving the products discussed [14, 48, 59, 60].

Another benefit arising from the use of probiotic bacteria to manufacture dry-fermented meat products is reduction of fat oxidation and proteolytic reactions. Primary and secondary products resulting from degradation of lipids and proteins have significant impact on deterioration of sensory quality (i.e. negative aftertastes: bitter, of old fat) but also of features such as colour and texture. Additionally, they affect the health safety and shorten the use by date of the meat products discussed [18, 61–63]. Research on autoxidation of the fat in ripening products clearly proves that probiotic strains protect lipids from oxidation during storage which is indicated by substantially lower values of TBARS parameter in comparison to the control sample [64, 65].

Proteolysis is one of the most important biochemical processes in dry-aged meat products where proteins are metabolized and broken down to polypeptides, peptides and free amino acids [62, 66]. Protein breakdown takes place with the participation of microbiological enzymes, which in turn leads to deamination and decarboxylation. These reactions occur faster at low pH values. The basic products of protein decarboxylation in meat are cadaverine, putrescine, tyramine and histamine. Large concentration of biogenic amines in meat products may result in adverse symptoms in consumers, such as increase in blood pressure, increase in rate and strength of heart contraction and problems with the central nervous system, including migraines. Additionally, it may cause stomachaches, vomiting or severe sweating [56]. It has been observed that the proper choice of probiotic strains limits proteolytic changes in dry-aged meat products [15, 26, 67]. This relation has been observed in studies [66] and [23] which examined dry-aged pork tenderloin with addition of *L. casei* ŁOCK 0900 strain with documented probiotic and very good technological properties. Controlling and proper conduct of the process of fermentation and ageing ensure low concentration of biogenic amines in raw cold-meat products, thereby preventing poisoning [15].

It is currently believed that dry-fermented meat products are an appropriate medium for probiotic bacteria. Many studies have shown that growth and survival rate of probiotic LAB in dry-fermented sausages are possible [18, 60]. However, the previous attempts to manufacture meat product in controlled process of fermentation and ageing conducted by proven and selected probiotic strains mainly pertain to sausages [1, 10, 23, 33, 54, 57, 68, 69]. Moreover, there are few research works published which will unequivocally confirm the technological suitability of probiotic cultures and their healthy impact on human body caused by regular consumption of such meat products [70–72].

Probiotic strains used in the production of dry-aged meat products must demonstrate suitable technological properties without departing from the traditional starter cultures used in meat processing. Therefore, the idea to use probiotic starter cultures in meat processing industry raises many issues from the technological, microbiological and analytical perspective (**Table 2**).

The task consisting in introducing the probiotic starter cultures to meat is not easy to perform, as these bacteria which are in fact the intestinal bacteria do not demonstrate very good technological properties. It was determined that from 50 to 500 million of lactic acid bacteria, including mainly *L. sakei* and *L. curvatus*, may be placed into one gram of the product discussed. Therefore, the raw meat material itself constitutes a problem, because spontaneous growth of LAB may occur there.

Secondly, inoculation of the probiotic bacteria is performed to the raw material which is not sterile as is the case of fermented milk products or fermented juices [73, 74]. Thirdly, certain analytic difficulties also emerge here. Identification of selected probiotic strains in meat with the use of traditional microbiological methods is not complete, because only the general number of LAB is assayed. Only advanced identification methods based on genetic analysis of nucleotide sequences typical for given bacterial strain may ensure that all of them will be assayed [54].

Numerous authors of available literature focus on the survival rate of probiotic starter bacteria added to dry-fermented meat products. The factors limiting and even inhibiting the growth of the discussed microbes in meat environment include mainly the native microflora but also low water activity and the content of sugars naturally occurring in meat, as well as technological additives: sodium chloride, nitrates and other curing agents [15].

Low content of simple sugars in fresh meat, necessary for lactic acid bacteria, including probiotic ones, to conduct metabolic change, also poses a significant problem (4.5–7 mM/g of raw material). Therefore, microorganisms discussed start to use amino acids as an alternative source of carbon which starts the spoilage process of meat and results in intensive bitter taste. For this reason, saccharides are added in amount of 0.4–0.8% during the production of aged meat products [13, 48].

There is also a technological difficulty in inoculating bacterial strain (form, number, application method) to cured element to an unground meat in particular. Starter cultures are most often manufactured in lyophilized or frozen form. In the case of dry-fermented sausages, they are inoculated to the sausage meat, usually after they are mixed with cold water or curing brine. Adding starter cultures to tenderloin or ham is significantly more difficult, as they are also posed by varied consistency of different muscles. They result, i.e. from the presence of fat at the meat's surface which may uneven drying up and thereby excessive or inhibited growth of microorganisms [15].

One of the major technological problems involves no detailed procedure for production of probiotic meat products developed. This primarily requires determination of optimal temperature for fermentation and ageing, which will allow probiotic strains to grow and dominate natural microbiota in the meat. Fermentation and ageing of meat products are mainly conducted in the temperature within the range of 15–26°C. Lower temperature allows to obtain high-quality product with a long ageing period and use by date. In contrast, the use of higher temperature decreases the duration of fermentation; however there is a risk that microorganisms responsible for product's spoilage will grow in the meat [13, 15].

Additionally, one of the important technological criteria to be met by a probiotic strain includes stability during storage, i.e. capability to retain the number of 6.00–7.00 log cfu/g in the product in the last use by date [70, 71].

Another aspect of the selection of bacterial cultures pertains mainly to their beneficial impact on sensory quality and also moderate acidifying activity, low thermal activity within range of 0–15°C, antagonism with respect to undesired microbes and food pathogens as well as resistance to bacteriophages [18, 56, 75].

Probiotic microorganisms selected to the production of aged meat products must meet not only the necessary requirements of safety and functionality but also the technological criteria discussed above.

3. Technological and health aspects of probiotic meat products

3.1. Influence of probiotic bacteria on lipid oxidation

The shelf life of fermented meat products is generally not limited by bacterial deterioration but by chemical spoilage [76]. It is oxidation stability that is the main restriction on the shelf life of probiotic meat products [77]. Processed products, which are minced, mixed with salt and heated, expose muscle tissue to oxidative stress responsible for loss of quality and lead to oxidative flavours and loss of haem iron and vitamins and finally cause discoloration [77]. Oxidation of lipids can also have a negative effect on nutritional value and may be responsible for the production of toxic compounds. In Ref. [76], they have reported that enzymatic hydrolysis during fermentation accelerates lipid peroxidation. In addition, a strong correlation between lipid and myoglobin oxidation, especially in fresh meat, has been documented by scientists [78]. In [78], they have reported that secondary lipid oxidation products (2-heptenal, 2-nonenal, 4-hydroxy-2-nonenal) promote pigment oxidation. However, there is also strong evidence that haem pigments may initiate lipid oxidation through the reaction of hydrogen peroxide with metmyoglobin to form ferryl and perferrylmyoglobin, which have powerful prooxidant effects on lipids. In probiotic meat product, the fact that the high 20–30% concentration of fat (dry-fermented ham, neck, sausage) does not limit the adaptive capacity of probiotic bacteria in fermented meat products is interesting. Probiotic bacteria can stabilize the oxidation process taking during the maturing and prolonged storage period. In Ref. [79], they found that neither the presence nor the level of probiotic *Bifidobacterium animalis* ssp. *lactis* BB-12 has a negative influence on colour and oxidative stability of dry-cured neck during 12 months of ageing. The authors observed the significantly ($P < 0.05$) lower TBARS values in neck B1 and B2 (1.54 and 1.69 mg MDA/kg) compared to the values with spontaneously added LAB (2.26 mg MDA/kg). In [80], they pointed out that inoculation with *L. fermentum* HL57 potential probiotic strain increased the amount of malondialdehyde in Iberian dry-fermented sausages resulting in a negative colour and taste. The interaction of myoglobin with H_2O_2 activates metmyoglobin, which may be a ferrylmyoglobin radical that is very unstable and can transform rapidly into the peroxyl radical form. On the other hand, in research [81], they proposed that *L. casei*, *L. plantarum*, *L. curvatus* and *L. sakei* strains actively contribute to the hydrolysis of sarcoplasmic proteins such as myoglobin. Also in Ref. [82], they found that some strains of lactic acid bacteria demonstrated antioxidative activity with inhibition rates of ascorbate autoxidation in the range of 7-12%. In another paper the same authors presented that six strains of *L. acidophilus* and two strains of *B. longum* demonstrated an inhibitory effect on linoleic acid peroxidation [83]. The inhibitory rates of linoleic acid peroxidation ranged from 33 to 46% when 1 mL of intracellular cell-free extract was tested [83]. Authors of the Ref. [18] found out that the addition of probiotic strain *L. casei* ŁOCK 0900 changed physicochemical profile of dry-fermented sausages. Sausages with lower probiotic bacteria inoculation (6.0 log cfu/g) had better quality, inclusive colour and lipid oxidative stability (lower peroxide value, conjugated dienes and TBARS value) than those with 6.3 log cfu/g of probiotic strain. Based on research [18], it can be concluded that dry-fermented sausages produced with probiotic *L. casei* 0900 ŁOCK are oxidatively stable and the stability of the fat does not limit the shelf life of probiotic-treated dry-fermented sausages. The study suggests that the probiotic strain can be used in the production of edible sausage. The study conducted by authors of [84] proved that the use of potential probiotic *L. acidophilus* Bauer in dry-fermented pork neck production process decreases the hydroperoxide concentration at a level comparable to synthetic antioxidant.

Studies of the effects of the probiotic *L. rhamnosus* LOCK 0900 strain with green tea extract on the oxidative stability of ageing dry-cured pork loin showed that adding the probiotic strain with natural antioxidant increased the antioxidant potential of meat product by lowering the oxidation-reduction potential and TBARS values and improving the part of red in the general tone of colour [13].

The results presented by authors of Ref. [85] clearly demonstrated that the use of probiotic strains mixture (*L. casei* LOCK 0900, *L. casei* LOCK 0908 and *Lactobacillus paracasei* LOCK 0919) is possible in manufacturing process of organic dry-fermented sausages without nitrate and/or nitrite. The uncured fermented sausages with probiotic strains have appropriate oxidative stability and are shelf-stable during 180 days of storage period [85].

Examples of starter cultures that represent significant influences on fermented meat products regarding lipid oxidation, proteolysis, biogenic amine formation and sensorial quality were collected in **Table 3**.

Starter culture	Product	Influence	Literature
L. rhamnosus LOCK900 (Formerly *Lactobacillus casei* ŁOCK 0900)	Dry-fermented sausage	The probiotic strain can be used in the production of edible sausage Dry-fermented sausage produced with probiotic is oxidatively stable during storage	[18]
	Dry-fermented pork loin	Pork loin inoculation with a probiotic strain has different free amino acid concentrations, the taste	[92]

Starter culture	Product	Influence	Literature
		and flavour attributes	
	Dry-fermented pork loin	Inoculation with a probiotic strain proved to be a protective measure against the formation and accumulation of biogenic amine	[91]
L. acidophilus Bauer	Dry-fermented pork neck	Probiotic strain decreases the hydroperoxide concentration at a level comparable to synthetic antioxidant *L. acidophilus* Bauer has antioxidant properties	[84]
L. rhamnosus LOCK900 (Formerly *Lactobacillus casei* ŁOCK 0900)	Dry-cured pork loin	Addition of probiotic strain with green tea extract increased the antioxidant potential of meat product and improved the part of red in the general tone of colour	[13]
L. rhamnosus LOCK900, *L. rhamnosus* LOCK908 and *L. casei* LOCK919 (Formerly *L. casei* ŁOCK 0900, *L. casei* ŁOCK 0908 and *L. paracasei* ŁOCK 0919)	Uncured fermented pork sausage (organic sausage)	The uncured fermented sausages with probiotic strain mixture have appropriate oxidative stability and are shelf-stable during 180 days of storage period	[85]

Table 3. Influence of probiotic starter cultures on lipid oxidation, proteolysis, biogenic amine formation and sensorial quality in meat processing.

3.2. Influence of probiotic bacteria on proteolysis and biogenic amine formation

Proteolysis results in generation of peptides, oligopeptides and finally free amino acids (FAAs). Proteolysis is one of the most important biochemical changes, which take place during ageing of fermented meat products. FAAs contribute to the basic taste and aroma of fermented meat products [86]. However, an excessive amount of FAAs seems to be responsible for the biogenic amine formation.

The biogenic amines (BAs) are the compounds in which one, two or three hydrogens of ammonia are replaced by alkyl or aryl groups. Tyramine and phenylethylamine have aromatic structure, while putrescine, cadaverine, spermine and spermidine have the aliphatic one. Heterocyclic structures were proved for histamine and tryptamine. Based on number of amine group, we can divide the BA into the monoamines (phenylethylamine, tyramine), diamines (cadaverine, putrescine) and polyamines (spermidine, spermine) [87]. Biogenic amines have been reported in variety of foods, such as fish, meat, cheese, vegetable and wine [88]. They can be formed but also degraded as a result of normal metabolism of living cells in plant, animal and microorganism. BA can be produced by two different pathways: firstly by the decarboxylation of free amino acids and secondly by the amination and transamination of aldehydes and ketones [15]. The control of biogenic amines formation mainly focused on the controlling the growth of biogenic amine-forming bacteria. Microorganisms have a different ability to synthesize decarboxylases. *Pseudomonas*, *Enterobacteriaceae*, enterococci and lactobacilli were found to have a high decarboxylase activity [88]. Within the same species, the presence, the activity and the specificity of decarboxylases are strain dependent. Bacterial amino acid decarboxylases usually have an acidic pH optimum 4.9–5.3, because the BA productions have been recognized as defence microbial mechanisms against an acidic environment [88, 89]. On the other hand, rapid and intense acidifications of environment reduce the growth of *Enterobacteriaceae* and enterococci. The factors that could significantly influence the BA formations in fermented meat are pH value, redox potential, environment microorganisms, starter culture, temperature of maturing, salt concentration, additives, water activity and hygienic quality of meat [89]. Authors of paper [90] proved that when salt concentration increased from 0 to 6%, the rate of BA production of *Lactobacillus delbrueckii* subsp. *bulgaricus* decreased. Other authors proved that concentration of sodium chloride at the level from 3.5 to 5.5% inhibited the histamine formation. Several studies showed that temperature of fermentation, maturing and storing have influence on BA accumulation in meat product [88]. Higher maturing temperature (20–25°C) could stimulate the growth of LAB which inhibits the amine-positive bacteria. The storing temperature below 4°C inhibits most of amine-positive bacteria except from psychrotrophic *Pseudomonas*, so the BA concentration in this kind of meat product is relatively low compared with product stored at 14–16°C. The addition of sugar (glucose, lactose) to fermented meat products has some influence on bacterial population dynamics and BA production. The absence of sugar stimulated the proteolysis and tyramine, cadaverine, putrescine and tryptamine formation. The preservative sodium nitrite could be added to fermented meat products because of their ability to reduce the putrescine and cadaverine accumulation. The addition of pure or mixture of various probiotic strains can decrease BA formation in fermented meat products. It is extremely important that probiotic starter culture should not form BA and have to be competitive in suppressing growth of amine-positive microbiota. In Ref. [91], they pointed out that pork loin inoculation with a probiotic strain *L. casei* ŁOCK 0900 has different free amino acid concentrations, which could influence the taste and flavour attributes. Also in [92], they presented evidence that some sorts of probiotic starter cultures (*L. casei* ŁOCK 0900, *Bifidobacterium bifidum*, *L. acidophilus* Bauer) have different abilities to create the high- or low-molecular-weight peptides and free amino acids. Another authors [93] found out that LAB reduced the pH values during ageing and thereby activated the endogenous acid protease (cathepsin B, L). Inoculation with a probiotic strain *L. casei* ŁOCK 0900 proved to be a protective measure against the formation and accumulation of cadaverine, putrescine, spermine and tryptamine. In Ref. [91] the author has not observed the correlation between the higher content of free amino acids (potential precursor of BA) and the level of biogenic amines. A 50% BA decrease was observed in comminuted fermented meat products with mixture of *L. curvatus* CTC371 and *S. xylosus* despite the increase of free amino acid availability. In Ref. [23] BA changes during maturation were presented. Potential probiotic pork loins were analysed in 4-, 8- and 16-month-old samples. The authors have not detected histamine and spermidine. Spermine was present at very low levels (4.0–5.8 mg/kg), while cadaverine (10.8–39.6 mg/kg) and tryptamine (17.8–49.2 mg/kg) were the most abundant BA. The level of all BA did not exceed the suggested toxic limits [23].

3.3. Bioactive peptides in probiotic fermented meat products

The proteolytic activity during meat processing generates a large amount of peptides and free amino acids because of calpain, cathepsin and peptidase enzymatic activity [86]. The most interesting peptides are those that can be considered as bioactive peptides because of their different health-care abilities like antihypertensive activity, antioxidant activity, antimicrobial activity, etc. The activities of bioactive peptides depend on their chemical structure (amino acids composition, kind of amino acid in N- and C-terminal), the length of molecule chain and their weight, charge character of amino acids and the hydrophobic/hydrophilic property. Meat has been reported to contribute to the generation of bioactive peptides. As such peptides, antihypertensive, opioid, immunostimulating, antimicrobial, antithrombotic, hypocholesterolemic, antioxidative and prebiotic activities have been studied. Angiotensin I-converting enzyme (ACE) plays an important physiological role in the regulation of blood pressure. Fermented food with probiotic bacteria, especially *Lactobacillus*, produce bioactive peptides known to inhibit the activity of angiotensin-converting enzyme (ACE) and thus alleviate high blood pressure (hypertension). Authors of the study [94] used calpis sour milk fermented with *Lactobacillus helveticus* and *Saccharomyces cerevisiae* and identified two peptides Ile-Pro-Pro and Val-Pro-Pro, both of which possessed ACE inhibitory activity in vitro. These two bioactive peptides were released from b-casein and k-casein by lactobacilli enzymes. In Ref. [95], hypertensive subjects were fed with milk fermented with *L. helveticus* LBK-16H containing bioactive peptides. After 21 weeks test subjects showed a significant lowering of their blood pressure. Even in antihypertensive peptides, it has been found that antioxidative (VW, DLYA, SLYA, DLQEKLE) and prebiotic (ELM) peptides are generated from meat protein by enzymatic digestion. In [96], they reported that bioactive peptides from hydrolysis of sarcoplasmic porcine proteins by the activity of *L. sakei* CRL 1862 and *L. curvatus* CRL 705 showed high ACE inhibitory activity. In [97], they pointed out that some peptides from Spanish dry-cured ham have DPPH radical-scavenging activity (39–92%) as well as superoxide ion-extinguishing ability with values ranging from 41.67 to 50.27% of the antioxidant activity, suggesting the presence of peptides with antioxidant activity. Moreover every sample exhibited pooled fractions corresponding to 1700 Da or lower were the most antihypertensive with a decrease of 38.38 mm Hg in systolic blood pressure [97]. The antioxidant activity of low-molecular-weight compounds isolated from Iberian-fermented sausage (chorizo) was tested in Ref. [98]. Authors did not observe many bioactive peptides; however plenty free amino acids, bacterial metabolites and β-alanyl-peptides have been identified. Bioactive peptides from meat and fermented meat products exhibit various biological activities which are favourable for human health.

4. Conclusion

In recent years, the possibility of development of probiotic meat products has been discussed in the field of meat science and industry. Probiotics in meat may exert their benefits by way of several mechanisms; therefore human clinical studies are needed to assess the health-promoting effect of probiotic dry-fermented meat products. So far, there is a little scientific evidence related to such studies. Therefore, further studies are required to demonstrate the clear benefits of probiotic meat products for human health.

On the other hand, the use of probiotic strain which possesses the ability to create the bioactive compounds is the challenge for research and meat industry and could develop novel functional meat products. Possible generation of bioactive peptides in dry meat products fermented by probiotics as starter cultures seems the most promising way for designing novel functional food. Therefore meat products with probiotics have a great future potential and it is expected that increasing interest will be shown in basic research and potential applications for designing new meat products.

Target products with probiotic bacteria are mainly dry sausages but also hams and loins, which are processed by fermentation without heat treatment. Technically, it has already become possible to produce probiotic meat products; moreover probiotic raw-fermented meat products exist on a German and Japanese market. However, the production of probiotic meat products requires overcoming certain technological limitations, such as the native microflora of meat, a need to use additives such as nitrites and salt and also low water activity and low content or absence of natural sugars. Probiotic bacteria strains that can be used in the manufacturing of dry-fermented meat products should be capable of surviving in conditions found in fermented products. Moreover, the product should maintain its sensory characteristics.

Additionally, since food safety is another critical aspect of food quality, efforts should also be directed to ensure that new functional meat products are safe. The dry-fermented meat products with probiotic starter cultures addition have to possess appropriate biogenic amine profile and should be oxidative and shelf-stable. Along with accumulation of scientific data, there is an urgent need to inform consumers of the exact physiological value of probiotic meat products. Without proof of product safety, most consumers would hesitate to adopt new foods in their diet.

Acknowledgements

The authors would like to express our appreciation to Professor Danuta Kołożyn-Krajewska and Professor Zbigniew Dolatowski for their support and constructive critiques during all studies on the possibility of the use of probiotic starter cultures in meat fermentation.

Author details

Katarzyna Neffe-Skocińska[1*], Karolina Wójciak[2] and Dorota Zielińska[1]

*Address all correspondence to: katarzyna_neffe_skocinska@sggw.pl

1 Department of Food Gastronomy and Food Hygiene, Warsaw University of Life Sciences (WULS), Warsaw, Poland

2 Department of Meat Technology and Food Quality, University of Life Sciences (LULS), Lublin, Poland

References

[1] Leroy F, Geyzen A, Janssens M, De Vuyst L, Scholliers P. Meat fermentation at the crossroads of innovation and tradition: a historical outlook. Trends in Food Science & Technology. 2013;31(2):130–137.

[2] Corthesy B, Gaskins HR, Mercenier A. Cross-talk between probiotic bacteria and the host immune system. Journal of Nutrition. 2007;137:781S–790S.

[3] FAO/WHO. Report of a joint FAO/WHO working group of drafting guidelines for the evaluation of probiotics in food: guidelines for the evaluation of probiotics in food, London; 2002.

[4] Kedia G, Wang R, Patel H, Pandiella SS. Use of mixed cultures for the fermentation of cereal-based substrates with potential probiotic properties. Process Biochemistry. 2002;42(1):65–70.

[5] Rozada-Sánchez R, Sattur AP, Thomas K, Pandiella SS. Evaluation of *Bifidobacterium* spp. for the production of a potentially probiotic malt-based beverage. Process Biochemistry. 2002;43(8):848–854.

[6] Kun S, Rezessy-Szabó JM, Nguyen QD, Hoschke Á. Changes of microbial population and some components in carrot juice during fermentation with selected *Bifidobacterium* strains. Process Biochemistry. 2008;43(8):816–821.

[7] Zielińska D, Kamińska A, Kołożyn-Krajewska D. Development of tofu production method with probiotic bacteria addition. The Journal of Microbiology, Biotechnology and Food Sciences. 2015;4(6):485.

[8] Klingberg TD, Axelsson L, Naterstad K, Elsser D, Budde BB. Identification of potential probiotic starter cultures for Scandinavian-type fermented sausages. International Journal of Food Microbiology. 2005;105(3):419–431.

[9] Macedo REFD, Pflanzer Jr SB, Terra NN, Freitas RJSD. Production of fermented sausage using probiotic *Lactobacillus* strains: quality characteristics. Food Science and Technology (Campinas). 2008;28(3):509–519.

[10] Pennacchia C, Vaughan EE, Villani F. Potential probiotic *Lactobacillus* strains from fermented sausages: further investigations on their probiotic properties. Meat Science. 2006;73(1):90–101.

[11] Rouhi M, Sohrabvandi S, Mortazavian AM. Probiotic fermented sausage: viability of probiotic microorganisms and sensory characteristics. Critical Reviews in Food Science and Nutrition. 2013;53(4):331–348.

[12] Rubio R, Aymerich T, Bover-Cid S, Guàrdia MD, Arnau J, Garriga M. Probiotic strains *Lactobacillus plantarum* 299V and *Lactobacillus rhamnosus* GG as starter cultures for fermented sausages. LWT-Food Science and Technology. 2013;54(1):51–56.

[13] Neffe-Skocińska K, Jaworska D, Kołożyn-Krajewska D, Dolatowski Z, Jachacz-Jówko L. The effect of LAB as probiotic starter culture and green tea extract addition on dry fermented pork loins quality. BioMed Research International. 2015. Available from: http://dx.doi.org/10.1155/2015/452757 [Accessed: 2015-01-01].

[14] Ammor MS, Mayo B. Selection criteria for lactic acid bacteria to be used as functional starter cultures in dry sausage production: an update. Meat Science. 2007;76(1):138–146.

[15] Kołożyn-Krajewska D, Dolatowski ZJ. Probiotic meat products and human nutrition. Process Biochemistry. 2012;47(12):1761–1772.

[16] Hugas M, Monfort JM. Bacterial starter cultures for meat fermentation. Food Chemistry. 1997;59(4):547–54.

[17] Erkkilä S, Petäjä E, Eerola S, Lilleberg L, Mattila-Sandholm T, Suihko ML. Flavour profiles of dry sausages fermented by selected novel meat starter cultures. Meat Science. 2001;58:111–116.

[18] Wójciak KM, Dolatowski ZJ, Kołożyn-Krajewska D, Trząskowska M. The effect of the *Lactobacillus casei* ŁOCK 0900 probiotic strain on the quality of dry-fermented sausage during chilling storage. Journal of Food Quality. 2012;35,353-365.

[19] Steinkraus K. Handbook of Indigenous Fermented Foods, revised and expanded. 2nd ed. CRC Press; 1995. 121p.

[20] Bassi D, Puglisi E, Cocconcelli PS. Comparing natural and selected starter cultures in meat and cheese fermentations. Current Opinion in Food Science. 2015;2:118–122.

[21] Pereira CI, Crespo MT, Romao MV. Evidence for proteolytic activity and biogenic amines production in *Lactobacillus homohiochii*. International Journal of Food Microbiology. 2001;68(3):211–216.

[22] Bover-Cid S, Miguelez-Arrizado MJ, Latorre Moratalla LL, Vidal Carou MC. Freezing of meat raw materials affects tyramine and diamine accumulation in spontaneously fermented sausages. Meat Sciences. 2006;72(1):62–68.

[23] Stadnik J, Dolatowski ZJ. Biogenic amines content during extended ageing of dry-cured pork loins inoculated with probiotics. Meat Science. 2012;91:374–377.

[24] Incze K. Fermented meat products. Fleischwirtschaft. 2002;4:112–117.

[25] Lücke FK. Utilization of microbes to process and preserve meat. Meat Science. 2000;56(2):105–115.

[26] Castellano P, Aristoy MC, Sentandreu MA, Vignolo G, Toldra F. *Lactobacillus sakei* CRL1862 improves safety and protein hydrolysis in meat systems. Journal of Applied Microbiology. 2012;113(6):1407–1416.

[27] Rubio R, Jofré A, Aymerich T, Guàrdia MD, Garriga M. Nutritionally enhanced fermented sausages as a vehicle for potential probiotic lactobacilli delivery. Meat Science. 2014;96(2):937–942.

[28] Jaworska D, Neffe K, łożyn-Krajewska D, Dolatowski Z. Survival during storage and sensory effect of potential probiotic lactic acid bacteria *Lactobacillus acidophilus* Bauer and *Lactobacillus casei* Bif3'/IV in dry fermented pork loins. International Journal of Food Science & Technology. 2011;46(12):2491–2497.

[29] Simion AMC, Vizireanu C, Alexe P, Franco I, Carballo J. Effect of the use of selected starter cultures on some quality, safety and sensorial properties of Dacia sausage, a traditional Romanian dry-sausage variety. Food Control. 2014;35(1):123–131.

[30] Cenci-Goga BT, Rossitto PV, Sechi P, Parmegiani S, Cambiotti V, Cullor JS. Effect of selected dairy starter cultures on microbiological, chemical and sensory characteristics of swine and venison (Dama dama) nitrite-free dry-cured sausages. Meat Science. 2012;90(3):599–606.

[31] Sameshima T, Magome C, Takeshita K, Arihara K, Itoh M, Kondo Y. Effect of intestinal *Lactobacillus* starter cultures on the behaviour of *Staphylococcus aureus* in fermented sausage. International Journal of Food Microbiology. 1998;41(1):1–7.

[32] Schillinger U, Lücke FK. Antibacterial activity of *Lactobacillus sakei* isolated from meat. Applied and Environmental Microbiology. 1989;55(8):1901–1906.

[33] Papamanoli E, Tzanetakis N, Litopoulou-Tzanetaki E, Kotzekidou P. Characterization of lactic acid bacteria isolated from a Greek dry-fermented sausage in respect of their technological and probiotic properties. Meat Science. 2003;65(2):859–867.

[34] Holzapfel WH, Geisen R, Schillinger U. Biological preservation of foods with reference to protective cultures, bacteriocins and food-grade enzymes. International Journal of Food Microbiology. 1995;24(3):343–362.

[35] Leroy F, De Vuyst L. Lactic acid bacteria as functional starter cultures for the food fermentation industry. Trends in Food Science & Technology. 2004;15(2):67–78.

[36] Gaenzle MG, Hertle C, van der Vossen JMBM, Hammes WP. Effect of bacteriocin-producing lactobacilli on the survival of *Escherichia coli* and *Listeria* in a dynamic model of the stomach and the small intestine. International Journal of Food Microbiology. 1999;48(1):21–35.

[37] Condon S. Responses of lactic acid bacteria to oxygen. FEMS Microbiology Reviews. 1987;3(3):269–280.

[38] Cintas LM, Rodriguez JM, Fernandez MF, Sletten K, Nes IF, Hernandez PE, Holo H Isolation and characterization of pediocin L50, a new bacteriocin from *Pediococcus acidilactici* with a broad inhibitory spectrum. Applied and Environmental Microbiology. 1995;61(7):2643–2648.

[39] Cleveland J, Montville TJ, Nes IF, Chikindas ML. Bacteriocins: safe, natural antimicrobials for food preservation. International Journal of Food Microbiology. 2001;71(1):1–20.

[40] Diep DB, Nes IF. Ribosomally synthesized antibacterial peptides in Gram positive bacteria. Current Drug Targets. 2002;3(2):107–122.

[41] Ennahar S, Sonomoto K, Ishizaki A. Class IIa bacteriocins from lactic acid bacteria: antibacterial activity and food preservation. Journal of Bioscience and Bioengineering. 1999;87(6):705–716.

[42] Hugas M, Garriga M, Aymerich MT, Monfort JM. Inhibition of *Listeria* in dry fermented sausages by the bacteriocinogenic *Lactobacillus sakei* CTC494. Journal of Applied Microbiology.1995;79(3):322–330.

[43] De Martinis EC, Franco BD. Inhibition of *Listeria monocytogenes* in a pork product by a *Lactobacillus sakei* strain. International Journal of Food Microbiology. 1998;42(1):119–126.

[44] Campanini M, Pedrazzoni I, Barbuti S, Baldini P. Behaviour of Listeria monocytogenes during the maturation of naturally and artificially contaminated salami: effect of lactic-acid bacteria starter cultures. International Journal of Food Microbiology. 1993;20(3):169–175.

[45] Dicks LMT, Mellett FD, Hoffman LC. Use of bacteriocin-producing starter cultures of *Lactobacillus plantarum* and *Lactobacillus curvatus* in production of ostrich meat salami. Meat Science. 2004;66(3):703–708.

[46] Teixeira de Carvalho AA, Aparecida de Paula R, Mantovani HC, Alencar de Moraes C. Inhibition of *Listeria monocytogenes* by a lactic acid bacterium isolated from Italian salami. Food Microbiology. 2006;23(3):213–219.

[47] Vignolo GM, Suriani F, Holgado APDR, Oliver G. Antibacterial activity of *Lactobacillus* strains isolated from dry fermented sausages. Journal of Applied Microbiology. 1993;75(4),344-349.

[48] Työppönen S, Petäjä E, Mattila-Sandholm T. Bioprotectives and probiotics for dry sausages. International Journal of Food Microbiology. 2003;83(3):233–244.

[49] De Carvalho KG, Bambirra F, Kruger M, Barbosa M, Oliveira J, Santos A, Nicoli J, Bemquerer M, De Miranda A, Salvucci E, Sesma F, Franco B. Antimicrobial compounds produced by *Lactobacillus sakei* subsp. sakei 2a, a bacteriocinogenic strain

isolated from a Brazilian meat product. Journal Indian Microbiology Biotechnology. 2010;37:381–390.

[50] Hugas M, Garriga M, Pascual M, Aymerich MT, Monfort JM. Enhancement of sakacin K activity against *Listeria monocytogenes* in fermented sausages with pepper or manganese as ingredients. Food Microbiology. 2002;19(5):519–528.

[51] Schillinger U, Lücke FK. Antibacterial activity of *Lactobacillus sakei* isolated from meat. Applied and Environmental Microbiology. 1989;55(8):1901–1906.

[52] Lewus CB, Montville TJ. Detection of bacteriocins produced by lactic acid bacteria. Journal of Microbiological Methods. 1991:13(2), 145–150.

[53] Hammes WP, Hertel C. New developments in meat starter cultures. Meat Science. 1998;49:S125–138.

[54] Kröckel L. Use of probiotic bacteria in meat products. Fleischwirtschaft. 2006;86:109–113.

[55] Aro Aro JM, Nyam-Osor P, Tsuji K, Shimada K, Fukushima M, Sekikawa M. The effect of starter cultures on proteolytic changes and amino acid content in fermented sausages. Food Chemistry. 2010;119(1):279–285.

[56] Stadnik J. Biogenic amines in dry cured meat products. Food. Science. Technology. Quality. 2013;3(88):5–15.

[57] Ruiz-Moyano S, Martin A, Benito MJ, Hernandez A, Casquete R, Serradilla MJ, Córdoba MC. Safety and functional aspects of pre-selected lactobacilli for probiotic use in Iberian dry-fermented sausages. Meat Science. 2009;83:460–467.

[58] Deepika Priyadarshani WM, Rakshit SK. Screening selected strains of probiotic lactic acid bacteria for their ability to produce biogenic amines (histamine and tyramine). International Journal of Food Science and Technology. 2011;46(10):2062–2069.

[59] Coll Cárdenas F, Giannuzzi NE, Zaritzky NE. Mathematical modeling of microbial growth in ground beef from Argentina. Effect of lactic acid addition, temperature and packaging film. Meat Science. 2008;79:509–520.

[60] Rivera-Espinoza Y, Gallardo-Navarro Y. Non-dairy probiotic products. Food Microbiology. 2010;27:1–11.

[61] Toldrá F, Flores M. The role of muscle proteases and lipases in flavour development during the processing of dry-cured ham. Critical Reviews in Food Science and Nutrition. 1998;38:331–352.

[62] Flores M, Barat JM, Aristoy MC, Peris MM, Grau R, Toldr F. Accelerated processing of dry-cured ham. Part 2. Influence of brine thawing/salting operation on proteolysis and sensory acceptability. Meat Science. 2006;72:766–772.

[63] Singh VP, Pathak V, Verma AK. Fermented meat products: organoleptic qualities and biogenic amines – a review. American Journal of Food Technology. 2012;7:278–88.

[64] Estevez M, Cava R. Effectiveness of rosemary essential oil as an inhibitor of lipid and protein oxidation: contradictory effects in different types of frankfurters. Meat Science. 2006;72:348–55.

[65] Valencia I, Ansorena D, Astiasaran I. Stability of linseed oil and antioxidants containing dry fermented sausages: a study of the lipid fraction during different storage conditions. Meat Science. 2006;73:269–77.

[66] Okoń A, Dolatowski ZJ. Proteolysis of proteins in raw-ripening meat products using *Lactobacillus casei* ŁOCK 0900 probiotic strain. Food. Science. Technology. Quality. 2012;6(85):138–151.

[67] Bodmer S, Imark C, Kneubuhl M. Biogenic amines in foods: histamine and food processing. Inflammation Research. 1999;48:296–300.

[68] Pennacchia C, Ercolini D, Blaiotta G, Pepe O, Mauriello G, Villani F. Selection of *Lactobacillus* strains from fermented sausages for their potential use as probiotics. Meat Science. 2004;67:309–317.

[69] Arihara K. Strategies for designing novel functional meat products. Meat Science. 2006;74:219–229.

[70] Jahreis G, Vogelsang H, Kiessling G, Schubert R, Bunte C, Hammes WP. Influence of probiotic sausage (*Lactobacillus paracasei*) on blood lipids and immunological parameters of healthy volunteers. Food Research International. 2002;235:133–138.

[71] Klingberg TD, Budde BB. The survival and persistence in the human gastrointestinal tract of five probiotic lactobacilli consumed as freeze-dried cultures or as probiotic sausage. International Journal of Food of Microbiology. 2006;109:157–159.

[72] Jiménez-Colmenero F, Ventanas J, Toldrá F. Nutritional composition of dry-cured ham and its role in a healthy diet. Meat Science. 2010;84:585–593.

[73] Klingberg TD, Axelsson L, Naterstad K, Elsser D, Bude BB. Identification of potential starter cultures for Scandinavian-type fermented sausages. International Journal of Food of Microbiology. 2005;105:419–431.

[74] Heller KJ. Probiotic bacteria in fermented foods: product characteristics and starter organisms. American Journal of Clinical Nutrition. 2005;73:374S-379S.

[75] Khan MI, Arshad MS, Anjum FM, Sameen A, Rehman A, Gill WT. Meat as a functional food with special reference to probiotic sausages. Food Research International. 2011;44:3125–3133.

[76] Nassu RT, Goncalves LAG, Da Silva MAAP, Beserra FJ. Oxidative stability of fermented goat meat sausage with different levels of natural antioxidant. Meat Science. 2003;63:43–49.

[77] Summo C, Caponio VM, Pasqualone A. Effect of vacuum-packaging storage on the quality level of ripened sausages. Meat Science. 2006;74:249–254.

[78] Faustman C, Liebler DC, Mcclure TD, SUN Q. Alpha, beta-unsaturated aldehydes accelerate oxymyoglobin oxidation. Journal of Agriculture and Food Chemistry, 1999;47:3140–3144.

[79] Libera J, Karwowska M, Stasiak DM, Dolatowski ZJ. Microbiological and physico-chemical properties of dry-cured neck inoculated with probiotic of *Bifidobacterium animalis* ssp. *lactis* BB-12. International Journal of Food Science and Technology. 2015;50:1560–1566.

[80] Ruiz-Moyano S, Martán A, Benito MJ, Hernández A, Casquete R, De Guia Córdoba M. Application of *Lactobacillus fermentum* HL57 and *Pediococcus acidilactici* SP979 as potential probiotics in the manufacture of traditional Iberian dry-fermented sausages. Food Microbiology. 2011;28:839–847.

[81] Fadda S, Sanz Y, Vignolo G, Aristoy M, Oliver G, Toldrá F. Hydrolysis of pork muscle sarcoplasmic proteins by *Lactobacillus curvatus* and *Lactobacillus sakei*. Applied and Environmental Microbiology. 1999;65:578–584.

[82] Lin MY, Yen CL. Antioxidative ability of lactic acid bacteria. Journal of Agriculture and Food Chemistry. 1999;47:1460–1466.

[83] Lin MY, Yen CL. Inhibition of lipid peroxidation by *Lactobacillus acidophilus* and *Bifidobacterium longum*. Journal of Agriculture and Food Chemistry. 1999;47:3661–3664.

[84] Libera J, Dolatowski ZJ. Effect of *Lactobacillus acidophilus* (Bauer) and *Bifidobacterium bifidum* on probiotic bacteria on changes in fat in dry-fermented meat products during storage. Food. Science. Technology. Quality. 2014;4(95):160–172.

[85] Wójciak KM, Karwowska M, Dolatowski ZJ. Fatty acid profile, colour and lipid oxidation of organic fermented sausage during chilling storage as influenced by acid whey and probiotic strains addition. Scientia Agricola. 2015;72(2):124–131.

[86] Toldrá F, Reig M. Innovation for healthier processed meats. Trends in Food Science and Technology. 2011;22:517–522.

[87] Spano G, Russo P, Lonvaud-Funel A, Lucas P, Alexandre H, Grandvalet C. Biogenic amines in fermented foods. European Journal of Clinical Nutrition. 2010;64:95–100.

[88] Suzzi G, Gardini F. Biogenic amines in dry fermented sausages: a review. International Journal of Food Microbiology. 2003;88:41–54.

[89] Chong CY, Abu Bakary F, Russly AR, Jamilah B, Mahyudin NA. The effects of food processing on biogenic amines formation. International Food Research Journal. 2011;18(3):867–876.

[90] Chander H, Batish VH, Babu, S, Singh RS. Factors affecting amine production by a selected strain of *Lactobacillus bulgaricus*. Journal of Food Science. 1989;54:940–942.

[91] Stadnik J, Dolatowski ZJ. Free amino acids and biogenic amines content during ageing of dry-cured pork loins inoculated with *Lactobacillus casei* ŁOCK 0900 probiotic strain. Food Science and Technology Research. 2015;21(2):167–174.

[92] Okoń A, Dolatowski ZJ. Effect of probiotic bacteria on free amino acid profile and sensory traits of raw-ripening pork sirloin during storage. Food. Science. Technology. Quality. 2014;3(94):92–107.

[93] Casaburi A, Di Monaco R, Cavella S, Toldrá F, Ercolini D, Villani F. Proteolytic and lipolytica starter cultures and their effect on traditional fermented sausages ripening and sensory traits. Food Microbiology. 2008;25(2):335–347.

[94] Nakamura Y, Yamamoto N, Sakai K, Takano T. Antihypertensive effect of sour milk and peptides isolated from it that are inhibitors to angiotensin I-converting enzyme. Journal of Dairy Science. 1994;78:1253–1257.

[95] Seppo L, Jauhiainen T, Poussa T, Korpela R. A fermented milk high in bioactive peptides has a blood pressure-lowering effect in hypertensive subjects. The American Journal of Clinical Nutrition. 2003;77:326–330.

[96] Castellano P, Aristoy MC, Sentandreu MA, Vignolo G, Toldrá F. Peptides with angiotensin I converting enzyme (ACE) inhibitory activity generated from porcine skeletal muscle proteins by the action of meat-borne *Lactobacillus*. Journal of Proteome Research. 2013;89:183–190.

[97] Escudero E, Aristoy MC, Nishimura H, Arihara K, Toldrá F. Antihypertensive effect and antioxidant activity of peptide fractions extracted from Spanish dry-cured ham. Meat Science. 2012;91:306–311.

[98] Broncano JM, Otte J, Petrón MJ, Parra V, Timón ML. Isolation and identification of low molecular weight antioxidant compounds from fermented "chorizo" sausages. Meat Science. 2012;90:494–501.

Chapter 15

Pectic Oligosaccharides and Other Emerging Prebiotics

Beatriz Míguez, Belén Gómez, Patricia Gullón,
Beatriz Gullón and José Luis Alonso

Additional information is available at the end of the chapter

http://dx.doi.org/10.5772/62830

Abstract

A prebiotic is a selectively fermented ingredient that results in specific changes in the composition and/or activity of the gastrointestinal microbiota, thus conferring benefit(s) upon host health. The most widely accepted prebiotics are lactulose, inulin, fructooligosaccharides (FOS), galactooligosaccharides (GOS), and the human milk oligosaccharides (HMO). However, there is a growing list of potential prebiotics although the evidence for these, especially in humans, is not as well established as for FOS and GOS. Some of them are already commercialized but others such as polydextrose (PDX), pectic oligosaccharides (POS), bacterial exopolysaccharides (EPS), polysaccharides derived from algae and sugar alcohols are still in the early stages of development. This chapter summarizes the scientific literature regarding the manufacture and the evaluation of the properties of this group "emerging prebiotics".

Keywords: emerging prebiotics, pectic oligosaccharides, polydextrose, algae-derived oligosaccharides, bacterial exopolysaccharides, sugar alcohols

1. Introduction

The consumption of prebiotics is being specially considered as a good health-improving strategy; they have been recently defined as "nondigestible compounds that through its metabolization by microorganisms in the gut, modulate the composition and/or the activity of the gut microbiota, thus conferring physiological benefit effects on the host health" [1].

The microbial communities that inhabit the human intestinal tract constitute a complex association, comprising more than 1000 species and around 10^{14} microorganisms, mainly anaerobic (>99.9%). **Figure 1** shows the human gastrointestinal tract, indicating the different levels of microorganisms and the main bacterial groups. Along the jejunum, and particularly in the ileum, there is a gradual increase in the number and diversity of bacteria, and finally, the majority of gastrointestinal microbes are housed in the colon [2].

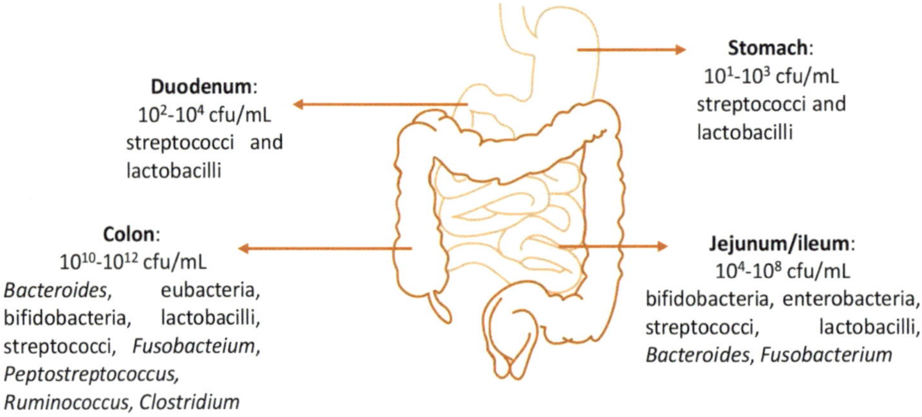

Figure 1. The human gastrointestinal tract (CFU, colony-forming units).

However, scientific works on this field suggest that the gut microbiota is not only a simply collection of microorganisms, but also reflects an interrelationship between the different groups that might work together for the benefit of the host [2]. In addition, the microbiota also establishes a close symbiosis with the host: humans provide the nutrients and the appropriate conditions for its development, and it performs three essential primary functions: metabolic, trophic, and defensive [3]. In fact, there is a long list of pathologies which are linked to the alteration of the gut microbiota, including hepatic encephalopathy, diarrhea, diabetes, obesity, colon cancer, IBS, IBD, gastrointestinal infections, and necrotizing enterocolitis [4, 5].

The composition of the gut microbiota is influenced by a variety of factors that include: (i) the microbial species which are acquired at birth, (ii) host genetics, (iii) age [6–8], (iv) diseases and antibiotic usage [9, 10], (v) the stress [11], and (vi) the diet. In fact, the diet is probably the most important factor and several studies are focused on the modulation of the gut microbiota by the consumption of functional foods, such as prebiotics [12–14].

For considering a food ingredient as a prebiotic, it must fulfill the following requirements [15]: (i) it cannot be hydrolyzed or absorbed in the upper gastrointestinal tract, (ii) it has to encourage the development of beneficial bacteria such as bifidobacteria and lactobacilli, and (iii) it must induce beneficial physiological effects on the host health, so that well-conducted human trials are required.

In addition to the generally identified as beneficial bacteria (bifidobacteria, lactobacilli, and even, eubacteria), a recent review by Hill et al. [16] indicates that the species *Akkermansia muciniphila* and *Faecalibacterium prausnitzii*, and others such as *Roseburia* spp. and *Eubacterium hallii*, which could be useful to alleviate gut inflammation, to induce and regulate of the immune system or to improve the intestinal barrier function.

http://dx.doi.org/10.5772/62830

The most widely accepted prebiotics are lactulose, inulin, fructooligosaccharides (FOS), galactooligosaccharides (GOS), and the human milk oligosaccharides (HMO). However, there is a growing list of potential prebiotics and some of them are already commercialized and others, like polydextrose (PDX), pectic oligosaccharides (POS), bacterial exopolysaccharides (EPS), polysaccharides derived from algae and sugar alcohols that are still in the early stages of study [15]. This chapter summarizes the scientific literature regarding the manufacture and evaluation of this group of emerging prebiotics.

2. Pectic oligosaccharides (POS)

POS have been recently classified as emerging prebiotics and their potential is currently being evaluated.

2.1. Raw materials for POS production

POS are oligosaccharides that can be obtained by partial hydrolysis of pectins, which are heteropolysaccharides with a highly complex structure.

Pectins are mainly made up by a backbone of galacturonic acid units (GalA) connected by α-(1,4) links that can be randomly acetylated at the O-2 and/or O-3 positions and methylated at C-6. This fraction is known as "smooth region," and it is occasionally interrupted by the "hairy region," where side chains, formed by a variety of neutral sugars, can be found. **Figure 2** shows the major structural fragments of pectin:

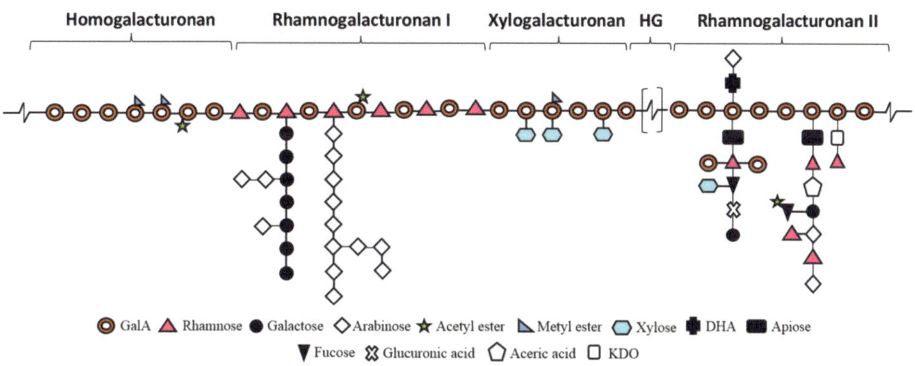

Figure 2. Simplified structure of pectin.

a. Homogalacturonan (HG). HG is a linear polymer consisting of a chain with an estimated length of 72–100 GalA units that represent, approximately, 60% of the total pectin [17]. Acetylation and methylation degrees (DA and DM, respectively) vary according to the origin and the development stage of the plant [18].

b. Xylogalacturonan (XG). XG is a chain of GalA residues partially substituted by D-xylose residues connected by β-(1,3) links at C-3 and/or C-2 positions.

c. Rhamnogalacturonan I (RG-I). It represents up to 7–14% of the pectins [19] and contains alternating units of α-(1,4)-galacturonosyl and α-(1,2)-rhamnosyl. In many cases, rhamnose residues show side chains as substituents on the O-4 position, made up of arabinan and/ or arabinogalactan I and II, although lower concentrations of xylose or glucose can be also found [18].

d. Rhamnogalacturonan II (RG-II). RGII is a region characterized by a length of 7–9 GalA units, where complex branches made up of 12 types of monosaccharides (as a maximum) can exist, including some minority monomers such as apiose, fucose, acetic acid, DHA, or KDO [20].

Pectin has a great number of applications including its use as ingredient for medicaments for treating gastrointestinal disorders, diabetes, high blood pressure, or hypercholesterolemia [21–23].

Currently, citrus pulp and apple pomace are the major sources of pectin, but this polymer can also be found in other agro-products such as sugar beet pulp [24].

2.2. Manufacture and purification

Several methods have been used for POS production from both agro-industrial byproducts and purified pectins, including partial enzymatic hydrolysis, acid hydrolysis, hydrothermal treatments, dynamic high-pressure microfluidization, or photochemical reaction in media containing TiO_2 [24].

Chemical methods include the acidic or basic hydrolysis of α and β-glucosidic links of the principal chains of HG, RG-I, and RG-II and their side chains. These methodologies include hydrothermal treatments and processes where external acids are added. In both cases, hydronium ions act as catalytic species [24]. A variety of raw materials such as orange albedo, apple pulp, or deesterified beet pulp have been treated to obtain POS, using acids such as HNO_3, HCl, or TFA [24], although alkalis (KOH) can also be employed [25]. POS mixtures have been obtained from lemon and orange peel wastes [26–28], dried apple pomace [29], sugar beet pulp [30], or alperujo [31] using stainless steel reactors, whereas Sato et al. [32] employed both a batch and a continuous tubular flow reactor to produce arabinooligosaccharides (AraOS) and feruloylated AraOS from beet fiber.

As an alternative, pectin-degrading enzymes constitute a group of enzymes that catalyze the degradation of the pectic polymers in plant cells. Although pectins have a complex structure, they can be modified by diverse enzymes, including hydrolases, lyases, and esterases [33].

Several raw materials with different characteristics have been enzymatically treated, such as bergamot peel [34], gum tragacanth [35, 36], ginseng pectin [37], orange peel wastes [38], lemon peel wastes [39], sugar beet [40, 41], apple pectin [42], or medicinal herbs [43].

Both mono-active and commercial mixtures can be used for pectin depolymerization; however, mono-active enzymes target only specific structures, causing the release of more defined oligosaccharides than when commercial enzyme mixtures or chemical treatments are employed [44]. Mixture of several preparations have been widely employed for POS production [38, 41, 45–48]. A comparable yield respect to acidic treatments can be achieved using enzyme preparations [42].

In addition, enzymes can be also advantageous for the alteration of the methylation or acetylation degree of the polymer [44].

On the other hand, chemical and enzymatic hydrolysis have been combined to depolymerize pectin [49] or to obtain different pectin fractions, such as POS and neutral and acidic xylooligosaccharides [31]. Other technologies that have been combined are enzymatic and microwave-assisted alkaline extraction [48], hydrothermal and acid treatment for polygalacturonic acid hydrolysis [50], subcritical water and ultrasonic-assisted treatments [51].

Finally, physical technologies (for instance, the dynamic high-pressure microfluidization under acidic conditions) have been emerged as innovative [52].

After production, purification stages are usually needed to obtain a product suitable to be used as food ingredient. The most common purification technique is the membrane filtration. A process involving diafiltration followed by concentration was performed by Gómez et al. [26] to purify pectic oligosaccharides from autohydrolysis liquors obtained from lemon peel wastes, yielding a refined product with about 98 wt% of oligomers which contained oligogalacturonides (with DP in the range of 2–18) and AraOS (with DP in the range of 2–8). A similar approach was performed by Gómez et al. [27] achieving a refined final product containing 90% of the target product, where there were identified AraOS (DP 3–21), GalOS (DP 5–12), and OGalA (DP 2–12), with variable DM and also long-chain products.

Rubio-Senent et al. [53] isolated fractions (MW > 3 kDa) which were rich in pectic material from an alperujo aqueous hydrolysate by ultrafiltration thought 3 kDa regenerated cellulose.

Ultrafiltration and diafiltration (50 kDa cut-off) were employed by Sulek et al. [54] to isolate AraOS, which were further fractionated into a stirred membrane reactor equipped with a 1 kDa MWCO.

This methodology has also been employed to sequentially fractionate oligosaccharides by its molecular weight [55].

Other alternatives were also used in this field; Lama-Muñoz et al. [31] fractionated and purified neutral and POS by adsorption XAD chromatography (Amberlite XAD-16 resin), and the gel Sephadex G-75 was selected by Lee et al. [56] to purify POS from Korean Citrus Hallabong peels.

2.3. Prebiotic potential of POS

POS have been suggested as a new class of prebiotics, which are capable of exerting a number of health-promoting effects, including [24] stimulation of apoptosis in human colonic adenocarcinoma cells, potential for cardiovascular protection *in vivo*, reduction of damage by heavy metals, antiobesity effects, antitoxic, antiinfection, antibacterial, and antioxidant properties.

The main derived products from the intestinal bacterial fermentation of POS, as well as from other dietary fiber, are the SCFA (acetate, propionate, and butyrate). SCFA exert several beneficial effects including: (i) a key role in the prevention and treatment of the metabolic syndrome, bowel disorders, and cancer [57–59]; (ii) protection against diet-induced obesity and regulation of the gut hormones [60]; or (iii) a positive effect on the treatment of ulcerative colitis, Crohn's disease, and antibiotic-associated diarrhea and obesity [61–63]. Particularly, butyrate is the major energy source for the colonocytes, propionate has a role in gluconeogenesis processes, and acetate is used for the lipogenesis [64].

The following paragraphs summarize the results derived from the recent *in vitro* and *in vivo* studies carried out employing POS as substrate:

a) In vitro assays

Citrus peel wastes and sugar beet pulp were subjected to hydrothermal treatment and the resulting liquors refined by membrane filtration. The final POS mixtures were then fermented by human fecal samples leading to an increase of the bacterial population of up to eight different groups. Specifically, POS from sugar beet pulp showed the highest bifidogenic potential and the maximum SCFA concentration. Meanwhile, the largest increase in *Lactobacillus* population was observed using POS from orange peel wastes as a carbon source, whereas the best results for other bacterial groups such as *Eubacterium, Faecalibacterium*, or *Roseburia* were observed for POS from lemon peels wastes [27, 65]. In the same way, POS derived from sugar beet (enriched in AraOS) were used as substrates in *in vitro* fermentation assays of POS leading to increases in bifidobacteria populations (which preferred low molecular weight fractions) without stimulating the growth of *Clostridium* [66–68]. In a recent study with POS from sugar beet pulp containing GalOS, AraOS, and mixtures of acidic oligosaccharides (mainly made up of RG and HG oligosaccharides), no a clear bifidogenic effect was observed, whereas important increases of *Faecalibacterium* were reported. Moreover, the SCFA concentrations were found higher in experiments with POS than with FOS [69].

Regarding apple pectin, a variety of works were reported concluding that POS might be an interesting prebiotic candidate with slightly improved physiological properties if they are compared to commercial ones. In this context, Gulfi et al. [70] indicated that pectin hairy regions from ripe apples revealed to be a very readily fermentable substrate for human colonic bacteria, showing a substantial impact on pH and SCFA production. Suzuki et al. [71] found that AraOS from apple pectin, especially those that consist of more than three units, are more selectively utilized by *Bifidobacterium adolescentis, B. longum*, and *Bacteroides vulgatus* than FOS and XOS. Meanwhile, Chen et al. [52] reported the ability of apple-derived POS for promoting the bifidobacteria and lactobacilli growth and for decreasing numbers of bacteroides and clostridia, whereas the fermentation of refined POS mixture from apple pomace with human feces resulted in an increase in the populations of *Bifidobacterium, Eubacterium rectale* and *Lactobacillus*, but also of *Clostridium* and *Bacteroides* [72].

Some authors as Mandalari et al. [12] employed other types of pectin sources, demonstrating that almond seeds, which contain arabinose-rich pectin, exhibited potential for their use as a novel sources of prebiotics, increasing the populations of bifidobacteria and *Eubacterium rectale* with the subsequent increase in butyrate concentrations. Guevara-Arauza et al. [73] observed that POS from nopal act as prebiotics, reducing putrefactive ammonium production, increasing SCFA production, and sustaining bifidogenic effects over longer periods of time.

In addition, in order to elucidate structure–function relationships in POS, Onumpai et al. [74] compared the fermentation properties of pectin fractions and their parent pectins using a pH-controlled fecal fermentation system. All of the tested carbohydrates increased the populations of bacteroides, but just galactan- and arabinan-derived oligosaccharides increased the bifidobacteria counts. On the other hand, methylated oligogalacturonides, compared to the parent polysaccharide and to other pectic fractions, caused a significant increase in the *Faecalibacterium prausnitzii* populations [74].

b) In vivo assays

Despite the advances in *in vitro* models, the *in vivo* studies involving the use of animals and especially of humans provide the best models for studying the changes in the microbiota populations. However, they often require specialist facilities and are both expensive and time-consuming, limiting the number of this type of assays [75].

Jiao et al. [76] demonstrated that water-soluble oligosaccharides isolated from Panax ginseng significantly inhibited tumor growth in mice by enhancing their immune system. In this last year, native intact (TrPP) and modified, low molecular weight (MTrPP) forms of pectic polysaccharides isolated from turmeric were evaluated for ulcer-preventive potentials in *in vivo* rat models. MTrPP was rich in galacturonic acid (687 mg/g; TrPP-544 mg/g) and galactose (52.9%; TrPP-21.7%) from HG and RG-I containing galactan. The results suggested that MTrPP possess significantly improved ulcer-preventive properties than TrPP (inhibiting ulcer scores up to 85%), revealing that the fine structural features of pectin are crucial in delivering its therapeutic benefits against gastric ulcer [77].

Regarding the clinical assays, Fanaro et al. [78] observed increased counts of bifidobacteria and lactobacilli by the administration of POS as a component of infant formulae. Similarly, Magne et al. [79] detected increased proportions of bifidobacteria in the mixture GOS/FOS/POS respect to the mixture GOS/FOS, as well as the proportions of *Bacteroides* and *Clostridium coccoides* decreased. Moreover, the use of neutral and acidic oligosaccharides to preterm infants (mixtures of POS, GOS and FOS) showed a trend toward a lower incidence of serious endogenous infection and serious infectious episodes [80]. Finally, the intake of POS in a mixture with short-chain GOS and long-chain FOS by volunteers who were in the earlier stages of HIV-1 infection, resulted in the modulation of gut microbiota by increasing the bifidobacteria numbers and by decreasing the counts of pathogens [81].

3. Polydextrose (PDX)

3.1. Structure and manufacture

PDX is an artificial highly branched polysaccharide synthesized conventionally by random polycondensation of glucose with sorbitol and a food grade acid (e.g., citric acid) as catalyst, at a high temperature and under partial vacuum [82]. Recently, other methods have been explored as the synthesis by microwave irradiation [83]. PDX is composed of a mixture of glucose oligomers, with an average degree of polymerization (DP) of 12, ranging from DP 2–120 [84, 85] and contains all different combinations of α- and β-(1,2), (1,3), (1,4), and (1,6) glycosidic linkages, but α-(1,6) linkages are predominant [85, 86]. PDX is regarded as a resistant polysaccharide [87] and it is widely used in the food industry as a low-energy bulking agent (1 kcal/g) and as a sugar or fat replacer [86].

3.2. Prebiotic effects

Due to its complex structure and to the nature of its glycosidic bonds, PDX is resistant to mammalian digestive enzymes in the upper gastrointestinal tract. For this reason, PDX reaches the colon intact where it is partially fermented by gut microbiota, stimulating selectively target bacterial groups [84, 85, 88]. These two characteristics, indigestibility and selective fermentability, support that the PDX has been identified as a source of prebiotic fiber with several health-promoting effects [89], including:

- Improvement of the bowel function, by promoting the growth of beneficial bacteria (e.g., bifidobacteria and lactobacilli) while preventing the growth of harmful ones (such as clostridia and bacteroides), decrease of fecal pH and increase of the residual concentration of short chain fatty acids (SCFA) [88].
- Reduction of the risk of colon cancer development [88, 90].
- Modulation of the lipid metabolism, decreasing the total cholesterol and LDL cholesterol and increasing HDL cholesterol [84].
- Prevention of the adhesion of opportunistic pathogens related with meningitis and sepsis in neonates [91].
- Anti-inflammatory action [92] and positive effects on canine osteoarthritis [93].
- Reduction of the symptoms of human atopic eczema [94].
- Improvement of the absorption of magnesium, calcium and iron [95–97]. The studies related to the biological and prebiotics effects of PDX (observed *in vivo, in vitro* and human intervention assays) are summarized in **Table 1**.

Biological and prebiotic effects	Study type	References
Proliferation of *Lactobacillus* and *Bifidobacterium* species and decreases in *Bacteroides* species. Increases in concentrations of SCFA. Improvement of the bowel function and inhibition of the excessive glucose absorption in the small intestine	C.I.	[98]
Increases in *Ruminococcus intestinalis* and *Clostridium* clusters I, II, and IV that are butyrate-producing. Decreases in fecal water genotoxicity	C.I.	[88]

Biological and prebiotic effects	Study type	References
Reduction of LDL cholesterol and total cholesterol	C.I.	[99]
Infants fed with formulas with PDX had softer stools (similar to breastfed infants) in comparison with those who receive unsupplemented formulas	C.I.	[100]
Increases in bifidobacteria and stools weight. Decreased in fecal ammonia, phenol, indoles and BCFA (isobutyrate, isovalerate, and valerate)	C.I.	[101]
Reduction of the orofecal transit time, and improvement of stool consistency in persons suffering from constipation	C.I.	[102]
Increases in *Faecalibacterium prausnitzii* numbers	C.I.	[103]
Reduction in fecal pH and improvement of stool consistency	C.I.	[104]
Supplementation with GOS–polydextrose and *Lactobacillus rhamnosus* GG in preterm infants reduces the risk of rhinovirus infections in infants	C.I.	[105]
The intake of yogurt with polydextrose, *B. lactis* HN019, *and L. acidophilus* NCFM® improved constipation	C.I.	[106]
Reduction of the production of biogenic amines and BCFA in rats. Improvement of the immune function	A.S.	[107]
Increases in defecation without diarrhea	C.I.	[108]
Increases in populations of bifidobacteria with a similar pattern with breastfed infants	C.I.	[109]
Increases in the number of bifidobacteria and selective stimulation of *Bifidobacterium infantis* compared with other carbohydrates tested	*in vitro*	[110]
Increases in bifidobacteria and lactobacilli and SCFA production	*in vitro*	[111]
Increases in the concentration of acetate and propionate and reduction of BCFA concentration.	*in vitro* (C.M.)	[112]
Increases in the production of fecal SCFA, especially acetate and propionate, and decreased fecal indole	A.S. (dogs)	[113]
Reduction of the expression of mucosal COX-2 (closely related to the colorectal cancer)	A.S. (pigs)	[114]
Increases in the content of ileal lactobacilli and in the levels of propionic and lactic acid. Reduction of cytokine expression	A.S. (pigs)	[89]
Reduction of chronic visceral hypersensitivity in rats exposed to early-life painful stimulus	A.S. (rats)	[115]
Improved calcium absorption in postmenopausal rats	A.S. (rats)	[116]
Ability to inhibit adherence of *C. sakazakii* to gastrointestinal epithelial cells	*in vitro*	[91]
Positive effect in canine osteoarthritis	A.S. (dogs)	[93]
Reduction of symptoms of allergen-induced dermatitis	A.S.(mice)	[94]
Stimulation of apoptosis in colon cancer cells	*in vitro* (C.M.)	[90]

A.S., animal study; C.I., clinical intervention; C.M., colonic model.

Table 1. Results obtained in studies carried out using polydextrose as substrate.

4. Algae-derived oligosaccharides

4.1. Structure, sources, and production

Seaweeds are a source of bioactive compounds like sulphated polysaccharides, proteins, polyunsaturated fatty acids (PUFA), and polyphenols with potential beneficial health effects, such as antibacterial [115], anti-inflammatory [116, 117], antioxidant [118–120], antitumoral [121, 122], anticoagulant [123] antiadhesive [116], and apoptotic activities [124, 125] among others. The major polysaccharides which can be found in seaweeds are alginates, laminarins, fucans and cellulose in brown seaweeds, ulvan in green seaweeds, and agars and carrageenans in red seaweeds. Several extraction methods of bioactive sulphated polysaccharides from seaweeds have been investigated in recent years, including: diluted acid extraction [126, 127], hydrothermal processing [128], microwave-assisted extraction [129–131], ultrasound-assisted extraction [132], enzyme-assisted extraction [132, 133], or pressurized liquid extraction [134].

4.2. Prebiotic properties

In the last decade, seaweed polysaccharides have been considered as dietary fibers and have attracted much interest because of their potential use as prebiotics [135, 136]. In this sense, several studies have reported that seaweed polysaccharides resist the digestion in the upper of gastrointestinal tract, support the growth of lactic acid bacteria, reduce of harmful bacteria as well as modulate the intestinal metabolism through their effects on pH and SCFA concentration [137].

To date, several studies *in vitro* and *in vivo* were carried out to evaluate the potential prebiotic effects of seaweed polysaccharides. **Table 2** summarizes the results obtained. No human trials have been conducted yet using this type of substrates.

Product or seaweed	Biological and prebiotic effects	Study type	References
Chondrus crispus and Sarcodiotheca gaudichaudii	Increases in the numbers of *Bif. longum* and *Streptococcus salivarius* and reduction in the populations of *C. perfringens*. Increases in SCFAs concentration and i-butyric acid.	A.S. (hens)	[140]
Laminarin	Increases in the levels of SCFAs	*In vitro* (HGM)	[137]
Laminarin	Variations of mucus composition in jejunum, ileum, cecum, and colon	A.S. (rats)	[137]
Ascophyllum nodosum	Reduction in populations of *Escherichia coli*	*In vitro* (PGM)	[141]
Carrageenans	Increases in cecal moisture and in concentrations of acetic and propionic acid. Reduction in the levels of triglycerides and total cholesterol	A.S. (rats)	[142]
Alginate oligosaccharides	Increases in numbers of fecal *bifidobacteria* and *lactobacilli* and reduced counts of *bacteroides* respect to the FOS	A.S. (rats)	[143]
Alginate oligosaccharides	Stimulation of the growth of *Bifidobacterium bifidum* ATCC 29521 and *Bifidobacterium longum* SMU 27001	*In vitro*	[143]
Saccharina latissima	Increases in the concentrations of acetic and propionic acids	A.S (rats)	[144]
Laminarin and fucoidan	Reduction in the populations of *Enterobacteria* and increases in the populations of *Lactobacilli*	A.S. (pigs)	[145]
Porphyran	Increases in the content of propionic acid in the cecum. Decreases in the number of *Clostridium coccoides*.	A.S. (mice)	[146]
Carrageenan	Increases in the populations of *Bif. breve* and reduction in the populations of *Clostridium septicum* and *Streptococcus neumoniae*. Increases in the concentrations of SCFAs and immunoglobulin levels	A.S. (rats)	[147]
Fucoidan and laminarin	Increases in the counts of *Lactobacillus* and *Bifidobacterium* in the ileum	A.S. (piglet)	[148]
Low MW polysaccharides from agar and alginate	Increases in the number of *bifidobacteria*. No effect on the populations of *Lactobacilli, Bacteroides, Eubacterium rectale/C. coccoides*, and *C. histolyticum*	*In vitro* (HGM)	[149]
Fucoidan	Stimulation of apoptosis in HT-29 and HCT116 human colon cancer cells	*In vitro*	[150]
Himanthalia elongata	Increases in the acetic, propionic, and butyric acids concentrations. Improvement of the lipid profile	A.S. (rats)	[151]
Fucoidan	Inhibition of the adhesion of *Helicobacter pylori* to the gastric mucous	*In vitro*	[152]
C. crispus	Enhancement of the host immunity and reduction of the infection by *Pseudomonas aeruginosa*	*In vitro*	[153]

A.S., animal study; C.I., clinical intervention; C.M., colonic model; HGM, human gut microbiota; PGM, pig gut microbiota.

Table 2. Results obtained in studies carried out using polysaccharides and oligosaccharides derived from algae as substrates.

5. Bacterial exopolisaccharides

5.1. Structure, sources, and production

Bacteria can produce polysaccharides that usually play a protective role against environment pressures. As these polymers are excreted into the extracellular surrounding, they are known as EPS. They can occur in two forms (capsules or biofilm) [150, 151] and are classified in two groups according to their composition:

- homo-EPSs made up of a single type of monosaccharide such as fructans, α-D-glucans, β-D-glucans, dextran, curdlan, alternan, mutan, reuteran, or levan [152–154].

- hetero-EPSs composed of different types of monosaccharides, mainly D-glucose, D-galactose, L-rhamnose, and their derivatives, such as xanthan, gellan, alginate, hyaluronan, succinoglycan, kefiran, emulsan, galactoPol, or FucoPol [152–154]. The heteropolysaccharides are the most abundant bacterial EPSs.

The critical factors for maximum EPSs production are carbon and nitrogen sources, mineral requirements, oxygen and aeration rate, temperature and pH [155], among others. Sugars are the most commonly carbon sources used for the production of bacterial EPSs. However, cheaper substrates, such as agro-food or industrial wastes and byproducts are suitable carbon sources for EPSs production [153]. EPSs synthesis is generally favored by the presence of the carbon source in excess, and the production of most bacterial EPSs occurs under aerobic conditions [153].

On the other hand, the methods for EPSs extraction have a crucial influence as their physicochemical properties could be affected by the isolation and purification techniques [154]. It can be carried out by two methods: (i) by solvent precipitation when they are in slim form and (ii) by alkaline extraction prior centrifugation and alcohol precipitation when they are in form of capsule. The recovery is performed by solvent precipitation [155].

5.2. Biological properties

The EPSs have been proved to have functional roles in human or animal health including immunomodulatory properties, antiviral, antioxidant, antimutagenecity, antihypertensive, antiulcer, and antitumor activities, and have also been used as food additives for texture improvement, as gelling agents or emulsifiers [152, 155, 156]. Moreover, EPSs may induce other positive physiological responses including lower cholesterol levels, reduced formation of pathogenic biofilms, modulation of adhesion to epithelial cells, and increased levels of bifidobacteria, showing a prebiotic potential [157].

The use of bacterial EPSs as prebiotic substrates has been scarcely investigated [151]. **Table 3** shows the results from some *in vitro* and *in vivo* assays that have explored the prebiotic potential of this kind of substrates. Up to date, not human interventions with bacterial EPSs have been carried out.

EPS type	Producer strain	Biological and prebiotic effects	Study type	References
Levan	*Lactobacillus sanfranciscensis* LTH1729, *Lactobacillus sanfranciscensis* LTH2590	Bifidogenic effect; enhanced growth *Eubacterium biforme*	*In vitro* (HGM)	[162]
EPS (type not identified)	*Weissella cibaria A2, Weeissella confusa A9, Lactobacillus plantarum A3 and Pediococcus.pentosaceus 5S4*	High resistance to gastric and intestinal digestions, enhancement of growth of *Bifibacterium bifidum* and some growth in case of *B. longum, B. adolescentis,* and *Lb. acidophilus*	*In vitro* (pure cultures)	[155]
EPS (type not identified)	*Weissella cibaria A2*	Enhanced growth of *Bifidobacterium* and *Lactobacillus /Enteroccoccus* groups, reduction of numbers of *Clostrida*. Increase in SCFA concentrations (acetate, propionate, butyrate)	*In vitro* (HGM)	[155]
EPS (type not identified)	*B. animalis, B. pseudocatenultum, B. longum*	Increases in SCFA concentration and moderate bifidogenic effect	*In vitro* (HGM)	[163]
Fructan	*Lactobacillus sanfranciscensis* TMW 1.392	Metabolized by *B. breve, B. bifidum, B. adolescentis,* and *B. infantis*	*In vitro* (pure cultures)	[164]

EPS type	Producer strain	Biological and prebiotic effects	Study type	References
Dextran	*Leuconostoc mesenteroides* NRRL B-1426	Low digestibility by simulated human gastric juice, high resistance to digestion by human a-amylases, stimulated the growth of *B. animalis, B. infantis, Lb. acidophilus*	*In vitro* (pure cultures)	[165]
Reuteran	*Lb. reuteri* TMW 1.656	Contribution to the prevention of enterotoxigenic *E. coli* adhesion to the intestinal mucosa	*In vivo* (weanling piglets)	[166]
EPS (type not identified)	*B. bifidum* WBIN03	Significant inhibition of enterobacteria, enterococci, and *Bacteroides fragilis*; significant enhancement of the amount of *Lactobacillus* and total anaerobes	*In vivo* (mice)	[167]

HGM, human gut microbiota.

Table 3. Results obtained in studies carried out using bacterial exopolysaccharides as substrates.

6. Sugar alcohols

6.1. Definition and production

Sugar alcohols are low digestible carbohydrates that are hydrogenated, which means that there is an alcohol group (>CH–OH) in place of the carbonyl group (>C=O) in the aldose and ketose moieties of mono-, di-, oligo- and polysaccharides [162]. They can be classified into three groups: (i) hydrogenated monosaccharides (erythritol, xylitol, sorbitol, manitol); (ii) hydrogenated disaccharides (lactitol, isomalt, maltitol), and (iii) hydrogenated polysaccharides (hydrogenated starch hydrolysates (HSHs), polyglycitols) [163].

Sugar alcohols occur naturally in certain fruits and vegetables, and some of them are even generated by the human body. However, huge amounts of sugar alcohols are manufactured for the food industry (**Table 4**) where they are used as replacers in foodstuffs performing functions such as flavor enhancer, humectant, sweetener, anticaking agent, bulking agent, glazing agent, stabilizer, thickener, emulsifier, and sequestrant [166].

Sugar alcohol	Natural source	Synthesis
Erythritol	Vegetables, fruits (melons, peaches, mushrooms, fermented foods (wine, beer, sake, soy sauce)	Fermentation of glucose using yeasts or lactic acid bacteria
Xylitol	Fruits, vegetables, berries, oats, mushrooms	Metal catalyzed hydrogenation of D-xylose Biotechnological production from corn cobs, waste of sugarcane, and other fibers using yeasts
Sorbitol	Apples, pears, apricots, nectarines, prunes, dates, raisins	Catalytic hydrogenation of glucose or dextrose using Ni catalyst at high Tª. Electrochemical reduction of dextrose at pH>7
Mannitol	Fruits, vegetables, brown seaweeds, wine	Fermentative process using lactic acid bacteria
Isomalt	–	Enzymatic transglucosidation of sucrose into maltulose and further hydrogenation
Lactitol	–	Catalytic hydrogenation of lactose using Raney nickel as catalyst
Maltitol	–	Catalytic hydrogenation of maltose or very high maltose glucose syrup
Polyglycitols/ HSHs	–	Partial hydrolysis of starch (from corn, potato or wheat) resulting in dextrins that undergoes subsequent hydrogenation

Table 4. Natural sources and industrial synthesis of sugar alcohols [170, 171]

6.2. Biological properties

Sugar alcohols are characterized by their lower blood glucose response, and they can be metabolized without insulin [166]. Although they are structurally similar to sugars, their nutritional value is lower than them because they are only partially absorbed by the body, and the absorbed portions are either poorly metabolized (e.g., erythritol) or excreted via the urinary tract. The unabsorbed polyols are partially fermented in the colon, and they can modulate beneficially the gut microbiota acting as prebiotics [109, 162]. **Table 5** lists the results obtained in several studies that have been carried out with sugar alcohols.

Sugar alcohol	Biological and prebiotic effects	Study type	References
Erythritol	Not change on bacterial population dynamics but significant increase in acetate	*In vitro* (human gut microbiota)	[113]
Sorbitol	Favors growth of autochthonous *Lactobacillus* species and increases colonic production of butyrate	*In vivo* (in rat)	[174]
Mannitol	Modification of large intestine fermentation to produce more butyrate and propionate	*In vivo* (in rat and pig model)	[175]
	Promotion of absorption and retention of Ca and Mg	*In vivo* (in rat)	[176]
	Lowering effect on body fat accumulation and reduction of the level of serum triglycerides	*in vivo* (in rat)	[177]
Isomalt	Significant increase in *bifidobacteria* and increase in butyrate, acetate and propionate	*In vitro* (human gut microbiota)	[113]
Lactitol	Ability to reduce circulating levels of NH3 and toxic microbial substances, the clinical utility of which is the treatment of hepatic encephalopathy	C.I.	[178]
	Reduction of levels of plasma endotoxin in chronic viral hepatitis through improving intestinal microbiota	C.I.	[179]
	Significant increases in counts of *Bifidobacterium* and both propionic and butyric acids and significant reduction of fecal pH with a consumption of 10 g/d	C.I.	[180]
	Fermentation by pure cultures of *Bifidobacterium lactis* Bi-07, *Lactobacillus acidophilus* NCFM, *Lactobacillis paracasei* Lpc-37, *Lactobacillus rhamnosus* HN001	*In vitro* (pure cultures)	[181]
	Increase fecal numbers of *L. acidophilus* NCFM. No significant changes in SCFA and fecal concentrations of spermicine and PGE2	C.I.	[182]
	Significant increase in *bifidobacteria* and increases in butyrate, acetate and propionate	*In vitro* (human gut microbiota)	[113]
Maltitol	Significant increase in *bifidobacteria*, minor increase in *Lactobacillus/enterococci*, and increases in major SCFA (acetate, propionate, and butyrate)	*In vitro* (human gut microbiota)	[113]
	Significant increases in *bifidobacteria, lactobacilli, clostridium histolyticum/perfringens* populations, *bacteroides, Fusobacterium prausnitzii, E. rectal, R. flavefaciens, Atopobium, R. bromii*, and in major SCFA (acetate, propionate, and butyrate)	C.I.	[183]

C.I., clinical intervention.

Table 5. Biological and prebiotic effects of sugar alcohols.

Acknowledgements

The authors acknowledge the financial support received from "Xunta de Galicia" (Project Ref. GRC2014/018 and "INBIOMED") and from the Spanish "Ministry of Economy and Competitivity" (Project "Advanced processing technologies for biorefineries," reference CTQ2014-53461-R). Both projects were partially funded by the FEDER Program of the European Union ("Unha maneira de facer Europa").

Author details

Beatriz Míguez[1,2], Belén Gómez[1,2], Patricia Gullón[3], Beatriz Gullón[4] and José Luis Alonso[1,2*]

*Address all correspondence to: xluis@uvigo.es

1 Chemical Engineering Department, Polytechnical Building, University of Vigo (Campus Ourense), Spain

2 CITI, Galicia Avenue, n° 2, Tecnopole, San Cibrao das Viñas, Spain

3 Chemical and Environmental Engineering Department, University of Basque Country, Square Europa, Spain

4 Department of Chemical Engineering, Institute of Technology, University of Santiago de Compostela, Spain

References

[1] Bindels LB, Delzenne NM, Cani PD, Walter J. Towards a more comprehensive concept for prebiotics. Nature Reviews Gastroenterology & Hepatology 2015;12:303–10. doi: 10.1038/nrgastro.2015.47.

[2] Binns N. Probiotics, prebiotics and the gut microbiota. ILSI Europe. Brussels, Belgium, 2013.

[3] Gotteland M. The role of the intestinal microbiota in the development of the obesity and the diabetes type-2. Chilean Journal of Endocrinology and Diabetes 2013; 6: 155-162.

[4] Guarner F. The colon as an organ: habitat of bacterial flora. Hospital Nutrition 2002; 17 Suppl 2: 7-10.

[5] Guarner F. Role of intestinal flora in health and disease. Hospital Nutrition 2007; 22 Suppl 2: 14-19.

[6] Woodmansey EJ. Intestinal bacteria and ageing. Journal of Applied Microbiology 2007;102:1178–86. doi:10.1111/j.1365-2672.2007.03400.x.

[7] O'Toole PW, Claesson MJ. Gut microbiota: Changes throughout the lifespan from infancy to elderly. International Dairy Journal 2010;20:281–91. doi:10.1016/j.idairyj. 2009.11.010.

[8] Claesson MJ, Jeffery IB, Conde S, Power SE, O'Connor EM, Cusack S, et al. Gut microbiota composition correlates with diet and health in the elderly. Nature 2012;488:178–84. doi:10.1038/nature11319.

[9] Ladirat SE. Galacto-oligosaccharides to counter the side effects of antibiotic treatments. Wageningen University. Wageningen, The Netherlands, 2014.

[10] Willing BP, Russell SL, Finlay BB. Shifting the balance: antibiotic effects on host-microbiota mutualism. Nature Reviews Microbiology 2011;9:233–43. doi:10.1038/ nrmicro2536.

[11] Prados-Bo A, Gómez-Martínez S, Nova E, Marcos A. Role of probiotics in obesity management. Nutrición Hospitalaria 2015;31 Suppl 1:10–8. doi:10.3305/nh. 2015.31.sup1.8702.

[12] Mandalari G, Nueno-Palop C, Bisignano G, Wickham MSJ, Narbad A. Potential prebiotic properties of almond (*Amygdalus communis* L.) seeds. Applied and Environmental Microbiology 2008;74:4264–70. doi:10.1128/AEM.00739-08.

[13] Samanta AK, Senani S, Kolte AP, Sridhar M, Sampath KT, Jayapal N, et al. Production and in vitro evaluation of xylooligosaccharides generated from corn cobs. Food and Bioproducts Processing 2012;90:466–74. doi:10.1016/j.fbp.2011.11.001.

[14] Cruz-Guerrero A, Hernández-Sánchez H, Rodríguez-Serrano G, Gómez-Ruíz L, García-Garibay M, Figueroa-González I. Commercial probiotic bacteria and prebiotic carbohydrates: a fundamental study on prebiotics uptake, antimicrobials production and inhibition of pathogens. Journal of the Science of Food and Agriculture 2014;94:2246–52. doi:10.1002/jsfa.6549.

[15] Corzo N, Alonso JL, Azpiroz F, Calvo MAA, Cirici M, Leis R, et al. Prebiotics; concept, properties and beneficial effects. Hospital Nutrition 2015;31: 99–118. doi:10.3305/ nh.2015.31.sup1.8715.

[16] Hill C, Guarner F, Reid G, Gibson GR, Merenstein DJ, Pot B, et al. Expert consensus document: The International Scientific Association for Probiotics and Prebiotics consensus statement on the scope and appropriate use of the term probiotic. Nature Reviews Gastroenterology & Hepatology 2014;11:506–14. doi:10.1038/nrgastro.2014.66.

[17] Voragen AGJ, Coenen GJ, Verhoef RP, Schols H a. Pectin, a versatile polysaccharide present in plant cell walls. Structural Chemistry 2009;20:263–75. doi:10.1007/ s11224-009-9442-z.

[18] Ele-Ekouna J-P, Pau-Roblot C, Courtois B, Courtois J. Chemical characterization of pectin from green tea (*Camellia sinensis*). Carbohydrate Polymers 2011;83:1232–9. doi: 10.1016/j.carbpol.2010.09.028.

[19] Jackson CL, Dreaden TM, Theobald LK, Tran NM, Beal TL, Eid M, et al. Pectin induces apoptosis in human prostate cancer cells: correlation of apoptotic function with pectin structure. Glycobiology 2007;17:805–19. doi:10.1093/glycob/cwm054.

[20] Westphal Y. Analytical profiling of plant cell wall polysaccharides. Wageningen University. Wageningen, The Netherlands, 2010.

[21] Paulsen BS, Barsett H. Polysaccharides I. In: Heinze T, editor. Advances in Polymer Science, vol. 186, Berlin/Heidelberg: Springer-Verlag; 2005, pp. 69–101. doi:10.1007/b136812.

[22] Yamada H, Kiyohara H. Immunomodulating Activity of Plant Polysaccharide Structures. In: Kamerling JP, Boons GJ, Lee YC, Suzuki A, Taniguchi N, Voragen AGJ, editors. Comprehensive Glycoscience. Volume 4 Cell Glycobiology and Development Health and Disease in Glycomedicine. Oxford: Elsevier; 2007, p. 663–694. doi: 10.1016/B978-044451967-2/00125-2.

[23] Matsumoto T, Moriya M, Sakurai MH, Kiyohara H, Tabuchi Y, Yamada H. Stimulatory effect of a pectic polysaccharide from a medicinal herb, the roots of *Bupleurum falcatum* L., on G-CSF secretion from intestinal epithelial cells. International Immunopharmacology 2008;8:581–8. doi:10.1016/j.intimp.2008.01.006.

[24] Gullón B, Gómez B, Martínez-Sabajanes M, Yáñez R, Parajó JC, Alonso JL. Pectic oligosaccharides: manufacture and functional properties. Trends in Food Science & Technology 2013;30:153–61. doi:10.1016/j.tifs.2013.01.006.

[25] Deng J, Shi ZJ, Li XZ, Liu HM. Soluble polysaccharides isolation and characterization from rabbiteye blueberry (*Vaccinium ashei*) fruits. BioResources 2013;8:405–19.

[26] Gómez B, Gullón B, Yáñez R, Parajó JC, Alonso JL. Pectic Oligosacharides from lemon peel wastes: production, purification, and chemical characterization. Journal of Agricultural and Food Chemistry 2013;61:10043–53. doi:10.1021/jf402559p.

[27] Gómez B, Gullón B, Remoroza C, Schols HA, Parajó JC, Alonso JL. Purification, characterization, and prebiotic properties of pectic oligosaccharides from orange peel wastes. Journal of Agricultural and Food Chemistry 2014;62:9769–82. doi:10.1021/jf503475b.

[28] Martínez-Sabajanes M, Yáñez R, Alonsó JL, Parajó JC. Chemical production of pectic oligosaccharides from orange peel wastes. Industrial and Engineering Chemistry Research 2010;49:8470–6. doi:10.1021/ie101066m.

[29] Wang X, Lü X. Characterization of pectic polysaccharides extracted from apple pomace by hot-compressed water. Carbohydrate Polymers 2014;102:174–84. doi:10.1016/j.carbpol.2013.11.012.

[30] Martínez-Sabajanes M, Gullón B, Schols HA, Alonso JL, Parajó JC. Assessment of the production of oligomeric compounds from sugar beet pulp. Industrial and Engineering Chemistry Research 2009;48:4681–7. doi:10.1021/ie8017753.

[31] Lama-Muñoz A, Rodríguez-Gutiérrez G, Rubio-Senent F, Fernández-Bolaños J. Production, characterization and isolation of neutral and pectic oligosaccharides with low molecular weights from olive by-products thermally treated. Food Hydrocolloids 2012;28:92–104. doi:10.1016/j.foodhyd.2011.11.008.

[32] Sato N, Takano Y, Mizuno M, Nozaki K, Umemura S, Matsuzawa T, et al. Production of feruloylated arabino-oligosaccharides (FA-AOs) from beet fiber by hydrothermal treatment. The Journal of Supercritical Fluids 2013;79:84–91. doi:10.1016/j.supflu.2013.01.012.

[33] Bonnin E, Garnier C, Ralet M-C. Pectin-modifying enzymes and pectin-derived materials: applications and impacts. Applied Microbiology and Biotechnology 2014;98:519–32. doi:10.1007/s00253-013-5388-6.

[34] Mandalari G, Nueno Palop C, Tuohy K, Gibson GR, Bennett RN, Waldron KW, et al. In vitro evaluation of the prebiotic activity of a pectic oligosaccharide-rich extract enzymatically derived from bergamot peel. Applied Microbiology and Biotechnology 2006;73:1173–9. doi:10.1007/s00253-006-0561-9.

[35] Coenen GJ, Kabel MA, Schols HA, Voragen AGJ. CE-MSn of complex pectin-derived oligomers. Electrophoresis 2008;29:2101–11. doi:10.1002/elps.200700465.

[36] Gavlighi HA, Meyer AS, Mikkelsen JD. Tragacanth gum: Functionality and prebiotic potential. Agro Food Industry Hi-Tech 2013;24:46–8.

[37] Yu L, Zhang X, Li S, Liu X, Sun L, Liu H, et al. Rhamnogalacturonan I domains from ginseng pectin. Carbohydrate Polymers 2010;79:811–7. doi:10.1016/j.carbpol.2009.08.028.

[38] Martínez-Sabajanes M, Yáñez R, Alonso JL, Parajó JC. Pectic oligosaccharides production from orange peel waste by enzymatic hydrolysis. International Journal of Food Science & Technology 2012;47:747–54. doi:10.1111/j.1365-2621.2011.02903.x.

[39] Gómez B, Yáñez R, Parajó JC, Alonso JL. Production of pectin-derived oligosaccharides from lemon peels by extraction, enzymatic hydrolysis and membrane filtration. Journal of Chemical Technology and Biotechnology 2016;91:234–247. doi:10.1002/jctb.4569.

[40] Concha J, Weinstein C, Zúñiga ME. Production of pectic extracts from sugar beet pulp with antiproliferative activity on a breast cancer cell line. Frontiers of Chemical Science and Engineering 2013;7:482–9. doi:10.1007/s11705-013-1342-5.

[41] Martínez-Sabajanes M, Gullón B, Yáñez R, Alonso JL, Parajó JC. Direct enzymatic production of oligosaccharide mixtures from sugar beet pulp: experimental evalua-

tion and mathematical modeling. Journal of Agricultural and Food Chemistry 2009;57:5510–7. doi:10.1021/jf900654g.

[42] Wikiera A, Mika M, Starzyńska-Janiszewska A, Stodolak B. Application of Celluclast 1.5L in apple pectin extraction. Carbohydrate Polymers 2015;134:251–7. doi:10.1016/j.carbpol.2015.07.051.

[43] Sakurai MH, Matsumoto T, Kiyohara H, Yamada H. B-cell proliferation activity of pectic polysaccharide from a medicinal herb, the roots of *Bupleurum falcatum* L. and its structural requirement. Immunology 1999;97:540–7. doi:10.1046/j.1365-2567.1999.00774.x.

[44] Holck J, Hotchkiss AT, Meyer AS, Mikkelsen JD, Rastall RA. Production and bioactivity of pectic oligosaccharides from fruit and vegetable biomass. In: Moreno FJ, Sanz ML, editors. Food Oligosaccharides: Production, Analysis and Bioactivity, Chichester, UK: John Wiley & Sons, Ltd; 2014, p. 76–87. doi:10.1002/9781118817360.

[45] Concha Olmos J, Zúñiga Hansen ME. Enzymatic depolymerization of sugar beet pulp: Production and characterization of pectin and pectic-oligosaccharides as a potential source for functional carbohydrates. Chemical Engineering Journal 2012;192:29–36. doi:10.1016/j.cej.2012.03.085.

[46] Combo AMM, Aguedo M, Quiévy N, Danthine S, Goffin D, Jacquet N, et al. Characterization of sugar beet pectic-derived oligosaccharides obtained by enzymatic hydrolysis. International Journal of Biological Macromolecules 2013;52:148–56. doi:10.1016/j.ijbiomac.2012.09.006.

[47] Ravn HC, Bandsholm Sørensen O, Meyer AS. Time of harvest affects the yield of soluble polysaccharides extracted enzymatically from potato pulp. Food and Bioproducts Processing 2015;93:77–83. doi:10.1016/j.fbp.2013.11.006.

[48] Khodaei N, Karboune S. Enzymatic generation of galactose-rich oligosaccharides/oligomers from potato rhamnogalacturonan I pectic polysaccharides. Food Chemistry 2016;197:406–14. doi:10.1016/j.foodchem.2015.10.122.

[49] Wikiera A, Mika M, Starzyńska-Janiszewska A, Stodolak B. Development of complete hydrolysis of pectins from apple pomace. Food Chemistry 2015;172:675–80. doi:10.1016/j.foodchem.2014.09.132.

[50] Manderson K, Pinart M, Tuohy KM, Grace WE, Hotchkiss AT, Widmer W, et al. In vitro determination of prebiotic properties of oligosaccharides derived from an orange juice manufacturing by-product stream. Applied and Environmental Microbiology 2005;71:8383–9. doi:10.1128/AEM.71.12.8383-8389.2005.

[51] Chen H, Fu X, Luo Z. Properties and extraction of pectin-enriched materials from sugar beet pulp by ultrasonic-assisted treatment combined with subcritical water. Food Chemistry 2015;168:302–10. doi:10.1016/j.foodchem.2014.07.078.

[52] Chen J, Liang R, Liu W, Li T, Liu C, Wu S, et al. Pectic-oligosaccharides prepared by dynamic high-pressure microfluidization and their in vitro fermentation properties. Carbohydrate Polymers 2013;91:175–82. doi:10.1016/j.carbpol.2012.08.021.

[53] Rubio-Senent F, Rodríguez-Gutiérrez G, Lama-Muñoz A, Fernández-Bolaños J. Pectin extracted from thermally treated olive oil by-products: Characterization, physico-chemical properties, in vitro bile acid and glucose binding. Food Hydrocolloids 2015;43:311–21. doi:10.1016/j.foodhyd.2014.06.001.

[54] Sulek K, Vigsnaes LK, Schmidt LR, Holck J, Frandsen HL, Smedsgaard J, et al. A combined metabolomic and phylogenetic study reveals putatively prebiotic effects of high molecular weight arabino-oligosaccharides when assessed by in vitro fermentation in bacterial communities derived from humans. Anaerobe 2014;28:68–77. doi: 10.1016/j.anaerobe.2014.05.007.

[55] Gavlighi HA, Michalak M, Meyer AS, Mikkelsen JD. Enzymatic depolymerization of gum tragacanth: bifidogenic potential of low molecular weight oligosaccharides. Journal of Agricultural and Food Chemistry 2013;61:1272–8. doi:10.1021/jf304795f.

[56] Lee EH, Park H-R, Shin M-S, Cho SY, Choi H-J, Shin K-S. Antitumor metastasis activity of pectic polysaccharide purified from the peels of Korean Citrus Hallabong. Carbohydrate Polymers 2014;111:72–9. doi:10.1016/j.carbpol.2014.04.073.

[57] Harig JM, Soergel KH, Komorowski RA, Wood CM. Treatment of diversion colitis with short-chain-fatty acid irrigation. New England Journal of Medicine 1989;320:23–8.

[58] Donohoe DR, Garge N, Zhang X, Sun W, O'Connell TM, Bunger MK, et al. The microbiome and butyrate regulate energy metabolism and autophagy in the mammalian colon. Cell Metabolism 2011;13:517–26. doi:10.1016/j.cmet.2011.02.018.

[59] Fukuda S, Toh H, Hase K, Oshima K, Nakanishi Y, Yoshimura K, et al. Bifidobacteria can protect from enteropathogenic infection through production of acetate. Nature 2011;469:543–7. doi:10.1038/nature09646.

[60] Lin H V, Frassetto A, Kowalik EJ, Nawrocki AR, Lu MM, Kosinski JR, et al. Butyrate and propionate protect against diet-induced obesity and regulate gut hormones via free fatty acid receptor 3-independent mechanisms. Plos One 2012;7:e35240. doi: 10.1371/journal.pone.0035240.

[61] Di Sabatino A, Morera R, Ciccocioppo R, Cazzola P, Gotti S, Tinozzi FP, et al. Oral butyrate for mildly to moderately active Crohn's disease. Alimentary Pharmacology & Therapeutics 2005;22:789–94. doi:10.1111/j.1365-2036.2005.02639.x.

[62] Binder HJ. Role of colonic short-chain fatty acid transport in diarrhea. Annual Review of Physiology 2010;72:297–313. doi:10.1146/annurev-physiol-021909-135817.

[63] Chambers ES, Viardot A, Psichas A, Morrison DJ, Murphy KG, Zac-Varghese SEK, et al. Effects of targeted delivery of propionate to the human colon on appetite regula-

tion, body weight maintenance and adiposity in overweight adults. Gut 2015;64:1744–54. doi:10.1136/gutjnl-2014-307913.

[64] Scott KP, Gratz SW, Sheridan PO, Flint HJ, Duncan SH. The influence of diet on the gut microbiota. Pharmacological Research 2013;69:52–60. doi:10.1016/j.phrs.2012.10.020.

[65] Gómez B, Gullón B, Yáñez R, Schols H, Alonso JL. Prebiotic potential of pectins and pectic oligosaccharides derived from lemon peel wastes and sugar beet pulp: A comparative evaluation. Journal of Functional Foods 2016;20:108–21. doi:10.1016/j.jff.2015.10.029.

[66] Al-Tamimi MAHM, Palframan RJ, Cooper JM, Gibson GR, Rastall RA. In vitro fermentation of sugar beet arabinan and arabino-oligosaccharides by the human gut microflora. Journal of Applied Microbiology 2006;100:407–14. doi:10.1111/j.1365-2672.2005.02780.x.

[67] Holck J, Lorentzen A, Vigsnæs LK, Licht TR, Mikkelsen JD, Meyer AS. Feruloylated and nonferuloylated arabino-oligosaccharides from sugar beet pectin selectively stimulate the growth of *Bifidobacterium* spp. in human fecal in vitro fermentations. Journal of Agricultural and Food Chemistry 2011;59:6511–9. doi:10.1021/jf200996h.

[68] Gullón B, Martínez-Sabajanes M, Sanz Y, Alonso JL, Parajó JC. Pectic-oligosaccharides from sugar beet pulp: membrane purification and preliminary evaluation of its prebiotic potential. 6th International CIGR Technical Symposium—Towards a Sustainable Food Chain: Food Process, Bioprocessing and Food Quality Management, 2011.

[69] Leijdekkers AGM, Aguirre M, Venema K, Bosch G, Gruppen H, Schols HA. In vitro fermentability of sugar beet pulp derived oligosaccharides using human and pig fecal inocula. Journal of Agricultural and Food Chemistry 2014;62:1079–87. doi:10.1021/jf4049676.

[70] Gulfi M, Arrigoni E, Amadò R. In vitro fermentability of a pectin fraction rich in hairy regions. Carbohydrate Polymers 2007;67:410–6. doi:10.1016/j.carbpol.2006.06.018.

[71] Suzuki Y, Tanaka K, Amano T, Asakura T, Muramatsu N. Utilization by intestinal bacteria and digestibility of arabino-oligosaccharides in vitro. Journal of the Japanese Society for Horticultural Science 2004;73:574–9.

[72] Gullón B, Gullón P, Sanz Y, Alonso JL, Parajó JC. Prebiotic potential of a refined product containing pectic oligosaccharides. LWT—Food Science and Technology 2011;44:1687–96. doi:10.1016/j.lwt.2011.03.006.

[73] Guevara-Arauza JC, de Jesús Ornelas-Paz J, Pimentel-González DJ, Rosales Mendoza S, Soria Guerra RE, Paz Maldonado LMT. Prebiotic effect of mucilage and pectic-derived oligosaccharides from nopal (*Opuntia ficus-indica*). Food Science and Biotechnology 2012;21:997–1003. doi:10.1007/s10068-012-0130-1.

[74] Onumpai C, Kolida S, Bonnin E, Rastall RA. Microbial utilization and selectivity of pectin fractions with various structures. Applied and Environmental Microbiology 2011;77:5747–54. doi:10.1128/AEM.00179-11.

[75] Macfarlane GT, Macfarlane S. Models for intestinal fermentation: association between food components, delivery systems, bioavailability and functional interactions in the gut. Current Opinion in Biotechnology 2007;18:156–62. doi:10.1016/j.copbio.2007.01.011.

[76] Jiao L, Zhang X, Li B, Liu Z, Wang M, Liu S. Anti-tumour and immunomodulatory activities of oligosaccharides isolated from Panax ginseng C.A. Meyer. International Journal of Biological Macromolecules 2014;65:229–33. doi:10.1016/j.ijbiomac.2014.01.039.

[77] Harsha MR, Chandra Prakash S, Dharmesh SM. Modified pectic polysaccharide from turmeric (*Curcuma longa*): a potent dietary component against gastric ulcer. Carbohydrate Polymers 2016;138:143–55. doi:10.1016/j.carbpol.2015.11.043.

[78] Fanaro S, Jelinek J, Stahl B, Boehm G, Kock R, Vigi V. Acidic oligosaccharides from pectin hydrolysate as new component for infant formulae: effect on intestinal flora, stool characteristics, and pH. Journal of Pediatric Gastroenterology and Nutrition 2005;41:186–90. doi:10.1097/01.mpg.0000172747.64103.d7.

[79] Magne F, Hachelaf W, Suau A, Boudraa G, Bouziane-Nedjadi K, Rigottier-Gois L, et al. Effects on faecal microbiota of dietary and acidic oligosaccharides in children during partial formula feeding. Journal of Pediatric Gastroenterology and Nutrition 2008;46:580–8. doi:10.1097/MPG.0b013e318164d920.

[80] Westerbeek EA, van den Berg JP, Lafeber HN, Fetter WP, Boehm G, Twisk JW, et al. Neutral and acidic oligosaccharides in preterm infants: a randomized, double-blind, placebo-controlled trial. The American Journal of Clinical Nutrition 2010;91:679–86. doi:10.3945/ajcn.2009.28625.

[81] Gori A, Rizzardini G, van't Land B, Amor KB, van Schaik J, Torti C, et al. Specific prebiotics modulate gut microbiota and immune activation in HAART-naive HIV-infected adults: results of the "COPA" pilot randomized trial. Mucosal Immunology 2011;4:554–63. doi:10.1038/mi.2011.15.

[82] Craig SAS, Holden JF, Troup JP, Auerbach MH, Frier HI. Polydextrose as soluble fiber: Physiological and analytical aspects. Cereal Foods World 1998;43:370–6.

[83] Wang H, Shi Y, Le G. Rapid microwave-assisted synthesis of polydextrose and identification of structure and function. Carbohydrate Polymers 2014;113:225–30. doi:10.1016/j.carbpol.2014.07.012.

[84] Putaala H. Polydextrose in Lipid Metabolism. In: Valenzuela R, editor. Lipid Metabolism. Croatia: InTechOpen; 2013, p. 233-261. doi:10.5772/51791

[85] Röytiö H, Ouwehand AC. The fermentation of polydextrose in the large intestine and its beneficial effects. Beneficial Microbes 2014;5:305–13. doi:10.3920/BM2013.0065.

[86] Lahtinen SJ, Knoblock K, Drakoularakou A, Jacob M, Stowell J, Gibson GR, et al. Effect of molecule branching and glycosidic linkage on the degradation of polydextrose by gut microbiota. Bioscience, Biotechnology, and Biochemistry 2010;74:2016–21. doi: 10.1271/bbb.100251.

[87] Aidoo RP, Depypere F, Afoakwa EO, Dewettinck K. Industrial manufacture of sugar-free chocolates—applicability of alternative sweeteners and carbohydrate polymers as raw materials in product development. Trends in Food Science & Technology 2013;32:84–96. doi:10.1016/j.tifs.2013.05.008.

[88] Costabile A, Fava F, Röytiö H, Forssten SD, Olli K, Klievink J, et al. Impact of polydextrose on the faecal microbiota: a double-blind, crossover, placebo-controlled feeding study in healthy human subjects. The British Journal of Nutrition 2012;108:471–81. doi:10.1017/S0007114511005782.

[89] Herfel TM, Jacobi SK, Lin X, Fellner V, Walker DC, Jouni ZE, et al. Polydextrose enrichment of infant formula demonstrates prebiotic characteristics by altering intestinal microbiota, organic acid concentrations, and cytokine expression in suckling piglets. The Journal of Nutrition 2011;141:2139–45. doi:10.3945/jn.111.143727.

[90] Putaala H, Mäkivuokko H, Tiihonen K, Rautonen N. Simulated colon fiber metabolome regulates genes involved in cell cycle, apoptosis, and energy metabolism in human colon cancer cells. Molecular and Cellular Biochemistry 2011;357:235–45. doi: 10.1007/s11010-011-0894-2.

[91] Quintero M, Maldonado M, Perez-Munoz M, Jimenez R, Fangman T, Rupnow J, et al. Adherence inhibition of *Cronobacter sakazakii* to intestinal epithelial cells by prebiotic oligosaccharides. Current Microbiology 2011;62:1448–54. doi:10.1007/s00284-011-9882-8.

[92] Witaicenis A, Fruet AC, Salem L, Di Stasi LC. Dietary polydextrose prevents inflammatory bowel disease in trinitrobenzenesulfonic acid model of rat colitis. Journal of Medicinal Food 2010;13:1391–6.

[93] Beynen AC, Saris DHJ, de Jong L, Staats M, Einerhand AWC. Impact of dietary polydextrose on clinical signs of canine osteoarthritis. American Journal of Animal and Veterinary Sciences 2011;6:93–9. doi:10.3844/ajavsp.2011.93.99.

[94] Weise C, Ernst D, van Tol EAF, Worm M. Dietary polyunsaturated fatty acids and non-digestible oligosaccharides reduce dermatitis in mice. Pediatric Allergy and Immunology 2013;24:361–7. doi:10.1111/pai.12073.

[95] Mineo H, Hara H, Kikuchi H, Sakurai H, Tomita F. Various indigestible saccharides enhance net calcium transport from the epithelium of the small and large intestine of rats in vitro. Journal of Nutrition 2001;131:3243–6.

[96] Freitas dos Santos E, Hitomi Tsuboi K, Araújo MR, Ouwehand AC, Adami Andreollo N, Kenji Miyasaka C. Dietary polydextrose increases calcium absorption in normal rats. ABCD Surgery Brazilian Archives of Digestive Surgery. 2009; 22: 201–205.

[97] Freitas dos Santos E, Hitomi Tsuboi K, Rachel Araujo M, Almeida Falconi M, Ouwehand AC. Ingestion of polydextrose increase the iron absorption in rats submitted to partial gastrectomy. Acta Cirurgica Brasileira 2010; 25: 518-524.

[98] Ashley C, Johnston WH, Harris CL, Stolz SI, Wampler JL, Berseth CL. Growth and tolerance of infants fed formula supplemented with polydextrose (PDX) and/or galactooligosaccharides (GOS): double-blind, randomized, controlled trial. Nutrition Journal 2012;11:38. doi:10.1186/1475-2891-11-38.

[99] Boler BMV, Serao MCR, Bauer LL, Staeger MA, Boileau TW, Swanson KS, et al. Digestive physiological outcomes related to polydextrose and soluble maize fibre consumption by healthy adult men. The British Journal of Nutrition 2011;106:1864–71. doi:10.1017/S0007114511002388.

[100] Hengst C, Ptok S, Roessler A, Fechner A, Jahreis G. Effects of polydextrose supplementation on different faecal parameters in healthy volunteers. International Journal of Food Sciences and Nutrition 2009;60 Suppl 5:96–105. doi: 10.1080/09637480802526760.

[101] Hooda S, Boler BMV, Serao MCR, Brulc JM, Staeger MA, Boileau TW, et al. 454 pyrosequencing reveals a shift in fecal microbiota of healthy adult men consuming polydextrose or soluble corn fiber. The Journal of Nutrition 2012;142:1259–65. doi: 10.3945/jn.112.158766.

[102] Timm DA, Thomas W, Boileau TW, Williamson-Hughes PS, Slavin JL. Polydextrose and soluble corn fiber increase five-day fecal wet weight in healthy men and women. The Journal of Nutrition 2013;143:473–8. doi:10.3945/jn.112.170118.

[103] Luoto R, Ruuskanen O, Waris M, Kalliomäki M, Salminen S, Isolauri E. Prebiotic and probiotic supplementation prevents rhinovirus infections in preterm infants: a randomized, placebo-controlled trial. The Journal of Allergy and Clinical Immunology 2014;133:405–13. doi:10.1016/j.jaci.2013.08.020.

[104] Magro DO, de Oliveira LMR, Bernasconi I, Ruela Mde S, Credidio L, Barcelos IK, et al. Effect of yogurt containing polydextrose, *Lactobacillus acidophilus* NCFM and *Bifidobacterium lactis* HN019: a randomized, double-blind, controlled study in chronic constipation. Nutrition Journal 2014;13:75. doi:10.1186/1475-2891-13-75.

[105] Peuranen S, Tiihonen K, Apajalahti J, Kettunen A, Saarinen M, Rautonen N. Combination of polydextrose and lactitol affects microbial ecosystem and immune responses in rat gastrointestinal tract. The British Journal of Nutrition 2004;91:905–14. doi: 10.1079/BJN20041114.

[106] Ribeiro TCM, Costa-Ribeiro H, Almeida PS, Pontes MV, Leite MEQ, Filadelfo LR, et al. Stool pattern changes in toddlers consuming a follow-on formula supplemented with

polydextrose and galactooligosaccharides. Journal of Pediatric Gastroenterology and Nutrition 2012;54:288–90. doi:10.1097/MPG.0b013e31823a8a4c.

[107] Scalabrin DMF, Mitmesser SH, Welling GW, Harris CL, Marunycz JD, Walker DC, et al. New prebiotic blend of polydextrose and galacto-oligosaccharides has a bifidogenic effect in young infants. Journal of Pediatric Gastroenterology and Nutrition 2012;54:343–52. doi:10.1097/MPG.0b013e318237ed95.

[108] Probert HM, Apajalahti JHA, Rautonen N, Stowell J, Gibson GR. Polydextrose, lactitol, and fructo-oligosaccharide fermentation by colonic bacteria in a three-stage continuous culture system. Applied and Environmental Microbiology 2004;70:4505–11. doi: 10.1128/AEM.70.8.4505-4511.2004.

[109] Beards E, Tuohy K, Gibson G. Bacterial, SCFA and gas profiles of a range of food ingredients following in vitro fermentation by human colonic microbiota. Anaerobe 2010;16:420–5. doi:10.1016/j.anaerobe.2010.05.006.

[110] Mäkeläinen HS, Mäkivuokko HA, Salminen SJ, Rautonen NE, Ouwehand AC. The effects of polydextrose and xylitol on microbial community and activity in a 4-stage colon simulator. Journal of Food Science 2007;72:M153–9. doi:10.1111/j.1750-3841.2007.00350.x.

[111] Beloshapka AN, Wolff AK, Swanson KS. Effects of feeding polydextrose on faecal characteristics, microbiota and fermentative end products in healthy adult dogs. The British Journal of Nutrition 2012;108:638–44. doi:10.1017/S0007114511005927.

[112] Fava F, Mäkivuokko H, Siljander-Rasi H, Putaala H, Tiihonen K, Stowell J, et al. Effect of polydextrose on intestinal microbes and immune functions in pigs. The British Journal of Nutrition 2007;98:123–33. doi:10.1017/S0007114507691818.

[113] Kannampalli P, Pochiraju S, Chichlowski M, Berg BM, Rudolph C, Bruckert M, et al. Probiotic *Lactobacillus rhamnosus* GG (LGG) and prebiotic prevent neonatal inflammation-induced visceral hypersensitivity in adult rats. Neurogastroenterology and Motility 2014;26:1694–704. doi:10.1111/nmo.12450.

[114] Legette LL, Lee W, Martin BR, Story JA, Campbell JK, Weaver CM. Prebiotics enhance magnesium absorption and inulin-based fibers exert chronic effects on calcium utilization in a postmenopausal rodent model. Journal of Food Science 2012;77:H88–94. doi:10.1111/j.1750-3841.2011.02612.x.

[115] [117] González del Val A, Platas G, Basilio A, Cabello A, Gorrochategui J, Suay I, et al. Screening of antimicrobial activities in red, green and brown macroalgae from Gran Canaria (Canary Islands, Spain). International Microbiology 2001;4:35–40. doi:10.1007/s101230100006.

[116] Cumashi A, Ushakova NA, Preobrazhenskaya ME, D'Incecco A, Piccoli A, Totani L, et al. A comparative study of the anti-inflammatory, anticoagulant, antiangiogenic, and

antiadhesive activities of nine different fucoidans from brown seaweeds. Glycobiology 2007;17:541–52. doi:10.1093/glycob/cwm014.

[117] Kang JY, Khan MNA, Park NH, Cho JY, Lee MC, Fujii H, et al. Antipyretic, analgesic, and anti-inflammatory activities of the seaweed *Sargassum fulvellum* and *Sargassum thunbergii* in mice. Journal of Ethnopharmacology 2008;116:187–90. doi:10.1016/j.jep.2007.10.032.

[118] Chandini SK, Ganesan P, Bhaskar N. In vitro antioxidant activities of three selected brown seaweeds of India. Food Chemistry 2008;107:707–13. doi:10.1016/j.foodchem.2007.08.081.

[119] Rupérez P, Ahrazem O, Leal JA. Potential antioxidant capacity of sulfated polysaccharides from the edible marine brown seaweed *Fucus vesiculosus*. Journal of Agricultural and Food Chemistry 2002;50:840–5. doi:10.1021/jf010908o.

[120] Balboa EM, Moure A, Domínguez H. Valorization of *Sargassum muticum* biomass according to the biorefinery concept. Marine Drugs 2015;13:3745–60. doi:10.3390/md13063745.

[121] Maruyama H, Tamauchi H, Hashimoto M, Nakano T. Antitumor activity and immune response of Mekabu fucoidan extracted from Sporophyll of *Undaria pinnatifida*. In Vivo 2003;17:245–9.

[122] Ye H, Wang K, Zhou C, Liu J, Zeng X. Purification, antitumor and antioxidant activities in vitro of polysaccharides from the brown seaweed *Sargassum pallidum*. Food Chemistry 2008;111:428–32. doi:10.1016/j.foodchem.2008.04.012.

[123] Pereira MG, Benevides NMB, Melo MRS, Valente AP, Melo FR, Mourão PAS. Structure and anticoagulant activity of a sulfated galactan from the red alga, *Gelidium crinale*. Is there a specific structural requirement for the anticoagulant action? Carbohydrate Research 2005;340:2015–23. doi:10.1016/j.carres.2005.05.018.

[124] Kwon M-J, Nam T-J. Porphyran induces apoptosis related signal pathway in AGS gastric cancer cell lines. Life Sciences 2006;79:1956–62. doi:10.1016/j.lfs.2006.06.031.

[125] Aisa Y, Miyakawa Y, Nakazato T, Shibata H, Saito K, Ikeda Y, et al. Fucoidan induces apoptosis of human HS-sultan cells accompanied by activation of caspase-3 and down-regulation of ERK pathways. American Journal of Hematology 2005;78:7–14. doi:10.1002/ajh.20182.

[126] Anastyuk SD, Imbs TI, Shevchenko NM, Dmitrenok PS, Zvyagintseva TN. ESIMS analysis of fucoidan preparations from *Costaria costata*, extracted from alga at different life-stages. Carbohydrate Polymers 2012;90:993–1002. doi:10.1016/j.carbpol.2012.06.033.

[127] Ale MT, Mikkelsen JD, Meyer AS. Designed optimization of a single-step extraction of fucose-containing sulfated polysaccharides from *Sargassum* sp. Journal of Applied Phycology 2012;24:715–23. doi:10.1007/s10811-011-9690-3.

[128] Balboa EM, Rivas S, Moure A, Domínguez H, Parajó JC. Simultaneous extraction and depolymerization of fucoidan from *Sargassum muticum* in aqueous media. Marine Drugs 2013;11:4612–27. doi:10.3390/md11114612.

[129] Rodriguez-Jasso RM, Mussatto SI, Pastrana L, Aguilar CN, Teixeira JA, Aguilar CN. Microwave-assisted extraction of sulfated polysaccharides (fucoidan) from brown seaweed. Carbohydrate Polymers 2011;86:1137–44. doi:sulfated polysaccharides.

[130] Lorbeer AJ, Lahnstein J, Fincher GB, Su P, Zhang W. Kinetics of conventional and microwave-assisted fucoidan extractions from the brown alga, *Ecklonia radiata*. Journal of Applied Phycology 2015;27:2079–87. doi:10.1007/s10811-014-0446-8.

[131] Yuan Y, Macquarrie D. Microwave assisted extraction of sulfated polysaccharides (fucoidan) from *Ascophyllum nodosum* and its antioxidant activity. Carbohydrate Polymers 2015;129:101–7. doi:10.1016/j.carbpol.2015.04.057.

[132] Rodrigues D, Sousa S, Silva A, Amorim M, Pereira L, Rocha-Santos TAP, et al. Impact of enzyme- and ultrasound-assisted extraction methods on biological properties of red, brown, and green seaweeds from the central west coast of Portugal. Journal of Agricultural and Food Chemistry 2015;63:3177–88. doi:10.1021/jf504220e.

[133] Athukorala Y, Jung W-K, Vasanthan T, Jeon Y-J. An anticoagulative polysaccharide from an enzymatic hydrolysate of *Ecklonia cava*. Carbohydrate Polymers 2006;66:184–91. doi:10.1016/j.carbpol.2006.03.002.

[134] Shang YF, Kim SM, Lee WJ, Um B-H. Pressurized liquid method for fucoxanthin extraction from *Eisenia bicyclis* (Kjellman) Setchell. Journal of Bioscience and Bioengineering 2011;111:237–41. doi:10.1016/j.jbiosc.2010.10.008.

[135] Devillé C, Gharbi M, Dandrifosse G, Peulen O. Study on the effects of laminarin, a polysaccharide from seaweed, on gut characteristics. Journal of the Science of Food and Agriculture 2007;87:1717–25. doi:10.1002/jsfa.2901.

[136] O'Sullivan L, Murphy B, McLoughlin P, Duggan P, Lawlor PG, Hughes H, et al. Prebiotics from marine macroalgae for human and animal health applications. Marine Drugs 2010;8:2038–64. doi:10.3390/md8072038.

[137] Gupta S, Abu-Ghannam N. Bioactive potential and possible health effects of edible brown seaweeds. Trends in Food Science & Technology 2011;22:315–26. doi:10.1016/j.tifs.2011.03.011.

[138] Gómez-Ordóñez E, Jiménez-Escrig A, Rupérez P. Effect of the red seaweed *Mastocarpus stellatus* intake on lipid metabolism and antioxidant status in healthy Wistar rats. Food Chemistry 2012;135:806–11. doi:10.1016/j.foodchem.2012.04.138.

[139] Wang Y, Han F, Hu B, Li J, Yu W. In vivo prebiotic properties of alginate oligosaccharides prepared through enzymatic hydrolysis of alginate. Nutrition Research 2006;26:597–603. doi:10.1016/j.nutres.2006.09.015.

[140] Jiménez-Escrig A, Gómez-Ordóñez E, Tenorio MD, Rupérez P. Antioxidant and prebiotic effects of dietary fiber co-travelers from sugar Kombu in healthy rats. Journal of Applied Phycology 2012;25:503–12. doi:10.1007/s10811-012-9884-3.

[141] Lynch MB, Sweeney T, Callan JJ, O'Sullivan JT, O'Doherty J V. The effect of dietary Laminaria-derived laminarin and fucoidan on nutrient digestibility, nitrogen utilisation, intestinal microflora and volatile fatty acid concentration in pigs. Journal of the Science of Food and Agriculture 2010;90:430–7. doi:10.1002/jsfa.3834.

[142] Kitano Y, Murazumi K, Duan J, Kurose K, Kobayashi S, Sugawara T, et al. Effect of dietary porphyran from the red alga, *Porphyra yezoensis*, on glucose metabolism in diabetic KK-Ay mice. Journal of Nutritional Science and Vitaminology 2012;58:14–9. doi:10.3177/jnsv.58.14.

[143] Liu J, Kandasamy S, Zhang J, Kirby CW, Karakach T, Hafting J, et al. Prebiotic effects of diet supplemented with the cultivated red seaweed Chondrus crispus or with fructo-oligo-saccharide on host immunity, colonic microbiota and gut microbial metabolites. BMC Complementary and Alternative Medicine 2015;15:279. doi:10.1186/s12906-015-0802-5.

[144] Murphya P, Dal Bello F, O'Doherty J, Arendt EK, Sweeney T, Coffey A. The effects of liquid versus spray-dried *Laminaria digitata* extract on selected bacterial groups in the piglet gastrointestinal tract (GIT) microbiota. Anaerobe 2013;21:1–8. doi:10.1016/j.anaerobe.2013.03.002.

[145] Ramnani P, Chitarrari R, Tuohy K, Grant J, Hotchkiss S, Philp K, et al. In vitro fermentation and prebiotic potential of novel low molecular weight polysaccharides derived from agar and alginate seaweeds. Anaerobe 2012;18:1–6. doi:10.1016/j.anaerobe.2011.08.003.

[146] Kim EJ, Park SY, Lee J-Y, Park JHY. Fucoidan present in brown algae induces apoptosis of human colon cancer cells. BMC Gastroenterology 2010;10:96. doi: 10.1186/1471-230X-10-96.

[147] Villanueva M-J, Morcillo M, Tenorio M-D, Mateos-Aparicio I, Andrés V, Redondo-Cuenca A. Health-promoting effects in the gut and influence on lipid metabolism of *Himanthalia elongata* and *Gigartina pistillata* in hypercholesterolaemic Wistar rats. European Food Research and Technology 2013;238:409–16. doi:10.1007/s00217-013-2116-5.

[148] Shibata H, Iimuro M, Uchiya N, Kawamori T, Nagaoka M, Ueyama S, et al. Preventive effects of *Cladosiphon fucoidan* against *Helicobacter pylori* infection in *Mongolian gerbils*. Helicobacter 2003;8:59–65. doi:10.1046/j.1523-5378.2003.00124.x.

[149] Liu J, Hafting J, Critchley AT, Banskota AH, Prithiviraj B. Components of the cultivated red seaweed *Chondrus crispus* enhance the immune response of *Caenorhabditis elegans* to *Pseudomonas aeruginosa* through the pmk-1, daf-2/daf-16, and skn-1 pathways.

Applied and Environmental Microbiology 2013;79:7343–50. doi:10.1128/AEM.01927-13.

[150] Donot F, Fontana A, Baccou JC, Schorr-Galindo S. Microbial exopolysaccharides: Main examples of synthesis, excretion, genetics and extraction. Carbohydrate Polymers 2012;87:951–62. doi:10.1016/j.carbpol.2011.08.083.

[151] Hongpattarakere T, Cherntong N, Wichienchot S, Kolida S, Rastall RA. In vitro prebiotic evaluation of exopolysaccharides produced by marine isolated lactic acid bacteria. Carbohydrate Polymers 2012;87:846–52. doi:10.1016/j.carbpol.2011.08.085.

[152] Harutoshi T. Exopolysaccharides of Lactic Acid Bacteria for Food and Colon Health Applications. In: Kongo JM, editor. Lactic Acid Bacteria—R & D for Food, Health and Livestock Purposes, InTechOpen; 2013, p. 515–38. doi:10.5772/50839.

[153] Freitas F, Alves VD, Reis MAM. Advances in bacterial exopolysaccharides: from production to biotechnological applications. Trends in Biotechnology 2011;29:388–98. doi:10.1016/j.tibtech.2011.03.008.

[154] Mishra A, JHA B. Microbial exopolysaccharides, in the prokaryotes. In: Rosenberg E, DeLong EF, Lory S, Stackebrandt E, Thompson F, editors. Applied Bacteriology and Biotechnology, Berlin, Heidelberg: Springer-Verlag; 2013, p. 179–92. doi: 10.1007/978-3-642-31331-8_25.

[155] Kumar AS, Mody K, Jha B. Bacterial exopolysaccharides—a perception. Journal of Basic Microbiology 2007;47:103–17. doi:10.1002/jobm.200610203.

[156] Madhuri K, Prabhakar K. Microbial exopolysaccharides: biosynthesis and potential applications. Oriental Journal of Chemistry 2014;30:1401–10. doi:10.13005/ojc/300362.

[157] Patel A, Prajapat JB. Food and health applications of exopolysaccharides produced by lactic acid bacteria. Advances in Dairy Research 2013;01. doi:10.4172/2329-888X.1000107.

[158] Korakli M, Ganzle MG, Vogel RF. Metabolism by bifidobacteria and lactic acid bacteria of polysaccharides from wheat and rye, and exopolysaccharides produced by *Lactobacillus sanfranciscensis*. Journal of Applied Microbiology 2002;92:958–65. doi: 10.1046/j.1365-2672.2002.01607.x.

[159] Kothari D, Tingirikari JMR, Goyal A. In vitro analysis of dextran from Leuconostoc mesenteroides NRRL B-1426 for functional food application. Bioactive Carbohydrates and Dietary Fibre 2015;6:55–61. doi:10.1016/j.bcdf.2015.08.001.

[160] Yang Y, Galle S, Le MHA, Zijlstra RT, Gänzle MG. Feed Fermentation with Reuteran- and Levan-producing *Lactobacillus reuteri* reduces colonization of weanling pigs by enterotoxigenic *Escherichia coli*. Applied and Environmental Microbiology 2015;81:5743–52. doi:10.1128/AEM.01525-15.

[161] Li S, Chen T, Xu F, Dong S, Xu H, Xiong Y, et al. The beneficial effect of exopolysaccharides from *Bifidobacterium bifidum* WBIN03 on microbial diversity in mouse

intestine. Journal of the Science of Food and Agriculture 2014;94:256–64. doi:10.1002/jsfa.6244.

[162] Livesey G. Health potential of polyols as sugar replacers, with emphasis on low glycaemic properties. Nutrition Research Reviews 2003;16:163–91. doi:10.1079/NRR200371.

[163] Grabitske HA, Slavin JL. Gastrointestinal effects of low-digestible carbohydrates. Critical Reviews in Food Science and Nutrition 2009;49:327–60. doi:10.1080/10408390802067126.

[164] Sarmiento-Rubiano LA, Zúñiga M, Pérez-Martínez G, Yebra MJ. Dietary supplementation with sorbitol results in selective enrichment of lactobacilli in rat intestine. Research in Microbiology 2007;158:694–701. doi:10.1016/j.resmic.2007.07.007.

[165] Maekawa M, Ushida K, Hoshi S, Kashima N, Ajisaka K, Yajima T. Butyrate and propionate production from D-mannitol in the large intestine of pig and rat. Microbial Ecology in Health and Disease 2005;17:169–76. doi:10.1080/08910600500430730.

[166] Grembecka M. Sugar alcohols—their role in the modern world of sweeteners: a review. European Food Research and Technology 2015;241:1–14. doi:10.1007/s00217-015-2437-7.

[167] Xiao J, Li X, Min X, Sakaguchi E. Mannitol improves absorption and retention of calcium and magnesium in growing rats. Nutrition (Burbank, Los Angeles County, California) 2013;29:325–31. doi:10.1016/j.nut.2012.06.010.

[168] Nishiyama A, Nishioka S, Islam SM, Sakaguchi E. Mannitol lowers fat digestibility and body fat accumulation in both normal and cecectomized rats. Journal of Nutritional Science and Vitaminology 2009;55:242–51. doi:10.3177/jnsv.55.242.

[169] Blanc P, Daures JP, Rouillon JM, Peray P, Pierrugues R, Larrey D, et al. Lactitol or lactulose in the treatment of chronic hepatic encephalopathy: results of a meta-analysis. Hepatology 1992;15:222–8.

[170] Chen C, Li L, Wu Z, Chen H, Fu S. Effects of lactitol on intestinal microflora and plasma endotoxin in patients with chronic viral hepatitis. The Journal of Infection 2007;54:98–102. doi:10.1016/j.jinf.2005.11.013.

[171] Finney M, Smullen J, Foster HA, Brokx S, Storey DM. Effects of low doses of lactitol on faecal microflora, pH, short chain fatty acids and gastrointestinal symptomology. European Journal of Nutrition 2007;46:307–14. doi:10.1007/s00394-007-0666-7.

[172] Mäkeläinen H, Saarinen M, Stowell J, Rautonen N, Ouwehand AC. Xylo-oligosaccharides and lactitol promote the growth of *Bifidobacterium lactis* and *Lactobacillus* species in pure cultures. Beneficial Microbes 2010;1:139–48. doi:10.3920/BM2009.0029.

[173] Ouwehand AC, Tiihonen K, Saarinen M, Putaala H, Rautonen N. Influence of a combination of Lactobacillus acidophilus NCFM and lactitol on healthy elderly:

intestinal and immune parameters. The British Journal of Nutrition 2009;101:367–75. doi:10.1017/S0007114508003097.

[174] Beards E, Tuohy K, Gibson G. A human volunteer study to assess the impact of confectionery sweeteners on the gut microbiota composition. The British Journal of Nutrition 2010;104:701–8. doi:10.1017/S0007114510001078.

[175] Jie Z, Bang-yao L, Ming-jie X, Hai-wei L, Zu-kang Z, Ting-song W, et al. Studies on the effects of polydextrose intake on physiologic functions in Chinese people. American Journal of Clinical Nutrition 2000;72:1503–9.

[176] Liu S, Tsai CE. Effects of biotechnically synthesized oligosaccharides and polydextrose on serum lipids in the human. Journal of the Chinese Nutrition Society 1995;20:1–12.

[177] Kulshreshtha G, Rathgeber B, Stratton G, Thomas N, Evans F, Critchley A, et al. Feed supplementation with red seaweeds, *Chondrus crispus* and *Sarcodiotheca gaudichaudii*, affects performance, egg quality, and gut microbiota of layer hens. Poultry Science 2014;93:2991–3001. doi:10.3382/ps.2014-04200.

[178] Dierick N, Ovyn A, De Smet S. In vitro assessment of the effect of intact marine brown macro-algae *Ascophyllum nodosum* on the gut flora of piglets. Livestock Science 2010;133:154–6. doi:10.1016/j.livsci.2010.06.051.

[179] Bello FD, Walter J, Hertel C, Hammes WP. In vitro study of prebiotic properties of levan-type exopolysaccharides from Lactobacilli and non-digestible carbohydrates using denaturing gradient gel electrophoresis. Systematic and Applied Microbiology 2001;24:232–7. doi:10.1078/0723-2020-00033.

[180] Salazar N, Gueimonde M, Hernández-Barranco AM, Ruas-Madiedo P, de los Reyes-Gavilán CG. Exopolysaccharides produced by intestinal Bifidobacterium strains act as fermentable substrates for human intestinal bacteria. Applied and Environmental Microbiology 2008;74:4737–45. doi:10.1128/AEM.00325-08.

[181] Patra F, Tomar SK, Arora S. Technological and functional applications of low-calorie sweeteners from lactic acid bacteria. Journal of Food Science 2009;74:R16–23. doi: 10.1111/j.1750-3841.2008.01005.x.

Chapter 16

Yeasts as Potential Source for Prebiotic β-Glucan: Role in Human Nutrition and Health

Pedro De Oliva-Neto, Sidmeire Santos Oliveira,
Estevão Zilioli and Márcia Zilioli Bellini

Additional information is available at the end of the chapter

http://dx.doi.org/10.5772/63647

Abstract

Yeasts are a potential source for prebiotic β-glucans. This polysaccharide is characterized by D-glucose monomers linked by β-glycosidic bonds. There are significant structural differences in β-glucans depending on the source and method in which they are obtaining. This polymer is a healthier food and feed additive. Numerous beneficial effects have been attributed to this polymer, in particular immunomodulatory action. Different studies confirm safe use and applicability of β-glucans in medicine for the treatment of diseases (cancer, infections, respiratory diseases) and reduction in glucose and cholesterol levels. Many advances in the processes to obtain β-glucans have been presented, including extraction, purification, and chemical modification, aiming the biological properties and yield. One limitation of their use is the cost, so a strategic discussion of the use of yeast biomass was performed for the production of β-glucans. An extensive and systematic review was undertaken to contribute to the science and technology to obtain β-glucans and their use in different applications.

Keywords: β-glucans, chemical properties, extraction, purification, immunostimulating properties

1. Introduction

One of the important biopolymers present in some cereals and fungi is the β-glucan. This polysaccharide plays an important role in the immune system, skin protection, among others. In addition to their cholesterol-lowering and potential cancer-preventing properties, β-glucans may be useful in controlling blood glucose levels. The β-D-glucans from yeast and some plants have been shown to have antitumor and antibacterial activity when injected or ingested by animals in experimentation [1–7].

Cereal grains, such as barley, oats, and rye, and fungi, such as *Aspergillus*, *Saccharomyces*, and *mushrooms*, contain β-D-glucans [8, 9]. The concentration of β-glucan in oats ranges from 1.9 to 8.0% [10, 11]. In barley grains, these values can reach 3.5–4.8% [12]. These variations are associated with genotype of grain and location and the environmental conditions in which the culture was grown and may result in variation in the quality of β-glucan. This problem is reduced if the source is from microorganisms, which are cultured in defined conditions, and they are not dependent from the location or the environmental conditions.

2. Chemical structure of β-glucans

Glucans are glucose polymers, classified according to their interchain linkage as being either α- or β-linked. β-glucans are a heterogeneous group of non-starch polysaccharides, consisting of D-glucose monomers linked by β-glycosidic bonds [13]. The central skeleton of the β-glucans is formed by linear monomers of D-glucose connected at position β-(1-3), with side chains attached to β-(1-6) or β-(1-4)-D-glucopyranosyl unit linkage (**Figure 1**). In yeast, the skeleton is branching at β-(1-6) and in plants and bacteria at β-(1-4) unit linkage [14–16]. In mushrooms, molecules with binding β-(1-6) and others with connections β-(1-6) and β-(1-4), whether or not linked to protein, were reported [17]. Significant structural differences in β-glucans are characterized by the glycosidic linkage ratios depending on both the source and method of isolation. In the cereal β-glucans, for example, the trisaccharide-to-tetrasaccharide ratios follow the order of wheat (4.2–4.5), barley (2.8–3.3), and oat (2.0–2.4) [18].

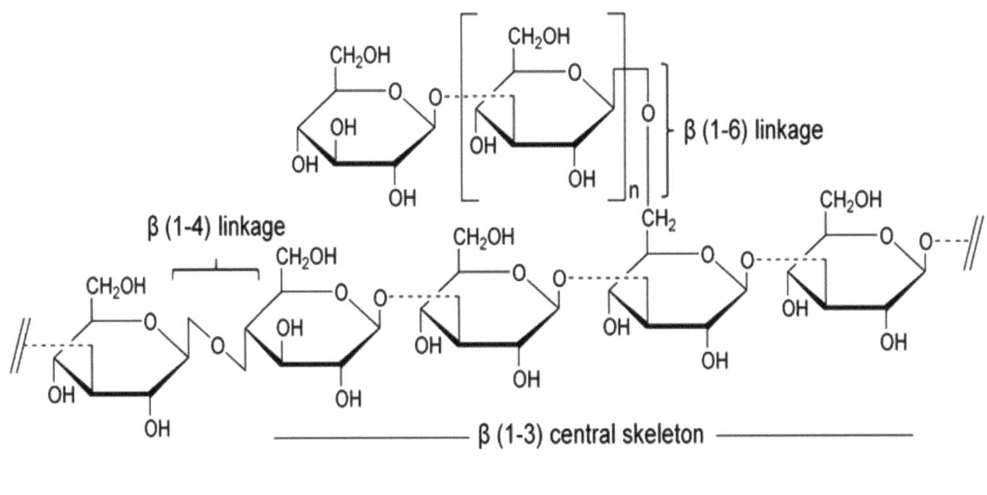

Figure 1. Polymer of β (1-3)-D-glycopyranosyl units with branching at β (1-6) and β (1-4)-D-glycopyranosyl units.

http://dx.doi.org/10.5772/63647

3. Biological properties and applications of β-glucans

In the last decades, the β-glucans have received special attention for its biological activity. Numerous beneficial effects have been attributed to this polymer, in particular due to its immunomodulatory potential. However, beyond the modulatory action of the immune system, several other activities related to β-glucans have been evaluated and proven, as their antitumoral, anti-inflammatory, antimutagenic, and antioxidant action, their hypoglycemic and hypocholesterolemic capacity, and also their protective effect against infections [19]. The β-glucans have a long scientific history, encompassing hundreds of studies. However, this molecule is not properly explored even in therapy, as an additive in food or feed, probably due to its relatively expensive price—about U$ 36/kg (brand Macrogard; Biorigin, Quatá, São Paulo, Brazil). Research involving the biological activity of this polymer originated in the 1940s, with the renowned scientist Pillemer and his colleagues, who obtained a crude-insoluble extract of the cell wall of the *Saccharomyces cerevisiae,* called zymosan, consisting of proteins, chitin, β-glucan, mannans, and lipids. According to the authors, this extract was able to stimulate the immune response in a non-specific manner [20]. Clinical studies in humans involving the β-glucans began in the 1970s, even before the evidence of their mode of action on the immune system, with reports of curing different types of cancer, including breast cancer, melanoma, and adenosquamous carcinoma of the lung after the application of extracts of β-glucans [21].

3.1. Immune system and immunomodulatory activity of β-glucans

The immune system operates seeking to protect the organism from infections that can be caused by various agents, including bacteria, viruses, fungi, and parasites. The cells and molecules of the immune system are highly specialized in the defense against infection. Individuals with a compromised immune defense system due to various factors, such as age, chronic infection, or malnutrition, are subject to several problems, including arthritis, reduced healing capacity, reduced proliferation of bone marrow cells with consequent low defense cell counts, anemia, and increased incidence of all types of microbial infections. Studies also show that one of the main elements of the process of aging is a decrease in the functional effectiveness of the immune system [22]. Among the immunologically competent cells, macrophages play a major role in the initiation and maintenance of immune response both innate and adaptive [15]. In addition to the functions of phagocytosis and the release of lysosomal enzymes, macrophages are also responsible for the release of a number of cytokines and inflammatory mediators can stimulate the immune system in general [22].

The β-glucan belongs to the class of substances BRMs, or a variety of different substances known as Biological Response Modifiers. being able to trigger a series of events in the immune response [23], increasing the immune defense of the host by activating the functions of cells of the immune system [20]. This polymer is currently considered as one of the most potent stimulators of the immune response, effective both orally or intravenously, completely non-toxic and safe [15]. The response of β-glucan in vertebrates begins with its recognition by receptors present on the cell surface of various immune cells, such as macrophages, neutrophils, dendritic cells, and natural killer cells (NK), and receptors have also been described presently as non-immune cells, endothelial cells, fibroblasts, alveolar epithelial, and Langerhans cells [20]. The various receptors present on the cell membranes of immune cells related to the recognition of β-glucan in vertebrates are dectin-1, complement receptor 3 (CR3), lactosylceramide receptor, Toll-like receptor 2 (TLR-2), and scavenger receptors [24, 25]. The dectin-1 is a type II transmembrane protein with receptor extracellular domain CDR which is responsible for carbohydrate recognition, and a cytoplasmic tail with immunoreceptor ITAM (tyrosine-based activating motif) involved in superoxide production by macrophages in response to the immunosystem defense. The dectin-1 can mediate diverse cellular responses, including phagocytosis and endocytosis. This protein may also induce the production of cytokines and inflammatory chemokines, such as tumor necrosis factor (TNF-α), macrophage inflammatory protein-2 (MIP-2), and interleukin-12 (IL-12) [16]. The receptor CR3 stimulates cytokine secretion by NK cells, especially in the presence of pathogens. This receptor acts as a cell adhesion molecule since it has a binding site for carbohydrates located on the terminal carbon, and thus a receptor for the phagocyte β-glucan [15].

3.2. Medical application: cancer

Anticarcinogenic substances are able to reduce, delay, or even prevent the development of malignancies [26]. Different studies have shown anticarcinogenic action of β-glucans and their derivatives [1, 2, 4]. At the end of 1970s, a study on mice with subcutaneous tumor implantation revealed that extracts containing high concentrations of β-glucan significantly reduced growth of mammary carcinomas and melanomas in animals treated and verified an increase in survival of these animals [27]. Kogan et al. [6] observed increased inhibition in the occurrence of lung metastases up to 94% in animals that received oral administration of β-glucan during treatment with cyclophosphamide for Lewis lung carcinoma. Several surveys show the effectiveness of antitumor action of β-glucans in chemotherapy and the improvement in the survival of patients with different types of cancer. A study involving women with malignant breast tumors confirmed the activation and proliferation of monocytes in peripheral blood of patients upon oral administration of β-glucan. According to the researchers, clinical improvement in the survival of patients with no evidence of any recurrent side effects was demonstrated [4]. The effective immune response against tumor cells mediated by β-glucans is based on the activation and expansion of several immune functions, among them the activation of cytotoxic T cells specifically attack cancer cells [28]. The CD4+ T lymphocytes play a role as modulators of immune cells to produce multiple cytokines. The latter are mediators essential for the generation of an effective immune response involving CD8+ T cells, which are necessary for the defense against tumor cells [1]. The effects of β-glucan in lymphocyte activation involving the antitumor immune response have been reported in experimental animal and human models. A study of 30 patients with advanced prostate cancer, who were treated by oral administration of a soluble fraction of β-glucan (carboxymethyl glucan), revealed that after administration there was a significant increase in CD3+, CD4+, and CD8+ in peripheral blood of patients and consequent stimulation of the immune system [2].

http://dx.doi.org/10.5772/63647

3.3. β-glucans applied in other diseases

Since β-glucans affect immune function stimulating various immune cell activations, studies were performed to demonstrate the effective application of this immunomodulatory compound in treatment of diseases. Patients with severe periodontitis have failed for the recruitment and activation of macrophages [29]. β-glucans induce macrophage activation and establishment of Th1, and their use may be responsible for the inhibition of tissue destruction in periodontal disease. The use of β-glucan in dental treatment has been systematically evaluated in recent years. Studies with animals showed a significantly reduced periodontal bone loss after oral administration of β-(1-3),(1-6) glucan [30]. Acar et al. [31] investigated the effects of non-surgical periodontal therapy (NPT) with an adjunctive use of systemic β-glucan on clinical, microbiological, and gingival parameters. Their findings showed that β-glucan might increase the concentration of TGF-β1, thereby augmenting periodontal healing potential. Proposals for treating allergic diseases using β-glucans have also been reported. A new therapeutic strategy for allergic diseases using β-glucan was proposed, with beneficial action in restoring the function of type 2 T-helper cells. Through the application of subcutaneous injections in child patients, β-glucan was demonstrated to be able to modulate allergic sensitization in patients, greatly improving their quality of life [32]. Furthermore, the antibacterial, antiviral, and antifungal properties of β-glucan and its derivatives are also reported. Different studies have shown the protective effect of β-glucan to *Staphylococcus aureus* [33], *Pneumocystis carinii*, *Leishmania donovani*, and *Influenza virus* [22]. The protective effect of β-glucan from *S. cerevisiae* against DNA damage and cytotoxicity in wild-type (k1) and repair-deficient xrs5 CHO cells were evaluated by Oliveira et al. [34].

3.4. Food and feed applications of β-glucans

The search for higher human living standards and greater longevity has generated the need for the development of nutritional alternatives that result in improved general health which means more enjoyment of life, less diseases and less time, and money required for medical needs. In this context, special foods enriched with molecules with health benefits are been developed. Some studies dealing with the enormous benefits of β-glucan as a nutritional supplement [31, 35–37]. Used as adjunctive to the positive effects of antioxidants, lipid balance enhancers, antibiotics, and other therapeutics, the β-glucans are currently considered a true antiaging supplement. These properties are associated with several studies which have shown biological activity of β-glucan, describing its action modulating the immune system and antitumor action [1, 3].

3.4.1. β-glucan in the human diet

In recent years, there has been increasing interest in the effect of the use of β-glucan as a dietary supplement. Different studies seek to prove the use of this polysaccharide in the diet has several health benefits. The beneficial effects of consistent intake of β-glucan and its action in reducing cholesterol levels in the blood have been systematically studied. A study of 20 hypercholesterolemic patients, who received daily dietary supplement containing 5.8 g of β-glucan for 4 weeks, reported a 9% decrease in cholesterol level in the intervention group, while there was no difference in the placebo (maltodextrin) group [7]. Nicolosi et al. [38] observed a significant reduction in total and LDL cholesterol in hypercholesterolemic obese patients after 8 weeks of intake of orange juice supplemented with β-glucan. The action of β-glucan on cholesterol reduction can be explained in terms of the reduction in bile reabsorption or the increase in viscosity in the small intestine. However, a more likely explanation relates to the size of the molecule and its subsequent absorption by the intestine. According to Kim et al. [37], molecules of small size, which are consequently less viscous, are less effective in lowering cholesterol. Studies with β-glucan of low molecular size (370,000–1,000,000) reported this polysaccharide ineffective in reducing the cholesterol level [39], whereas Braaten et al. [7] reported a significant reduction in cholesterol levels in the blood of patients who included β-glucan of molecular size above 1.2 million in their diet. β-glucans become a great special food in a diet designed to adjunct in diabetic patients. The action of this polymer in lowering blood glucose level is also reported in the literature. Research has demonstrated the antidiabetic effect of IL-1 cytokine, which increases insulin production, resulting in the lowering of blood glucose levels [40, 41]. Since the β-glucan acts on the activation of macrophages, and these are considered the major source of IL-1 in the human body, this polymer becomes useful in diets designed for diabetic patients. According to Regand et al. [42], the physiological activity of β-glucan in reducing glycemic responses has been mostly attributed to its effect in increasing viscosity in the upper digestive tract. The introduction of β-glucan in the diet may decrease the incidence of colds, respiratory diseases, in addition to alleviating the symptoms caused by these diseases, since this polymer increases the body's potential to defend against invading pathogens [31]. A study with seventy-five marathon runners showed that daily administration of β-glucan can prevent upper respiratory tract (URTI) symptoms and improve overall health and mood following a competitive marathon [36]. More recently, a study of 162 healthy participants with recurring infections who received a diet supplemented with β-(1-3),(1-6) glucan showed a reduction in the number of symptomatic common cold infections by 25% and the mean symptom score was 15% lower compared to the control group [35].

3.4.2. *β-glucan additives in animal feed*

β-glucan has been prominent among the ingredients used as supplements in animal feed in order to reduce the risk of chronic diseases both in mammals and in fish and birds [43], since they are able to absorb mycotoxins, thus decreasing their toxic effect and mediating their removal from the body [44]. Different food supplements containing β-glucan are available for commercial use for animals. Among them, Bio-Mos® is used in the prevention of infectious diseases of various origins and MTB100® in the elimination of the mycotoxins and inhibition of their toxic effect, both manufactured by Alltech Inc. (Nicholasville, KY). Animals treated with foods supplemented with β-glucan exhibit greater resistance to pathogenic microorganisms, and bacteria or viruses requiring lower dosages of antibiotics or antivirals to deal with infections [5].

http://dx.doi.org/10.5772/63647

4. Production of purified β-glucan

4.1. β-glucan extraction and purification by yeast cells

Many processes and raw materials of obtaining β-glucans have been described, but the challenge is finding the best extraction leading to high purity with the great immunostimulant and antitumor action, periodontal therapy, among others. After the discovery of the benefits of β-glucan for animals and humans, various processes of purification and isolation of this polysaccharide have been developed [44]. The research for new methods of obtaining β-glucan is being conducted prioritizing a non-aggressive extraction, which preserves the most of the original structure of the macromolecule. Currently, β-glucan used as additive in feed is produced by the cultivation of *S. cerevisiae* or as residue from the fuel ethanol or beer industry. In this respect, just the Brazilian production of sugar cane in the 2012/2013 harvest was 589 million tons of cane and 23.64 billion liters in ethanol was produced [45–47] with expectation of growing. The trading of β-glucan could be increased, since the yeast extraction from the fuel ethanol distilleries up to 5% per day or 7.5 kg powder yeast per m^3 ethanol/day would be possible, which could reach at least 177,300 ton of yeast/day, only in the Brazilian fuel ethanol industry.

4.1.1. Lysis of yeast cell

The basic process of β-glucan extraction involves the lysis of cells (chemical, biochemical, mechanical, or by autohydrolysis), separation of cell wall (centrifugation or filtration), extraction, and purification (precipitation and centrifugation). The yeast cells are normally processed to produce β-glucan, mannan, and yeast extract. One important aspect of the technology to produce β-glucan and other valuable products from yeasts is the method of cell wall lysis. Yeast autolysis is used in the industrial processes due to the low cost, fractionation efficiency, and quality of products obtained. Firstly, the fresh yeast cells are autolysed, and the cell wall is separated by centrifugation.

The yeast cell wall has a thickness of 100–200 nm, and the wall is not only for protection and structural function but is also metabolically important [48]. The thickness and structure of the wall could vary depending on several factors like the strain, the industrial process of yeasts, and culture conditions. The concentration of β-glucans also depends on these parameters since the wall is used for the β-glucan extraction. The outer layer of mannoproteins retains the periplasmic proteins conferring resistance to the cells of yeasts and acts as a barrier to external attack of enzymes and some other molecules [49]. The layer of glucan is more internal and linked with chitin in adjacent layers to the plasma membrane and confers rigidity and the cell shape [50].

Autolysis is an irreversible process caused by intracellular enzymes of yeast under stress conditions, such as temperature, pH, yeast concentrations unsuitable for the survival of the cells. This process is based mainly on heat treatment and causes lysis of the cells from activation of a group of intracellular enzymes that breaks the wall [51]. According to Nagodawithana [51], lysis occurs primarily because of the enzymes β-(1-3) glucanase and protease. Enzymes β-(1-6) glucanases and mannanases participate in solubilizing the matrix of the cell wall, and over forty enzymes have been identified in *S. cerevisiae* containing a major role in the autolytic process. Probably due to metabolic differences between different strains of *S. cerevisiae*, several studies disagree on the physicochemical conditions more appropriate for the autolysis of the cells vary from 45 to 55°C in 3–7 days of treatment [52]. The optimization of autolysis of *Saccharomyces cerevisiae* from a brewery was studied aiming at the maximum ribonucleic acid extraction and yeast extract production [52]. The best conditions for yeast autolysis were 55.2°C, pH = 5.1 and 9.8% NaCl in 24 h of processing. In these conditions, the RNA extraction yield was 89.7%, resulting in 51.3% of dehydrated yeast extract with 57.9% protein, and 48.7% cellular wall with 21.7% protein. The thermal shock at 60°C per 15 min prior to autolysis provided an increase in this yield of 89.7–91.4%. The optimized autolysis including NaCl plasmolysis was efficient, economic, and fast, thus usable for industrial purposes. Currently, yeast residues are exported as yeast flour for feed at low prices by the countries which are producers of fuel ethanol and beer. The improvement of the technology of fractionation and purification in other products like β-glucan, RNA, mannan, mannoprotein, and others is strategic since more valuable products can be produced. This is in accordance with the concept of biorefinery, that is, co-production of biofuels, bioenergy, and marketable chemicals from renewable biomass [53].

Thereafter, the β-glucan is extracted from autolysed yeast cells by hot alkaline hydrolysis (NaOH) and purified by citric acid precipitation. Another combination of alkali and inorganic acid to extract β-(1-3) glucan was performed by Sandula et al., [54], followed the method described by Machová et al., [55] to obtain water-insoluble β-(1-3) glucan from *S. cerevisiae*. In this method, 6% NaOH solution at 60°C was also used; however, the extraction was done by 4% phosphoric acid at room temperature [56]. The effects of drying were evaluated in three different processes (lyophilization, spray drying, and solvent precipitation) on the physical properties and immunoregulatory effect of β-glucan of *Saccharomyces*.

4.2. Chemical modification of β-1,3 glucan

The research of modification of β-1,3 glucan has been performed aiming to improve biological properties. Others steps to obtain modified glucan like methylation, permethylation, carboxymethylation, sulfoethylation, and ultrasonication Depending on the application or use of this molecule. Carboxymethylation of the glucans was made with glucan or chitin–glucan complex suspended in a mixture with 30% NaOH and isopropanol, and stirred at 10°C for 1 h. The degree of substitution of the carboxymethylated glucan was 0.56 or 0.91 for glucan and 0.43 for chitin–glucan complex, depending on the amount of monochloroacetic acid used [57]. The procedure of sulfoethylation of the glucans was performed using sodium β-chloroethylsulfonate in isopropanol solution [58], and permethylation of baker's yeast glucan was carried out according to Ciucanu & Kerek [59] using powdered NaOH. The immunomodulatory activity was detected in fibrillar (non-soluble) and partially hydrolyzed baker's yeast glucan as well as its soluble derivatives prepared by carboxymethylation and sulfoethylation. All these glucans showed anti-infective activity against *Klebsiella pneumoniae* after intravenous or subcutaneous prophylactic application to mice [60].

The evolution of β-(1,3) glucan use in the pharmaceutical and medical areas, as well as food and feed, depends on the development of more economical and efficient methods of extraction, purification, and chemical modification of this interesting molecule. Although their biological properties are amply evidenced, more studies are needed about its application, making this knowledge more available to benefit the health of human and animal.

5. Conclusion

β-(1-3) glucan is a promising healthier food and feed additive whose special properties certified ranging from the activation of the immune system, replacement of antibiotics in animal production, particularly for fish and pork, and various therapies: antitumor, allergic and respiratory diseases, periodontitis and peritonitis. This polymer has also proven to be available as food ingredient for the control of cholesterol and diabetes in special foods. Despite having started their studies for some decades, this molecule remains expensive and not widely available, with the technology dominated by a few producers.

The extraction methods using alkali and acid, with previous pre-treatments, and the step of purification and chemical modification, are needed to obtain β-glucan according to specific biological properties. The solubility, molecular size, level of protein, and degree of methylation are essential parameters to be considered for these properties. This work also highlighted some technological aspects of economic obtaining of β-glucan from yeast.

Author details

Pedro De Oliva-Neto[1*], Sidmeire Santos Oliveira[2], Estevão Zilioli[3] and Márcia Zilioli Bellini[3]

*Address all correspondence to: pedroolivaneto@gmail.com

1 São Paulo State University (UNESP)—School of Sciences and Languages of Assis, Assis, Brazil

2 Estácio de Sá Colleges, Ourinhos, SP, Brazil

3 Integrated Adamantinenses Colleges (FAI), Adamantina, Brazil

References

[1] Magnani, M., Castro-Gómez, R.J.H., Mori, M.P., Kuasne, H., Gregório, E.P., Libos Jr., F. & Cólus, I.M.S. (2011a). Protective effect of carboxymethyl-glucan (CM-G) against

DNA damage in patients with advanced prostate cancer. *Genetics and Molecular Biology, 34*(1), 131–135.

[2] Magnani, M., Castro-Gómez, R.J.H., Aoki, M.N., Gregório, E.P. & Libos Jr, F. Morimoto, H.K., Reiche, E.M.V. & Watanabe, M.A.E. (2011b). Analysis of peripheral T cells and the CC chemokine receptor (CCR5) delta32 polymorphism in prostate cancer patients treated with carboxymethyl-glucan (CM-G). *Natural Product Research: Formerly Natural Product Letters, 26*(10), 945–951.

[3] Murakawa, K., Fukunaga, K., Tanouch, M., Hosokawa, M., Hossan, Z. & Takahashi, K. (2007). Therapy of myeloma in vivo using marine phospholipid in combination with *Agaricus blazei* Murill as an immune respond activator. *Journal of Oleo Science, 56*(4), 179–188.

[4] Demir, G., Klein, H.O., Mandel-Molinas, N. & Tuzuner, N. (2007). β-glucan induces proliferation and activation of monocytes in peripheral blood of patients with advanced breast cancer. *International Immunopharm, 7*, 113–116.

[5] Xiao, Z., Trincado, C.A. & Murtaugh, M.P. (2004). β-Glucan enhancement of T cell IFN-gamma response in swine. *Veterinary Immunology and Immunopathology, 102*(3), 315–320.

[6] Kogan, G., Šandula, J., Korolenko, T.A., Falameeva, O.V., Poteryaeva, O.N., Zhanaeva, S.Ya., Levina, O.A., Filatova, T.G. & Kaledin, V.I. (2002). Increased efficiency of Lewis lung carcinoma chemotherapy with a macrophage stimulator—yeast carboxymethyl glucan. *International Immunopharmacol, 2*, 775–781.

[7] Braaten, J.T., Wood, P.J., Scott, F.W., Wolynetz, M.S., Lowe, M.K., Bradley-White, P. & Collins, M.W. (1994). Oat beta-glucan reduces blood cholesterol concentration in hypercholesterolemic subjects. *European Journal of Clinical Nutrition, 48*, 465–74.

[8] Genc, H., Ozdemir, M. & Demirbas, A. (2001). Analysis of mixed-linked (1→3), (1→4)-β-D-glucans in cereal grain from Turkey. *Food Chemistry, 73*, 221–224.

[9] Hegsted, M., Windhauser, M.M. & Lester, S.B. (1993). Stabilized rice bran and oat bran lower cholesterol *in* humans. *Nutrition Research, 13*(4), 387–398.

[10] Saastamoinem, M.; Plaami, S. & Kumpulainen, J. (1989). Pentosans and β glucan content of Finnish winter varieties as compared with rye six other countries. *Journal of Cereal Science, 10*, 199–207.

[11] Sayar, S.; Jannink, J.; White, P.J. (2005). *In Vitro* bile acid binding of flours from oat lines varying in percentage and molecular weight distribution of *β*-glucan. *J. Agric. Food Chem., 53*: 8797–8803.

[12] Engstrom, D.F., Mathison G.W. & Goonewardene, L.A. (1992). Effect of β-glucan, starch, and fibre content and steam vs. dry rolling of barley grain on its degradability and utilization by steers. *Animal Feed Science and Technology, 37*(2), 33–46.

[13] El Khoury, D., Cuda, C., Luhovyy, B.L. & Anderson, G.H. (2012). Beta glucan: health benefits in obesity and metabolic syndrome. *Journal of Nutrition and Metabolism, 2012*: 28. doi:10.1155/2012/851362.

[14] Magnani, M. & Castro-Gómez, R.J.H. (2008). β-glucan from *Saccharomyces cerevisiae*: constitution, bioactivity and obtaining. *Semina: Ciencias Agrarias, 29*(3), 631–650.

[15] Chan, G.C., Chan, W.K. Sze, D.M. (2009). The effects of β-glucan on human immune and cancer cells. *Journal of Hematology & Oncology, 2*, 25–36.

[16] Stone, B.A. & Clarke, A.E. (1992). Chemistry and biology of (1,3)-D-glucans. *La Trobe University*, Victoria, Australia Press.

[17] Camelini, C.M., Mendonça, M., Dias, P.F. & Maraschin, M. (2005). β-glucans from mushrooms. *Biotecnologia Ciencia e Desenvolvimento, 35*, 36–47.

[18] Li, W., Cui, S.W. & Kakuda, Y. (2005). Extraction, fractionation, structural and physical characterization of wheat β-D-glucans. *Carbohydrate Polymers, 63*, 408–416.

[19] Jantova, S., Bakos, D., Birosova, L. & Matejov, P. (2015). Biological properties of a novel coladerm-beta glucan membrane. In vitro assessment using human fibroblasts. *Biomed Papers of Medical Faculty of the University Palacky Olomouc, Czech Repub*, 159(1):67–76. doi: 10.5507/bp.2012.115.

[20] Brown, G.D. & Gordon, S. (2003). Fungal β-glucans and mammalian immunity. *Immunity, 19*(3), 311–315.

[21] Mansell, P.W.A., Ichinose, I.I., Reed, R.J., Krements, E.T., McNamee, R.B. & Di Luzio, N.R. (1975). Macrophage-mediated destruction of human malignant cells in vive. *Journal of the National Cancer Institute, 54*, 571–580.

[22] Akramienė, D., Kondrotas, A., Didžiapetrienė, J. & Kėvelaitis, E. (2007). Effects of β-glucans on the immune system. *Medicina (Kaunas), 43(8)*, 597–606.

[23] Bohn, J.A. & BeMiller, J.M. (1995). (1-3)-β-D-glucans as biological response modifiers: a review of structure-functional activity relationships. *Carbohydrate Polymers, 28 (1)*, 3–14.

[24] Kwiatkowski, S., Kwiatkowski, S.E. Yeast (*Saccharomyces cerevisiae*) Glucan Polysaccharides—Occurrence, Separation and Application in Food, Feed and Health Industries. (2012). In: D.N. Karunaratne (Ed.), *The Complex World of Polysaccharides*, (47–70), In Tech, Rijeka, Croatia. http://dx.doi.org/10.5772/48100.

[25] Battle, J., Ha, T., Li, C., Della Beffa, V., Rice, P., Kalbfleisch, J., Browder, W. & Williams, D. (1998). Ligand binding to the (1-3)-β-D-glucan receptor stimulates NFkB activation, but not apoptosis in U937 cells. *Biochemical and Biophysical Research Communications, 249(2)*, 499–504.

[26] Kuroda, Y. & Hara, Y. (1999). Antimutagenic and anticarcinogenic activity of tea polyphenols. *Mutation Research, 436*(1), 69–97.

[27] Di Luzio, N.R. (1983). Immunopharmacology of glucan: a broad spectrum enhancer of host defense mechanisms. *Trends in Pharmacological Sciences, 4*, 344–347.

[28] Manners, D.J., Mason, A.J. & Patterson, J.C. (1973). The structure of a 1,3 β-glucan from yeast cell walls. *Biochemistry Journal, 135*, 19–30.

[29] Chaple, C.C., Srivastrava, M. & Hunter, N. (1998). Failure of macrophage activation in destructive periodontal disease. *The Journal of Pathology, 186*, 281–286.

[30] Hartland, R.P., Vermeulen, C.A., Sietsma, J.H., Wessels, J.G.H. & Klis, F.M. (1994). The linkage of (1-3)-β-glucan to chitin during cell wall assembly in *Saccharomyces cerevisiae. Yeast (Chichester, England), 10*(12), 1591–1599.

[31] Acar, N.N., Noyan, U., Kuru, L., Kadir, T. & Kuru, B. (2012). Adjunctive Systemic Use of Beta-Glucan in the Nonsurgical Treatment of Chronic Periodontitis. In N. Budeneli (Ed.), *Pathogenesis and Treatment of Periodontitis*, (pp. 167–182). Shanghai: In Tech China.

[32] Sarinho, E., Medeiros, D., Schor, D., Silva, A.R., Sales, V., Motta, M.E., Costa, A., Azoubel, A. & Rizzo, J.A. (2009). Production of interleukin-10 in asthmatic children after beta-1-3-glucan. *Allergol Immunopathol, 37*, 188–192.

[33] Di Luzio, N.R. & Williams, D.L. (1978). Protective effect of glucan against systemic *Staphylococcus aureus* septicemia in normal and leukemic mice. *Infection and Immunity, 20*, 804–810.

[34] Oliveira, R.J., Matuo, R., da Silva, A.F., Matiazi, H.J., Mantovani, M.S. & Ribeiro, L.R. (2007). Protective effect of β-glucan extracted from *Saccharomyces cerevisiae* against DNA damage and cytotoxicity in wild-type (k1) and repair-deficient xrs5 CHO cells. *Toxicology In Vitro: An International Journal Published in Association with BIBRA, 21*, 41–52.

[35] Auinger, A., Riede, L., Bothe, G., Busch, R. & Gruenwald, J. (2013). Yeast (1,3)-(1,6)-beta-glucan helps to maintain the body's defense against pathogens: a double-blind, randomized, placebo controlled, multicentric study in healthy subjects. *European Journal of Nutrition, 52*(8), 1913–1918.

[36] Talbott, S. & Talbott, J. (2009). Effect of Beta 1,3/1,6 Glucan on upper respiratory tract infection symptoms and mood state in marathon athletes. *Journal of Sports Science and Medicine, 8*, 509–515.

[37] Kim, S.Y., Song, H.J., Lee, Y.Y., Cho, K. & Roh, Y.K. (2006). Biomedical Issues of Dietary fiber –Glucan. *Journal of Korean Medical Science, 21*, 781–789.

[38] Nicolosi, R., Bell, S.J., Bistrian, B.R., Greenberg, I., Forse, R.A. & Blackburn, G.L. (1999). Plasma lipid changes after supplementation with β-glucan fiber from yeast. *American Journal of Clinical Nutrition, 70*(2), 208–212.

[39] Beer, M.U., Arrigoni, E. & Amado, R. (1995). Effects of oat gum on blood cholesterol levels in healthy young men. *European Journal of Clinical Nutrition, 49*, 517–22.

[40] Lang, C.H. & Dobrescu, C. (1989). Interleukin-l induced increases in glucose utilization are insulin mediated. *Life Sciences 45*(22), 27–34.

[41] Robertsen, B., Engstad, R.E. & Jorgensen, J.B. (1994). Beta-glucans as Immunostimulants in fish. *Modulators of Fish Immune Responses, 1,* Fair Haven, NJ, USA.

[42] Regand, A., Tosh, S.M., Wolever, T.M.S. & Wood, P.J. (2009). Physicochemical properties of β-glucan in differently processed oat foods influence glycemic response. *Journal of Agricultural and Food Chemistry, 57,* 8831–8838.

[43] Kogan, G. & Kocher, A. (2007). Role of yeast cell wall polysaccharides in pig nutrition and health protection. *Livestock Science, 109,* 161–165.

[44] Li, J., Li, D.F., Xing, J.J., Cheng, Z.B. & Lai, C.H. (2006). Effects of β-glucan extracted from *Saccharomyces cerevisiae* on growth performance, and immunological and somatotropic responses of pigs challenged with *Escherichia coli* lipopolysaccharide. *Journal of Animal Science, 84,* 2374–2381.

[45] MAPA—Brazilian Department of Agriculture, Livestock and Supply (2013). http://www.agricultura.gov.br/vegetal/safras-estoques. Access in the site: April 23, 2014.

[46] CONAB Brazilian National Company of Supply. (2013). Site: http://www.conab.gov.br/OlalaCMS/uploads/arquivos/13_04_09_10_30_34_boletim_cana_portugues_abril_2013_4o_lev.pdf. Access in the site: Access in: April, 2014.

[47] Aguiar, C. (2011). STAB congress of sugar and ethanol. *Management practices and Sustainability*. Access site: http://www.stab.org.br/12sba/5.CLEBERAGUIAR.SAOMANOEL.26.10.11hrs.pdf

[48] Dzienzak, J.D. (1987). Yeast and Yeast derivatives applications. *Food Technology, 41*(2), 122–125.

[49] Kopecká, M., Phaff, H.J. & Fleet, G.H. (1974). Demonstration of a fibrillar component in the cell wall of the yeast *Saccharomyces cerevisiae* and its chemical nature. *The Journal of Cell Biology, 62*(1), 66–76.

[50] Kapteyn, J.C., Ram, A.F., Gross, E.M., Kollar, R., Montijn, R.C., Van Den Ende, H., Llobel, A.A., Cabib, E. & Klis, F.M. (1997). Altered extent of cross-linking of β 1,6-glucosylated mannoproteins to chitin in *Saccharomyces cerevisiae* mutants with reduced cell wall β 1,3 glucan content. *Journal of Bacteriology,* 179(20), 6279–6284.

[51] Nagodawithana, T. (1992). Yeast-derived flavors and flavor enhancers and their probable mode of action. *Food Technology,* 46, 138–144.

[52] Oliveira, A.M. & Oliva-Neto, P. (2011). Improvement in RNA extraction from *S. cerevisie* by optimization in the autolysis and NH3 hydrolysis. *Brazilian Archives of Biology and Technology,* 54, 1007–1018.

[53] Cherubini, F. & Ulgiati, S. (2010), Crop residues as raw materials for biorefinery systems —A LCA case study. *Applied Energy, 87,* 47–57.

[54] Sandula, J., Kogan, G., Kacuráková, M. & Machová, E. (1999). Microbial (1-3)-β-D-glucan their preparation, physico-chemical characterization and immunomodulatory activity. *Carbohydrate Polymer, 38,* 247–253.

[55] Machová, E., Kogan, G. Alföldi, J., Soltes, L. & Sandula, J.(1995). Enzymatic and ultrasonic depolymerization of carboxymethylated β(1-3)-D-glucans derived from *S. cerevisiae. Journal of Applied Polymer Science, 55,* 699–704.

[56] Torronen, R., Kansanen, L., Uusitupa, M., Hanninen, O., Myllymaki, O., Harkonen, H. & Malkki, Y. (1992). Effects of an oat bran concentrate on serum lipids in free-living men with mild to moderate hypercholesterolaemia. *European Journal of Clinical Nutrition, 46,* 621–627.

[57] Jamas, S., Easson, D.D. & Ostroff, G.R. (1997). Glucan preparation. *US Patent 5622939.*

[58] Pastýr, J., Sandula, J., Master, L., Trnovec, T. & Benes, G. (1997). Preparation of water-soluble sulfoderivatives of microbial β(1-3)-D-glucans. Slovak Patent no. 278783.

[59] Ciucanu, I. & Kerek, F. (1984). A simple and rapid method for the permethylation of carbohydrates. *Carbohydr Res., 131,* 209–217.

[60] Kogan, G., Master, C., Sandula, J., Navarová, J. & Trnovec, T. (1989). Recent results on the structure and immunomodulating activities of yeast glucan. In V. Crescenzi, I.C.M. Dea, S. Pruletti, S.S. Stivala, I.W. Sutherland (Eds). *Biochemical and Biotechnological Advances in Industrial Polysaccharides.* Elsevier. New York.

Chapter 17

Prebiotics, Probiotics, Synbiotics and Functional Foods in Control and Treatment of Type II Diabetes Mellitus and Colorectal Cancer

Samuel Longoria-García, Ruth E. Belmares-Cerda,
Mildred I.M. Flores-Verástegui,
Juan C. Contreras-Esquivel,
Julio C. Montañez-Sáenz and
Mario Alberto Cruz-Hernández

Additional information is available at the end of the chapter

http://dx.doi.org/10.5772/63643

Abstract

Prebiotics, probiotics and synbiotics are components that enhance human health by several mechanisms. Patients suffering from type II diabetes mellitus (T2DM) and colorectal cancer have seen benefits when treated with a prebiotic, probiotic or synbiotic therapy. These benefits include the improvement of their lipid profile, oxidative stress status, as well as the modulation of the inflammatory and immune responses. The associated benefits of prebiotic, probiotic or synbiotic functional foods have been studied, showing promising results into the prevention or control of diabetes and colorectal cancer. This novelty research provides new evidence that the use of functional foods along with medical therapy could be used to further enhance patient's health.

Keywords: prebiotics, probiotics, synbiotics, T2DM, colorectal cancer

1. Introduction

Prebiotics, probiotics and synbiotics provide several health benefits to its consumer, such as better control of the glycemic index, blood triglycerides (TG) reduction, prevention of cancer, improvement of mineral absorption, among others [1–3]. Prebiotics, probiotics and synbiotics have been added to food products in order to develop functional foods that confer additional health benefits besides the nutritional ones. Due to the health benefits they provide, the market for functional foods has increased in the previous years, growing up to a 47.6 billion US$, and it is expected to continue growing during the following years [4].

The objective of this chapter was to show some of the latest work done regarding the use of prebiotics, probiotics and synbiotics in prevention and treatment of type II diabetes mellitus (T2DM) and colorectal cancer, along with clinical studies showing that functional foods enriched with at least one of these components show a health benefit to patients.

2. Diabetes

Diabetes is a disease in which the body cannot regulate the amount of sugar in blood, being two major types of the disease:

- Type I: there is little or none insulin production, and insulin injections are needed daily.
- Type II: insulin resistance is present and glucose is unable to enter the cells to be used stored or used as energy.

Symptoms of both types include fatigue, blurry vision and slower healing in bladder and kidney infections. For type I, insulin injection is currently the only treatment, as for type II, medication is used when needed. These therapeutic drugs include α-glucosidase inhibitors, sulfonylureas, biguanides, among others. However, for most cases of T2DM, weight loss, healthy diet as well as exercise are enough to control or put into remission the disease [5]. Due to the nature of T2DM, this type poses a real possibility of overcoming the disease and where most of research is done in order to prevent, control and cure the disease.

The epidemics of diabetes is growing alarmingly, and it is estimated that by 2030, 342 million people (4.8% world's population) will be suffering from this disease [6]. It is estimated that 4 million people die from its complications each year, costing around 3.9 billion US$ for Brazil, 0.8 billion US$ for Argentina, 2.0 billion US$ for Mexico, and up to 44 billion US$ for USA in 1994; in 2012, it was 245 billion US$ for USA [7,8].

2.1. T2DM prebiotic, probiotic and synbiotic clinical therapy

2.1.1. Proposed molecular mechanisms

The molecular mechanisms on how probiotics or prebiotics work is not fully understood yet; however, few proposed or suggested mechanisms have been presented. Since T2DM is at a higher risk of cardiovascular complications, improvement or control of the lipid profile associated with prebiotics and probiotics has been studied, and it has been suggested that this improvement is done by the production of short-chain fatty acids (SCFA), which act as inhibitors of lipid synthesis in liver [9].

Probiotics have also shown the ability to reduce reactive oxygen species (ROS) which, among other harmful effects, damage the intestinal barrier and allow bacterial translocation, which might lead to different infections and inflammation. *Bifidobacterium* has been associated with control of mild chronic inflammation, since it has been found that when levels of *Bifidobacterium* decrease, bacterial lipopolysaccharides (LPS) increase, and this is a characteristic of endotoxemia which leads to a higher concentration of pro-inflammatory cytokines [10]. Also, it has been shown that probiotic *Lactobacillus casei* regulates the release of LPS into blood via liver GlyRs upregulation [11].

Another proposed mechanism is that probiotics have the ability to modulate Th1 and Th2 pro-inflammatory responses, aiding in prevention of development of T2DM. Probiotic regulation of expression of *FoxA2* gene, whose product affected inulin sensitivity, has also been found. Also, a probiotic effect in Cl secretion and chloride channel protein expression in small intestine was determined. Chloride channel protein expression modulation has the effect of maintaining the normal function of tight junction barrier, decreasing bacterial translocation. All these results were observed in *L. casei*; further studies would be needed in order to associate similar effects for other probiotic strains [11]. However, these results show possible molecular mechanisms in which probiotics act on immune response.

Moving on to prebiotics, inulin, the most widely studied prebiotic, has shown the effect of glycemic index control by reducing the absorption rate of glucose and lipid profile control by decreasing the amount of serum triglycerides through the inhibition of glycerol-3-phosphate acyltransferase and fatty acid synthase as well as key enzymes in *de novo* lipid synthesis [12].

Extensive work has been done regarding the study of molecular mechanisms in which both prebiotics and probiotics function. Still, further studies are needed in order to establish a better understanding of the molecular mechanisms in which both enhance human health.

2.1.2. Recent studies done with T2DM

Several studies had been made with the use of prebiotics, probiotics or synbiotics into the treatment of T2DM. One of the first most recent studies uses probiotics as an aid in the treatment in diabetic rats along with gliclazide, an antidiabetic drug. Forty rats were divided into four groups: healthy, healthy probiotic, diabetic and diabetic probiotic. In the last two, diabetes was induced by alloxan solution injection (30 mg/kg). A mixture of *Lactobacillus acidophilus, B. lactis* and *Lactobacillus rhamnosus* was prepared in a formulation and administered along with the pharmaceutical to both healthy and diabetic male Wistar rats in a concentration of 10^{11} cells/g and 20 mg/kg, respectively. Probiotics were administered through gavage twice daily for 3 days for both health and diabetic groups and, after taking a baseline blood sample, gliclazide was administered by gavage as a single sample, taking blood sample doses from 5 min up to 600 min. Insulin concentrations in blood and blood glucose levels were measured for analysis. HPLC and MS were used to determine gliclazide serum concentration using a non-compartmental model. Parameters such as maximum concentration, time to maximum concentration, half-life and mean residence time were evaluated by an analysis of variance (ANOVA). The study showed that in groups with probiotic treatment, there was no difference in glucose levels in healthy rats, but there was a significant reduction in diabetic ones from 23.8 ± 3 mmol/l to 12.6 ± 4 mmol/l. The bioavailability of gliclazide in both healthy and diabetic rats was studied, and results showed that there was a reduction in bioavailability in healthy rats from (1.06 ± 0.30) × 10^4 μg/mL to (0.45 ± 0.14) × 10^4 μg/mL and an increase in diabetic ones from (0.80 ± 0.15) × 10^4 μg/mL to (1.00 ± 0.23) × 10^4 μg/mL [13]. However, alloxan-induced diabetes is considered to be suffering from type I diabetes.

A different study used oligofructose-enriched inulin in order to evaluate the effect on several T2DM markers such as triglycerides (TG), total cholesterol (TC), malondialdehyde (MDA), low-density lipoprotein cholesterol (LDL-C), among others. A randomized, triple-blind, placebo-controlled trail was conducted for 8 weeks in 70 diabetic female volunteers whose ages range from 25 to 65 years old and having diabetes diagnosed for more than 6 months; however, only 52 patients completed the study. Maltodextrin was used as placebo in the control group, while the oligofructose-enriched inulin for the intervention group, both doses consisted of 5 g of supplement to be eaten during breakfast and 5 g at dinner. An Analysis of Covariance (ANCOVA) was performed to identify differences between the two groups. Results show that there was a general decrease in lipid levels, such as TC, from 203.1 mg/dL to 175 mg/dL, and LDL-C from 116.3 mg/dL to 94.3 mg/dL. There was no significant decrease in TG, from 216.8 mg/dL to 176.9 mg/dL, nor in MDA which values ranged from 4.3 nmol/mL to 2.6 nmol/mL [14]. This study suggests that these prebiotics have potential in improving the lipid profile of patients with T2DM, and this would lead to a decrease in the cardiovascular risk associated with the disease.

Impaired glucose tolerance is a major risk factor involved in T2DM, and a study was made assessing the effect of a probiotic in a preventive and/or ameliorating way in male Sprague Dawley rats. *L. casei* was administered on a 10^9 CFU/d to 50 rats divided into five groups: normal control (NC), *L. casei* preventive (LP), *L. casei* therapeutic (LT), hyperinsulinemia model group at 9 weeks (HMI) and hyperinsulinemia model group at 13 weeks (HMII). During the course of the study, 14 weeks, they evaluated parameters such as blood glucose level, total bile acids levels and liver glycogen content along with the composition of intestinal predominate bacteria. The statistical analysis was performed using an ANOVA and Fisher's least significant difference (LSD) to compare among groups. This study suggests an increase in glucose tolerance as well as the number of *Lactobacillus* and *Bifidobacterium* present in colon, while decreasing *Clostridium*. *L. casei* ameliorated glucose tolerance in rats, and this is suggested by the decrease in glycogen content in liver, stopping an excessive stress with an increase in liver's glucose uptake due to the fact that over 70% of dietary fructose is metabolized by the liver leading to an improvement in health [15].

As mentioned earlier, it is suggested that lipid profile and oxidative stress are improved by probiotics. A single-blinded clinical trial was performed with 40 T2DM patients studying the effect of probiotics *L. acidophilus, Lactobacillus bulgaricus, L. casei* and *L. bifidum* in 1500 mg capsules twice daily during 6 weeks, while control group receives 1000 mg magnesium stearate capsules. Lipid profile and oxidative stress biomarkers such as TC, TG, LDL-C, among others were evaluated. For statistical analysis, paired *t*-test samples were used to compare continuous variables within groups, while comparison between different groups was done through two independent-samples *t*-tests. In the absence of normal distribution, Wilcoxon and Mann–Whitney *U*-tests were used. There was not any significant difference found between control group and probiotic treated group, and authors argue that it might have been due to the sample size or the short duration of the study [6]. These results pose controversial evidence between health enhancement properties of prebiotics, probiotics and synbiotics; however, further analyses into the sample size, duration of each trial, and dosage have to be taken into account in order to establish an objective conclusion as well as the duration of the study.

Further studies have been done in the topic of T2DM; however, there is no an extensive amount of literature available. A short summary of these is presented in **Table 1**.

Authors	Component	Host	Dosage/ length	Study's design
[16]*	Several *Bifidum* and *Lactobacillus* strains	T2DM patients	4 g sachets daily intake (2.5×10^9 CFU/g) 26 weeks	Single-center, double-blinded, randomized, placebo-controlled study with 60 patients
[11]	*L. casei*	Sprague Dawley Rats	4×10^9 CFU/d rat 2 weeks	1. Sixteen rats divided into high-fat fructose diet (HFS) and normal control (NC) 2. Twenty-seven rats divided into three groups: HSF, NC, and HSF with probiotics ANOVA followed by LSD
[17]*	Inulin oligofructose	Pre-diabetic patients	10 g daily 6.5 months	Randomized crossover controlled trial Kolmogorov–Smirnov goodness-of-fit test, Pearson correlation, and ANOVA
[18]	Several *Bifidum* and *Lactobacillus* strains	T2DM patients	Range from 1.5×10^9 to 7×10^9 CFU 15 months	Randomized double-blinded controlled clinical trial Kolmogorov–Smirnov test, Paired sample *t*-test, Student's *t*-test
[19]*	Inulin	Pre-diabetic patients	10 g inulin daily 6 weeks	Double-blinded, placebo-controlled, parallel group design Multiple-sample repeated-measures analysis of variance, ANCOVA
[20]	*L. acidophilus Bifidobacterium*	T2DM patients	10^9 CFU/day 7 months	Randomized double-blinded parallel group placebo-controlled trial Shapiro–Wilk

Authors	Component	Host	Dosage/ length	Study's design
	animalis			test, Student's *t*-test
[21]	*B. animalis* Polydextrose Antidiabetic drugs	Mice	10^9 CFU Polydextrose 0.25 g/day 4 weeks	1. Forty mice divided into four groups: diabetic control, *B. animalis* (B420) intake, metformin, metformin + B420 2. Forty-eight mice divided into six groups: non-diabetic control, diabetic control, sitagliptin (SITA), SITA + polydextrose (PD), SITA + B420, SITA + PD + B420 2 × 2 Factorial, Shapiro–Wilk, ANOVA, Tukey's HSD

* To our knowledge, results of clinical trial have not been published to the date of writing.

Table 1. Recent studies done with prevention or treatment of T2DM using prebiotics, probiotics or synbiotics.

2.2. Functional foods in T2DM

As mentioned above, T2DM can be controlled by a healthy diet. This has been used as a novelty approach into the treatment of the disease using prebiotic, probiotic or synbiotic functional foods, while evaluating the health benefits provided. Most of the functional foods studied are either yoghurts or breads.

A probiotic yogurt with *L. acidophilus* and *B. lactis* was used to evaluate the effect on the lipid profile of T2DM patients. This was a double-blinded randomized controlled clinical trial in which a total of 64 subjects were assigned to either a control group or a treatment group. Three-hundred grams of either control or probiotic yoghurt were consumed daily during the 6-week period the study lasted. It was determined that an average of 4.14×10^6 CFU/g for *L. acidophilus* and 3.61×10^6 CFU/g for *B. lactis* was the concentration on probiotic yoghurts when consumed by patients. For statistical analysis of the parameters measured, different tests were measured such as Kolmogorov–Smirnov, *t*-tests, chi-squared tests and Mann–Whitney *U*-test. It was found a decrease of 4.54% of total cholesterol and 7.45% decrease in LDL-C, while no significant effect was found on triglycerides and in high-density lipoprotein cholesterol (HDL-C). However, authors discussed certain limitations such as the short duration time and the lack of a control group who did not consumed yogurt at all [22]. This study suggests that the consumption of a probiotic yoghurt might help reduce cardiovascular risk in patients with T2DM.

One year later, results from another similar study were published in which a probiotic yogurt containing *L. acidophilus* and *B. lactis* was used to assess the effect on oxidative stress biomarkers of T2DM patients. Similarly, this was a double-blinded randomized controlled clinical trial, conformed by 64 patients in which patients were randomly assigned either a control or an intervention group. During 6 weeks, patients consumed 300 g a day of either a probiotic or conventional yoghurt. Probiotic yoghurt contained an average of 1.85×10^6 CFU/g of *L. acidophilus* and 1.79×10^6 CFU/g. of *B. lactis*. Some of the parameters measured were the glutathione peroxidase activity, MDA serum concentration and hemoglobin A1c. Several statistical tests were used such as Kolgomorov–Smirnov, independent-samples *t*-test, chi-square and Mann–Whitney *U*-tests. It was shown that the consumption of this yogurt decreased fasting blood glucose and increased erythrocyte superoxide dismutase and glutathione peroxidase activity. These results show the improvement in the oxidative stress status of patients and that this probiotic yogurt is a promising agent for diabetes management [23].

On another study, the evaluation of the lipid profile of T2DM patients while consuming a synbiotic bread containing *Lactobacillu sporogenes* and inulin was made. This study was a randomized double-blinded controlled clinical trial in which 78 subjects were randomly assigned to three groups: a control group consuming bread, a probiotic bread consuming probiotic bread with a bacteria concentration of 1×10^8 CFU and a synbiotic bread containing the probiotic and 0.07 g inulin per 1 g of bread. One hundred-twenty grams of bread were consumed daily for 8 weeks. For statistical analysis, tests such as Kolmogorov–Smirnov and ANOVA were used to identify significant differences. The best results were obtained with the synbiotic bread in which triacylglycerols (TAG), very low-density lipoprotein cholesterol (VLDL-C) and the ratio between total cholesterol and HDL-C were decreased significantly compared to the control group and the probiotic one. However, there was no effect on the fasting plasma glucose (FPS), total cholesterol (TC), LDL-C and non-HDL-C. These results show that this synbiotic bread enhances patient's health even further than probiotic or prebiotic ones [24].

On a different approach, *L. sporogenes* with inulin were used as synbiotic components in a different study. This clinical trial consisted of a randomized double-blinded crossover in which 62 patients consumed the product during 6 weeks. The dosage consumed by subjects daily was of 27×10^7 CFU and 1.08 inulin. Statistical analysis of the assessed variables was evaluated through Kolmogorov–Smirnov and paired *t*-tests. The assessed variables were consistent with other studies regarding the lipid profile. It was found that there was a significant decrease in insulin levels, serum hs-CRP, while there was an increase in uric acid levels, but no significant effect on LDL-C, serum triglycerides and HDL-C in patients with T2DM. These results also suggest that synbiotics have a positive effect in glycemic control [25]. However, the high dosage of probiotics should be taken into account when comparing with similar studies, and this dosage was the highest found in consulted literature.

In a different study, another synbiotic functional food was developed enriched with β-carotene, and this food contained inulin as a prebiotic and *L. sporogenes* as a probiotic. This was double-blinded controlled crossover clinical trial in which 102 patients were randomly allocated to a control food group or a synbiotic one for 6 weeks. Their daily dosage was 3×10^7 CFU, 0.3 g of inulin and 0.15 g β-carotene. Results show a decreased insulin's concentration, triglycerides, VLDL-C and TC/HDL-C, improving the lipid profile of patients and lower cardiovascular disease associated with T2DM; however, β-carotene should be taken into account when considering these results, and authors suggest a mechanism in which β-carotene impacts gene expression and gut microbiota–SCFA–hormone axis [26]. Nonetheless, previous studies show the health enhancing properties of probiotics and prebiotics, so this should not take any credit for these results.

To conclude with T2DM and functional foods, another synbiotic bread was developed using *L. sporogenes* and inulin to evaluate its effect of nitric oxide (NO) and MDA, biomarkers of oxidative stress and liver enzyme activities. A randomized double-blinded, placebo-controlled clinical was done, and 81 patients were divided into three groups: Group A consuming synbiotic bread, Group B consuming probiotic bread and Group C consuming control bread. All three groups consumed 120 g/day of bread, and dosages for treatment groups consisted of 3×10^8 CFU and 0.21 g inulin per day. Statistical analysis was done using Kolmogorov–Smirnov and ANOVA tests. It was observed that there was a significant increase in NO and MDA levels, while there was no effect on plasma total antioxidant capacity, plasma glutathione (GSH) and serum liver enzymes, among others. This study shows that the consumption of the synbiotic bread had positive effects on NO and MDA levels, improving the oxidative stress status of T2DM patients [27]. These results support the idea that functional foods might be useful as an aid in the treatment of T2DM. There were no significant differences in other variables such as GSH activity, blood pressure, serum liver enzymes, among others, which must be considered when taking a control of T2DM using functional foods.

3. Colorectal cancer

As any other cancer, colorectal is characterized by uncontrolled proliferation of cells which lead to the formation of tumors. Symptoms involve blood in stool, either diarrhea or constipation, fatigue, frequent gas pain cramps, among others. Colorectal cancer is the third most common cancer worldwide in men, just below lung and prostate cancers, and second most common in women just below breast cancer. There were 1.3 million new diagnosed cases of colorectal cancer in 2012 and it is expected that this figure will keep growing [28].

The cost of colorectal cancer in 2010 in the US was of 14.14 billion US$, while worldwide it is estimated to be of 99 billion US$ annually [29, 30].

3.1. Colorectal cancer prebiotic, probiotic and synbiotic clinical therapy

3.1.1. Proposed molecular mechanisms

Several molecular mechanisms in which probiotics and prebiotics work and help prevent as well as ameliorate health in colorectal cancer patients have been proposed, some are presented here. Probiotics cause the acidification of pH which has been shown to inhibit *Escherichia coli* and clostridia, subsequently causing the decrease in bacterial enzymes linked to conversion of procarcinogens into carcinogens such as β-glucuronidase. Probiotics isolated from "idly," a traditional cereal pulse from India, had the ability to exert desmutagenicity in various mutagens such as heterocyclic amines and aflatoxins. Also, bifidobacteria have shown binding properties on the carcinogens such as methylazoxymethanol and 3-amino-1,4-dimethyl-5H-pyrido[4,3-b]indole and the ability of removing them physically through feces, reducing the amount of absorption of this carcinogens in lumen and thus reducing the probabilities of developing cancer. Furthermore, *Bifidobacterium longum* showed reduction in expression of *ras*-p21 oncoprotein, and mutations in *ras* genes have been found to be present in colon adenomas, carcinomas and tumors. A general summary of mechanisms can be seen in **Figure 1** [31].

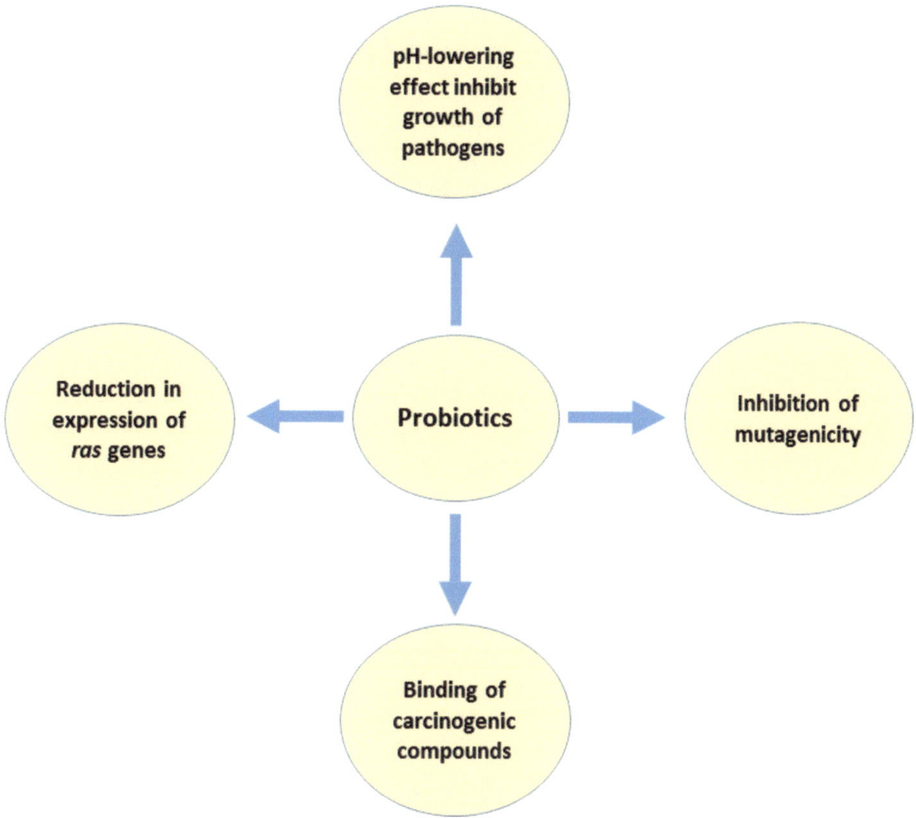

Figure 1. General anti-carcinogenic probiotic mechanisms in colorectal cancer.

Most of the studies done on the mechanism of prebiotics have been on oligofructose prebiotics such fructooligosaccharides and inulin. Oligofructose-enriched inulin has shown a decrease in the expression of enzymes linked to colorectal cancer such as glutathione S-transferase and nitric oxide synthase. Also, cyclooxygenase 2, an enzyme upregulated in cancers was in lower in prebiotic rats than in control rats. Fermentation in colon generates SCFA, butyrate being one of them. Sodium butyrate has been found to be a grown inhibitor and inducer of phenotype differentiation and apoptosis, reducing the risk factors of developing cancer [31].

While there are several proposed mechanisms with evidence suggesting them, for both probiotics and prebiotics, further studies must be done in order to provide uncontroversial evidence on the established pathways and provide better understanding of the molecular dynamics followed in the human colon.

3.1.2. Recent studies done with colorectal cancer

Several studies have been made in order to evaluate the effect on several variables associated with colorectal cancer. In a randomized double-blinded placebo-controlled trial, a synbiotic treatment containing *L. rhamnosus, B. lactis* and inulin was used in a study evaluating the effects on several markers of immune functions. During 12 weeks, 34 patients were randomly placed on either the control group or the treatment one. Control or placebo group consumed daily encapsulated maltodextrin and a 10 g sachet of maltodextrin, while the treatment group consumed 1×10^{10} CFU *L. rhamnosus* and 1×10^{10} CFU of *B. lactis* along with a 10 g sachet of inulin. Several parameters such as burst activity of monocytes and neutrophils, lytic activity of natural killer cells and production of interleukins (IL)-2, IL-10 and IL-12, among others were evaluated. The statistical analysis was done using Kolgomorov–Smirnov, ANOVA and Dunnett's tests. The synbiotic therapy only showed significant effect on an increased capacity of peripheral blood mononuclear cells to produce IFN-γ. These results do not show promising evidence, but it should be noted that authors measured immune response factors in blood. Authors even suggest future studies should aim gut-associated immune system. The main contribution of this study was to determine that the immune effects of a synbiotic treatment are kept in human colon [32].

A different approach has also been taken, and *Bifidobacterium adolescentis* extracts were used in a study to evaluate the antiproliferative effects on three human colon cancer cells: Caco-2, HT-29 and SW480, measuring the production of tumor necrosis factor-α (TNF-α) and NO. This study consisted in the isolation of *B. adolescentis* from 20 healthy Koreans 20–30 years old. Extracts were prepared in several concentrations ranging from 12.5 μg/mL up to 200 μg/mL and incubated with the different cell lines mentioned earlier. There was a significant decrease in the proliferation of the three human colon cancer cells, correlated with the increase in TNF-α and NO production, from 25 μg/mL to 200 μg/mL in a dose-dependent manner. There are no data shown for the increase in NO production. The increase in both of these immune response markers as well as the decrease in cancer cell proliferation show the potential of including *B. adolescentis* in therapy or diet diminishing cancer advance; however, studies should be done *in vivo*, without using an extract, and also in clinical trials before reaching a definitive conclusion [33].

Fructans and soybean meal (SM) were used to evaluate the effect on tumors. Some of the variables measured in colorectal cancer-induced rats with azoxymethane were GST activity and bacterial enzyme activity. Ninety Fisher 344 male rats were randomly assigned to nine groups, which difference was the diet. Control groups rats were fed with American Institute of Nutrition-93 Growth/Maintenance (AIN-93G/M) diet, and the eight groups were fed with the following diets: prebiotics 5%, prebiotics 10%, SM 5%, SM 10%, prebiotics 5% + SM 5%, 10% + SM 10%, 5% + SM 10% and 10% + SM 5%. Tumors present in control group were bigger in size than those fed with either fructans, soybean meal or both. GST activity was increased in two- to fourfold in rats fed with treatment diets compared to the control group, and β-glucosidase activity showed no significant difference between control group and treatment one, with the exception of a significant increase in rats fed with prebiotics 10% and rats fed with prebiotics and SM 10% + 5%. Overall there were better results obtained in prebiotics + SM consumption [34]. These results suggest that prebiotics can be used in treatment of colorectal cancer.

L. acidophilus has also shown properties in colon tumor suppression in rats. This probiotic was inoculated into female BALB/cByJ mice during 14 consecutive days at a concentration of 1 × 10^8 CFU/mouse. After 14 days, cancer cell implantation was done using CT-26 cells in a concentration of 5 × 10^6. And during the following 3 weeks, 1 × 10^9 CFU/mouse of *L. acidophilus* was inoculated. After 28 days of tumor induction, mice were killed and several variables were assessed, such as chemokine mRNA expression, tumor size and cell surface phenotypes. For the statistical analysis of results, one-way and two-way ANOVA tests were used. Tumors in rats that were pre-inoculated showed a 50.3% size reduction, and there was an enhanced tumor apoptosis and downregulation of CXCR4 mRNA expressions in colon. These results show that *L. acidophilus* is able to play a role in attenuating tumor growth as well as increasing apoptosis in tumor tissue [35]. This study contributes to the understanding in how probiotics regulate tumor proliferation in an *in vivo* system.

The effect of inulin and lactulose on procarcinogenic biomarkers in 1,2-dimethylhydrazine dihydrochloride (DMH)-induced rats has also been evaluated. Thirty-two male Sprague Dawley rats were divided into four groups: group I which is the control group received a single dose of EDTA saline solution per week, group II received a single dose of DMH per week, group III received a single dose of DMH + inulin 10 mg/0.1 mL and Group IV received DMH + lactulose 14 mg/0.1 mL. All doses were given during the course of 6 weeks. For groups III and IV, prebiotics were administered orally daily and on the 8th day, a single dose of DMH was administered. Three variables were measured among others, and these are as follows: nitroreductase, β-glucosidase and β-glucuronidase activities. Statistical analysis was done using one-way ANOVA and a post hoc LSD tests. Activity of β-glucuronidase (0.045 ± 0.006 μg/h/mg) and β-glucosidase (1.007 ± 0.115 μg/h/mg) was found to be decreased in the inulin + DMH group when compared to control (0.243 ± 0.059 μg/h/mg and 2.219 ± 0.745 μg/h/mg, respectively). Nitroreductase activity was increased in inulin + DMH (0.045 ± 0.005 μg/h/mg) compared to control (0.0162 ± 0.005 μg/h/mg) [36]. These results also suggest the colorectal cancer protection properties of inulin, which could be used in the prevention of developing colorectal cancer.

On similar study, thirty male and female Sprague Dawley rats were divided into three groups: a control group fed only with conventional feed, a DMH group and a DMH + inulin fed group. DMH and DMH + inulin group were treated with DMH at a dose of 21 mg/kg five times in weekly intervals, and DMH + inulin rats were fed with a dose of 80 g/kg of conventional feed during 28 weeks. For statistical analysis of the variables evaluated, a one-way ANOVA test was used. It was found that activity of β-glucuronidase decreased as well as the number of COX-2- and NFκB-positive cells along with a decrease in the expression of IL-2, TNF-α and IL-10. Moreover, there was a significant decrease in β-glucosidase activity (0.03 ± 0.02 μmol/min/g) when compared to the control group (0.08 ± 0.02 μmol/min/g), and also there was a significant decrease in coliforms (5.96 ± 0.22 log_{10} CFU/g) when compared to control (6.17 ± 0.56 log_{10} CFU/g) and DMH group 6.34 ± 0.25 log_{10} CFU/g). This decrease in coliforms explains the reduction in β-glucuronidase activity. Butyric and propionic acid levels were higher in DMH + inulin group, and these short-chain fatty acids have been associated with apoptosis and metastasis, carcinogen reduction, among others [37].

Several other studies have been made, and these are shown along with a brief summary of each in **Table 2**.

Authors	Component	Organism/cell line	Dosage/length	Study's design
[38]	*L. delbrueckii* fermentation supernatant	Colon cancer SW620	Several protein concentrations ranging from 0 up to 0.75 mg/mL 24 h	*L. delbrueckii* fermented MRS medium. Supernatant was incubated with SW620 cells and evaluated in viability essays Statistical analysis were done using one-way ANOVA and Bonferroni's multiple comparison test
[39]	*L. plantarum* *L. rhamnosus* supernatants	Caco-2 HT-29	2.5, 5 and 10 mg/mL 48 h	Probiotic fermented medium Supernatants was incubated with cancer cells and evaluated viability Statistical data were analyzed using one-way ANOVA
[40]	*L. casei*	C57BL/6 mice	1 × 10^8 CFU 10 weeks	Mice were administered probiotic and DMH, intestinal damage evaluation, cytokine analysis, gene expression analysis Bonferroni's multiple comparison test
[41]	Xylooligo saccharides (XOS)	Wistar rats	5% and 10% XOS 45 days	XOS diet in rats, bacterial analysis y cecal matter, biochemical assays, proliferation markers One-way ANOVA
[42]	*L. paracasei*	HT-29	0, 10, 50, 100, MOI 48 h	Calculation of multiplicity of infection (MOI), analysis cell distribution, RNA extraction, and semiquantitative RT-PCR One-way ANOVA and Duncan's post hoc tests

Table 2. Recent studies done regarding colorectal cancer using prebiotics or probiotics.

3.2. Functional foods in colorectal cancer

To the best of our knowledge, only a couple of studies have been made regarding prebiotic, probiotic or synbiotic functional foods for prevention, control or treatment of colorectal cancer.

A synbiotic food using oligofructose-enriched inulin and *L. rhamnosus* and *B. lactis* was developed and evaluated as a potential reduction risk agent in colorectal cancer patients. This

http://dx.doi.org/10.5772/63643

study was a randomized double-blinded placebo-controlled trial in which 37 colon cancer patients were divided into a control group or an intervention one. Intervention patients were given daily a synbiotic food during 12 weeks consisting of 12 g of inulin and 10^{10} CFU of probiotics. For statistical analysis of the data, a generalized linear modeling was used. It was found that the number of *Bifidobacterium* and *Lactobacillus* in feces was increased, while a decrease in the number of *Clostridium* was found. The effect of the synbiotic intervention on DNA damage, as well as the effect on epithelial barrier functions in tumor cell invasion, was also studied. It was found that intervention group had a significant decrease in the level of DNA damage (55.84 ± 21.21 tail lengths) compared to the placebo group (59.18 ± 15.94 tail lengths), but there was no significant difference between control (101.9 ± 6.6) and intervention group (104.9 ± 6.2). A decrease in the level of DNA suggests that there was a decrease in exposure of the colon epithelium to cytotoxic and genotoxic agents, along with decreased cancer cell proliferation. An improvement of the epithelial barrier function is associated with lower cancer risk, while in this study there was no significant difference, it has been seen that probiotics provide a better formation of this layer [43].

A study was done on 56 F344 rats using a probiotic fermented milk with *L. acidophilus, L. casei* and *L. rhamnosus*. The rats were divided into seven groups randomly: group 1 served as control by receiving 0.85% saline solution by gavage. Rats in groups 2–7 were injected with DMH 30 mg/kg once a week for 6 weeks; group 2 served as positive carcinogenic control, and groups 3 through 7 were supplemented with 2, 1.5, 1, 0.5 and 0.25 mL of probiotic milk containing at least 50×10^9 CFU during 12 weeks. Variables were observed and evaluated such as the activity of quinone reductase (QR), GST and β-glucuronidase. Statistical analysis of the data was done using one-way ANOVA test. It was found that G4 and G5 improved 154% and 109% compared to control group. QR activity was reduced significantly in all rats treated with DMH when compared to the control group. β-Glucuronidase activity showed a significant decrease by 49% compared to control group. This study shows that there is potential in probiotic functional foods in the prevention, control and treatment of colorectal cancer; however, further studies are needed in order to provide more information about this [44].

4. Conclusions and perspectives

The effect of prebiotics, probiotics and synbiotics over several health markers in T2DM and colorectal cancer patients has been shown through several studies discussed in this chapter. Some of the health benefits presented in this chapter for T2DM are the improvement of lipid and glycemic profile, increase in blood insulin concentration and modulation on the inflammatory response. For colorectal cancer, some of the health benefits presented in this chapter are the modulation of the immune response, antitumor activity and tumor size reduction. However, further research is needed in order to understand completely the specific molecular pathway of each component has.

The use of functional foods for prevention and control of T2DM is a promising opportunity which must be taken into account, after all, and one of the most common causes of this disease is obesity and poor diet. The design of functional foods with prebiotics, probiotics or synbiotics that will help enhance T2DM patient's health would be an aid in the fight against it; however, the elimination or substitution of antidiabetic drugs is not recommended or endorsed.

There is much to do in the research of prebiotic, probiotic or synbiotic functional foods for the prevention, control or treatment of colorectal cancer. There is evidence suggesting that therapy enhances patient's health, and this should encourage further research into the development of functional foods and their clinical studies in patients. If successful results during the following years are obtained, this could provide as an aid in the fight against colorectal cancer.

The use of functional foods should be used with caution and as a support to clinical therapy, not exclusively as an alternative. This combination could lead to further improvement in patient's health as some studies have found synergistic effect of probiotics along with medical drugs.

Author details

Samuel Longoria-García[1], Ruth E. Belmares-Cerda[1], Mildred I.M. Flores-Verástegui[2], Juan C. Contreras-Esquivel[1], Julio C. Montañez-Sáenz[1] and Mario Alberto Cruz-Hernández[2*]

*Address all correspondence to: myke13_80@hotmail.com

1 Department of Food Research, School of Chemical Sciences, Autonomous University of Coahuila, Saltillo, Coahuila, Mexico

2 Department of Food Science and Technology, Antonio Narro Autonomous Agricultural University, Buenavista Saltillo, Coahuila, Mexico

References

[1] Zannini E., Pontonio E., WatersD. M., Arendt E. K. Applications of microbial fermentations for production of gluten-free products and perspectives. Applied Microbiology and Biotechnology. 2012;93(2):473-485. DOI: 10.1007/s00253-011-3707-3

[2] Mensink M. A., Frijlink H.W., Van der Voort M.K., Hinrichs L.J. Inulin, a flexible oligosaccharide I: Review of its physicochemical characteristics. Carbohydrate Polymers. 2015;130DOI: 10.1016/j.carbpol.2015.05.026

[3] Mensink M.A., Frijlink H.W., Van der Voort M.K., Hinrichs L.J. Inulin, a flexible oligosaccharide. II: Review of its pharmaceutical applications. Carbohydrate Polymers. 2015;134:418-428. DOI: 10.1016/j.carbpol.2015.08.022

[4] Siró I., Kápolna E., Kápolna B., Lugasi A. Functional food. Product development, marketing and consumer acceptance—A review. Appetite. 2008;51(3):456-467. DOI: 10.1016/j.appet.2008.05.060

[5] Wisse B., Zieve D., Ogilvie I. Diabetes: MedlinePlus Medical Encyclopedia [Internet]. [Updated: 8/5/2014]. Available from: https://www.nlm.nih.gov/medlineplus/ency/article/001214.htm [Accessed: 02/01/2016]

[6] Mazloom Z., Yousefinejad A., Dabbaghmanesh, M. H. Effect of Probiotics on Lipid Profile , Glycemic Control , Insulin Action , Oxidative Stress , and Inflammatory Markers in Patients with Type 2 Diabetes : A Clinical Trial. Iranian Journal of Medical Sciences. 2013;38(1):38-43.

[7] WHO. WHO Diabetes: The cost of Diabetes [Internet].Available from: http://www.who.int/mediacentre/factsheets/fs236/en/ [Accessed: 2/01/2016]

[8] Yang W., Dall T.M., Halder P., Gallo P., Kowal S. L., Hogan P. F., et al. Economic costs of diabetes in the U.S. in 2012. Diabetes care. 2013;36(4):1033-1046. DOI: 10.2337/dc12-2625

[9] Brown A. C., Valiere A. Probiotics and Medical Nutrition Therapy. Nutrition Clinical Care. 2004;7(2):56-68. DOI: 10.1016/j.micinf.2011.07.011.Innate

[10] Gomes A. C., Bueno A. A., de Souza G. M., Mota J. F. Gut microbiota, probiotics and diabetes. Nutrition journal. 2014;13(60)DOI: 10.1186/1475-2891-13-60

[11] Zhang Y., Guo X., Guo J., He Q., Li H., Song Y., et al. Lactobacillus casei reduces susceptibility to type 2 diabetes via microbiota-mediated body chloride ion influx. Scientific reports. 2014;4:5654. DOI: 10.1038/srep05654

[12] Boeckner L. S., Schnepf M. I., Tungland B. C. Inulin: A review of nutritional and health implications. Advances in Food and Nutrition Research. 2001;43:1-63. DOI: 10.1016/S1043-4526(01)43002-6

[13] Al-Salami H., Butt G., Fawcett J.P., Tucker I.G., Golocorbin-Kon S., Mikov M. Probiotic treatment reduces blood glucose levels and increases systemic absorption of gliclazide in diabetic rats. European journal of drug metabolism and pharmacokinetics. 2008;33(2):101-106. DOI: 10.1007/BF03191026

[14] Aliasgharzadeh A., Khalili M., Mirtaheri E., Gargari B. P., Farhangi M. A., Babaei H., et al. A Combination of Prebiotic Inulin and Oligofructose Improve Some of Cardiovascular Disease Risk Factors in Women with Type 2 Diabetes: A Randomized Controlled Clinical Trial. Advanced Pharmaceutical Bulletin. 2015;5(4):507-514. DOI: 10.15171/apb.2015.069

[15] Zhang Y., Wang L., Zhang J., Li Y., He Q., Li H., et al. Probiotic Lactobacillus casei Zhang ameliorates high-fructose-induced impaired glucose tolerance in hyperinsulinemia rats. European Journal of Nutrition. 2014;53(1):221-232. DOI: 10.1007/s00394-013-0519-5

[16] Alokail M. S., Sabico S., Al-saleh Y., Al-daghri N. M., Alkharfy K. M., Vanhoutte P. M., et al. Effects of probiotics in patients with diabetes mellitus type 2 : study protocol for a randomized . Trials. 2013;14:195.

[17] Kellow N.J., Coughlan M.T., Savige G. S., Reid C. M. Effect of dietary prebiotic supplementation on advanced glycation, insulin resistance and inflammatory biomarkers in adults with pre-diabetes: a study protocol for a double-blind placebo-controlled randomised crossover clinical trial. BMC endocrine disorders. 2014;14(1):55. DOI: 10.1186/1472-6823-14-55

[18] Asemi Z., Sahar B., Shakeri H., Jamal A., Faraji A. Effect of multispecies probiotic supplements on serum minerals, liver enzymes and blood pressure in patients with type 2 diabetes. International Journal of Diabetes in Developing Countries. 2015;35(2): 90-95. DOI: 10.1159/000349922

[19] Mitchell C.M., Davy B.M., Halliday T.M., Hulver M.W., Neilson A.P., Ponder M.A., et al. The effect of prebiotic supplementation with inulin on cardiometabolic health: Rationale, design, and methods of a controlled feeding efficacy trial in adults at risk of type 2 diabetes. Contemporary Clinical Trials. 2015;45:328-337. DOI: 10.1016/j.cct.2015.10.012

[20] Tonucci, L. B., Olbrich dos Santos K. M., Licursi de Oliveira L., Rocha Ribeiro S.M., Duarte Martino H. S. Clinical application of probiotics in type 2 diabetes mellitus: A randomized, double-blind, placebo-controlled study. Clinical Nutrition. Forthcoming. DOI: 10.1016/j.clnu.2015.11.011

[21] Stenman L. K., Waget A., Garret C., Briand F., Burcelin R., Sulpice T., et al. Probiotic B420 and prebiotic polydextrose improve efficacy of antidiabetic drugs in mice. Diabetology & Metabolic Syndrome. 2015;7:75. DOI: 10.1186/s13098-015-0075-7

[22] Ejtahed H. S., Mohtadi-Nia J., Homayouni-Rad A., Niafar M., Asghari-Jafarabadi M., Mofid V., et al. Effect of probiotic yogurt containing Lactobacillus acidophilus and Bifidobacterium lactis on lipid profile in individuals with type 2 diabetes mellitus. Journal of dairy science. 2011;94(7):3288-3294. DOI: 10.3168/jds.2010-4128

[23] Ejtahed H. S., Mohtadi-Nia J., Homayouni-Rad A., Niafar M., Asghari-Jafarabadi M., Mofid V. Probiotic yogurt improves antioxidant status in type 2 diabetic patients. Nutrition. 2012;28(5):539-543. DOI: 10.1016/j.nut.2011.08.013

[24] Shakeri H., Hadaegh H., Abedi F., Tajabadi-Ebrahimi M., Mazroii N., Ghandi Y., et al. Consumption of synbiotic bread decreases triacylglycerol and VLDL levels while increasing HDL levels in serum from patients with type-2 diabetes. Lipids. 2014;49(7): 695-701. DOI: 10.1007/s11745-014-3901-z

[25] Asemi Z., Khorrami-Rad A., Alizadeh S.A., Shakeri H., Esmaillzadeh A. Effects of synbiotic food consumption on metabolic status of diabetic patients: A double-blind randomized cross-over controlled clinical trial. Clinical Nutrition. 2014;33(2):198-203. DOI: 10.1016/j.clnu.2013.05.015

[26] Asemi Z., Alizadeh S., Ahmad K., Goli M.,Esmaillzadeh A. Effects of beta-carotene fortified synbiotic food on metabolic control of patients with type 2 diabetes mellitus: A double-blind randomized cross-over controlled clinical trial. Clinical nutrition . Forthcoming. DOI: 10.1016/j.clnu.2015.07.009

[27] Bahmani F., Tajadadi-Ebrahimi M., Kolahdooz F., Mazouchi M., Hadaegh H., Jamal A., et al. The Consumption of Synbiotic Bread Containing Lactobacillus sporogenes and Inulin Affects Nitric Oxide and Malondialdehyde in Patients with Type 2 Diabetes Mellitus: Randomized, Double-Blind, Placebo-Controlled Trial. Journal of the American College of Nutrition. 2015;0(0):1-8. DOI: 10.1080/07315724.2015.1032443

[28] Ferlay J., Soerjomataram I., Ervik M., Dikshit R., Eser S., Mathers C., et al. Cancer Incidence and Mortality Worldwide: IARC CancerBase No. 11 [Internet]. 2012 . Available from: http://globocan.iarc.fr [Accessed: 2/01/2016]

[29] Mariotto A. B., Robin Yabroff K., Shao Y., Feuer E.J., Brown M.L. Projections of the cost of cancer care in the United States: 2010-2020. Journal of the National Cancer Institute. 2011;103(2):117-128. DOI: 10.1093/jnci/djq495

[30] The American Cancer Society. The Global Economic Cost of Cancer. In: LiveStrong, editor. The American Cancer Society; 2012. p. 1-14.

[31] Liong M. T. Roles of probiotics and prebiotics in colon cancer prevention: Postulated mechanisms and in-vivo evidence. nternational Journal of Molecular Sciences. 2008;9(5):854-863. DOI: 10.3390/ijms9050854

[32] Roller M., Clune Y., Collins K., Rechkemmer G., Watzl B. Consumption of prebiotic inulin enriched with oligofructose in combination with the probiotics Lactobacillus rhamnosus and Bifidobacterium lactis has minor effects on selected immune parameters in polypectomised and colon cancer patients. The British journal of nutrition. 2007;97(4):676-684. DOI: 10.1017/S0007114507450292

[33] Lee D. K., Jang S.,Kim M. J., Kim J. H., Chung M. J., Kim K. J., et al. Anti-proliferative effects of Bifidobacterium adolescentis SPM0212 extract on human colon cancer cell lines. BMC cancer. 2008;8:310. DOI: 10.1186/1471-2407-8-310

[34] Gourineni V. P., Verghese M., Boateng J., Shackelford L., Bhat N. K., Walker L. T. Combinational effects of prebiotics and soybean against azoxymethane-induced colon cancer in vivo. Journal of Nutrition and Metabolism. 2011;:868197. DOI: 10.1155/2011/868197

[35] Chen C.C., Lin W.C., Kong M.S., Shi H.N., Walker W.A., Lin C.Y., et al. Oral inoculation of probiotics Lactobacillus acidophilus NCFM suppresses tumour growth both in segmental orthotopic colon cancer and extra-intestinal tissue. British Journal of Nutrition. 2012;107(11):1623-1634. DOI: 10.1017/S0007114511004934

[36] Verma A., Shukla G. Administration of prebiotic inulin suppresses 1,2 dimethylhydrazine dihydrochloride induced procarcinogenic biomarkers fecal enzymes and

preneoplastic lesions in early colon carcinogenesis in Sprague Dawley rats. Journal of Functional Foods. 2013;5(2):991-996. DOI: 10.1016/j.jff.2013.02.006

[37] Hijová E., Szabadosova Vi., Štofilová J., Hrcková G. Chemopreventive and metabolic effects of inulin on colon cancer development. Journal of Veterinary Science. 2013;14(4): 387-393. DOI: 10.4142/jvs.2013.14.4.387

[38] Wan Ying., Xin Y., Zhang C., Wu D., Ding D., Tang L., et al. Fermentation supernatants of lactobacillus delbrueckii inhibit growth of human colon cancer cells and induce apoptosis through a caspase 3-dependent pathway. Oncology Letters. 2014;7(5):1738-1742. DOI: 10.3892/ol.2014.1959

[39] Sadeghi-Aliabadi H., Mohammadi F., Fazeli H., Mirlohi M. Effects of lactobacillus plantarum A7 with probiotic potential on colon cancer and normal cells proliferation in comparison with a commercial strain. Iranian Journal of Basic Medical Sciences. 2014;17(10):815-819.

[40] Lenoir M., del Carmen S., Cortes-Perez N.G., Lozano-Ojalvo D., Muñoz-Provencio D., Chain F., et al. Lactobacillus casei BL23 regulates Treg and Th17 T-cell populations and reduces DMH-associated colorectal cancer. Journal of Gastroenterology. 2016;1–12.DOI: 10.1007/s00535–015–1158–9.

[41] Aachary A.A., Gobinath D., Srinivasan K., Prapulla S. G. Protective effect of xylooligosaccharides from corncob on 1,2-dimethylhydrazine induced colon cancer in rats. Bioactive Carbohydrates and Dietary Fibre. 2015;5(2):146-152. DOI: 10.1016/j.bcdf.2015.03.004

[42] Huang L., Shan Y., He C., Ren M., Tian P., Song W. Effects of L. paracasei subp. paracasei X12 on cell cycle of colon cancer HT-29 cells and regulation of mTOR signalling pathway. Journal of Functional Foods. 2016;21:431-439. DOI: 10.1016/j.jff.2015.12.024

[43] Rafter J., Bennett M., Caderni G., Clune Y., Hughes R., Karlsson P. C., et al. Dietary synbiotics reduce cancer risk factors in polypectomized and colon cancer patients. American Journal of Clinical Nutrition. 2007;85(2):488-496. DOI: 85/2/488 [pii]

[44] Desrouillères K., Millette M., Vu K.D., Touja, R., Lacroix, M. Cancer preventive effects of a specific probiotic fermented milk containing Lactobacillus acidophilus CL1285, L. casei LBC80R and L. rhamnosus CLR2 on male F344 rats treated with 1,2-dimethylhydrazine. Journal of Functional Foods. 2015;17:816-827. DOI: 10.1016/j.jff.2015.06.035

Chapter 18

Probiotics, Prebiotics, and Biogenics for the Stomach

Yasuhiko Komatsu, Yuji Aiba, Yasuhiro Nakano and Yasuhiro Koga

Additional information is available at the end of the chapter

http://dx.doi.org/10.5772/62828

Abstract

Recently, many studies concerning probiotics, prebiotics, and biogenics have been performed, whereas only a few are related to the stomach (about 2% as publication number). In this chapter, we focus on recent studies on probiotics, prebiotics, and biogenics for the stomach and also describe our recent research on a novel strain of lactobacillus beneficial to stomach, *Lactobacillus johnsonii* No.1088 (LJ88). As probiotics for the stomach, some beneficial strains were summarized, and underlying mechanisms of anti-*Helicobacter pylori* activity were discussed. Prebiotics for the stomach were considered as a future potential target, since no indigenous bacteria beneficial to the stomach have been found to date. As biogenics, some plant-derived candidates were discussed. In this context, recent results on LJ88 lactobacillus were presented. Orally administered LJ88 inhibited *H. pylori* growth and the increase in the number of gastrin-producing cells, which side effect is caused by triple therapy for *H. pylori*. LJ88 had no resistance to typical antibiotics, and both living and heat-killed forms of it increased the number of bifidobacteria among human intestinal-microbiota in mice. These results suggest that LJ88 is a lactobacillus beneficial to both stomach and intestine as a probiotic and biogenic.

Keywords: Probiotics, Prebiotics, Biogenics, Stomach, *Helicobacter pylori*

1. Introduction

Historically, probiotics have been thought as agents beneficial to improve the microbial environment in the intestines, but some strains of lactic acid bacteria have been used as probiotics, with the claim of providing health benefits to the stomach.

Nestlé's *Lactobacillus L. johnsonii* La1 (LC1) [1–3] and Meiji's *Lactobacillus gasseri* OLL2716 [4–6] are typical strains said to be useful to reduce the number of *Helicobacter pylori* in stomach infections. Recently, we found a novel strain of lactic acid bacteria, *L. johnsonii* No.1088 (LJ88), which is extremely acid resistant and also has the ability to significantly reduce the number of infective *H.pylori* in the stomach [7]. Furthermore, LJ88 not only has anti-pylori activity but also reduces excessive gastric acid production [7]. So we are very interested in the beneficial effects of probiotics on stomach health. Likewise, those effects of "Prebiotics" are also of great interest.

In addition to living bacteria, i.e., "Probiotics", heat-killed "dead" bacteria retain some beneficial properties of probiotic bacteria. For example, the ability of heat-killed LJ88 to reduce excessive gastric acid production can be thought as having this property [7]. Such food ingredients that beneficially affect the host by "direct" stimulation, suppression, etc., were defined by Mitsuoka as "Biogenics" [8]. So we added this category to this chapter. So the title of the chapter was chosen to be "Probiotics, Prebiotics, and Biogenics for the Stomach".

In this chapter, we review the current status of probiotics, prebiotics, and biogenics for the stomach, and also discuss novel aspects of our lactic acid bacterium, LJ88, which is beneficial to the stomach.

2. Number of publications

Figure 1 depicts yearly changes up to 2014 in the number of publications related to "probiotics OR prebiotics OR biogenics" as a whole (A) and those related to the stomach (B), based on a PubMed search. The total number of publications shown in Figure 1A was 14,417, of which those including the word "stomach" (Figure 1B) were only 290 (about 2% of the total publications). As shown in Figure 1A, the number of publications in this area increased almost linearly from year 2000, reaching 1936 publications in 2014; whereas the subset related to the stomach hit its ceiling at about 30 publications/year (Figure 1B).

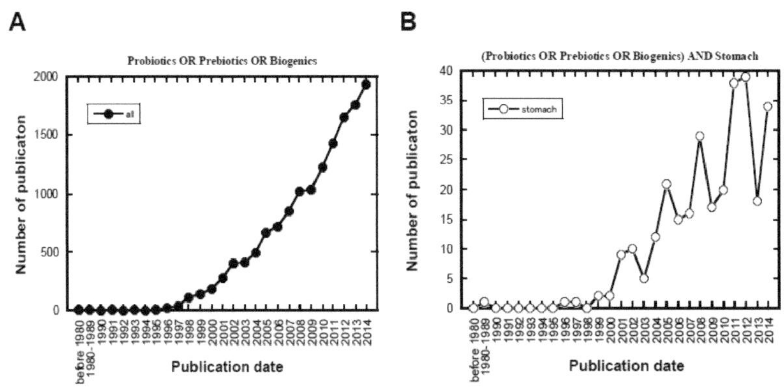

Figure 1. Yearly change in the number of publications related to probiotics/prebiotics/biogenics (A) and the subset of "A" related to the stomach (B).

As shown above, probiotics/prebiotics/biogenics involving the stomach is not a major area of this research field. However, since a variety of bacteria have been detected not only from feces or saliva but also from gastric fluid, although mainly as dead forms [9], it is thought that this area will expand in the future.

2.1. Anti-H. pylori activity of probiotics

2.1.1. Probiotics and virulent bacteria

Although a very recent definition of probiotics is "live microorganisms, which when consumed in adequate amounts, confer a health effect on the host" [10], probiotics have been thought as agents that improve the balance of microbiota mainly in the intestines. Typically, the ingestion of probiotics brings about an increase in the number of so-called "beneficial bacteria", e.g., bifidobacteria, and a decrease in the number of so-called "bad" bacteria, e.g., clostridia. Moreover, some probiotic strains have been reported to inhibit the growth of some virulent bacteria, resulting in prevention of and recovery from diarrhea.

As regards the stomach, *H. pylori* is the main virulent bacteria residing in the gastric mucosa, causing chronic gastritis and peptic ulcer. Also, *H. pylori* is now thought to be responsible for almost all cases of gastric cancer [11]. Some strains of probiotic bacteria have been reported to be effective in reducing the number of *H. pylori*, and also decreasing the extent of inflammation caused by infection by this bacterium.

2.1.2. Probiotic strains useful to reduce symptoms related to H. pylori infection

One of the well-known probiotic strains beneficial for the treatment of *H. pylori* infections is *L. johnsonii* La1, which was found and developed by a Swiss company, Nestlé, and has been widely used in fermented milk worldwide [1–3]. Another strain beneficial to *H. pylori*-infected subjects is *L. gasseri* OLL2716, found by Meiji, a Japanese company [4–6]. This strain is now used mainly in fermented milk in Japan as LG21 and promoted as "lactic acid bacteria combating risk" (a catchy tag from Meiji). In addition to these two strains of probiotic bacteria, some other strains have been reported to be effective in ameliorating symptoms derived from *H. pylori* infection, e.g., *Lactobacillus acidophilus* Strain LB [12], *Bacillus subtilis* 3 [13], *Weissella confusa* Strain PL9001 [14], *Lactobacillus delbrueckii subsp. bulgaricus* [15], and *Lactobacillus reuteri* [16].

2.1.3. L. johnsonii No. 1088 (LJ88) as a probiotic

Recently, we found a novel strain of lactobacillus, LJ88, in the gastric juice of a healthy human volunteer. When administered as a living form, LJ88 reduced the number of *H. pylori* in the stomach of human intestinal microbiota-bearing mice, as shown in **Figure 2** [7]. This anti-*H. pylori* effect of LJ88 can be brought not only by proliferating bacteria (Figure 2A) but also by its lyophilized form (Figure 2B), suggesting that this strain is useful both as fermented milk and also as the lyophilized form of a dietary supplement.

From Aiba et al. [7] with permission.

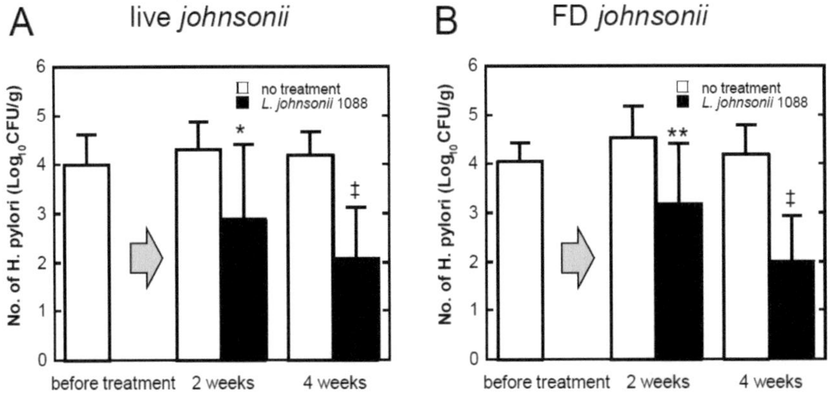

Figure 2. *Anti-H. pylori* effect of *L. johnsonii* No. 1088 (LJ88) in human intestinal microbiota-bearing mice. Mice with human intestinal microbiota were prepared by using germ-free mice and were then infected with *H. pylori* No. 130 (10^9 cfu/mice). *H. pylori*-bearing mice were orally and daily administered live LJ88 (A) or a comparable number of lyophilized cells (B) for two or four weeks. In mice treated with either live or the lyophilized (freeze-dried) form of LJ88, the number of *H. pylori* in the stomach was significantly decreased. Statistical significance was determined by use of Student's *t*-test ($*p < 0.05$, $**p < 0.01$, $‡p < 0.0001$ vs. no treatment for comparable time periods).

To evaluate the probiotic property of LJ88, we examined the sensitivity of LJ88 to different types of antibiotics. Mueller–Hinton agar plates containing 128, 64, 32, 16, 8, 4, 2, 1, 0.5, 0.25, 0.125, 0.0625, 0.031, 0.016, 0.008, 0.004, 0.002 or 0.001 μg/mL of different antibiotics (ampicillin, oxacillin, cefoxitin, gentamicin, clarithromycin, vancomycin, ciprofloxacin, and chloramphenicol) were prepared; and 5000 cfu of LJ88 (5 μL), after having been cultured in Mueller–Hinton broth for 24 h at 37 °C, was inoculated onto each plate. The minimum inhibitory concentrations (MICs) were determined after cultivation for 48 h at 37°C. The results are depicted in **Table 1**. As shown in **Table 1**, no resistance to any of the antibiotics used was observed, suggesting that LJ88 should be of no concern with respect to the transfer of drug-resistance genes to virulent bacteria.

Antibiotics	**MIC (μg/mL)**
ampicilin	0.004
oxacillin	0.125
cefoxitin	0.004
gentamicin	0.25
clarithromycin	0.5
vancomycin	0.016
ciprofloxacin	0.5
chloramphenicol	0.5

Table 1. MIC of various antibiotics against LJ88.

http://dx.doi.org/10.5772/62828

To know whether LJ88 is also beneficial to intestinal microbiota, we examined the effect of live LJ88 on the number of bifidobacteria and clostridia in the feces of human intestinal microbiota-bearing mice. These mice were established as described earlier [7]. In brief, 0.5 mL of human feces diluted 100-fold with water were administered to male germ-free Balb/c mice (4 weeks old). Then 10^9 cfu of LJ88 was orally administered once a day for 2 weeks. The amount of lactobacilli, bifidobacteria, and clostridia in the feces of mice were determined before and after LJ88 administration. The results are shown in **Figure 3**. Although lactobacilli were not detected before administration of LJ88, about 10^8 cfu/g of lactobacilli appeared after its administration (Figure 3A), which might reflect the administered LJ88. In association with the administration of LJ88, the number of bifidobacteria and clostridia increased and decreased, respectively (Figure 3B and C). Since bifidobacteria are reportedly beneficial to human health due to their ability to regulate intestinal microbial homeostasis [17], the bifidobacteria-increasing effect of LJ88 is thought to be one of its beneficial effects on the intestines. Although not all of the species belonging to clostridia are virulent, some of them are known to be harmful to human health, e.g. *Clostridium difficile* [18], *Clostridium perfringens* [19], etc. So the effect LJ88 of reducing the number of clostridia in the intestines is another beneficial property of LJ88. These data taken together suggest that LJ88 is a probiotic strain of lactobacilli beneficial to both stomach and intestines.

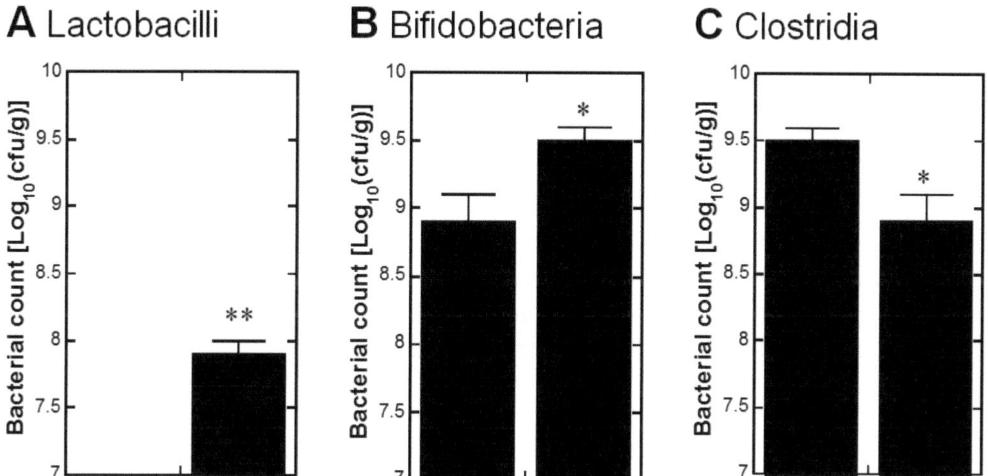

Figure 3. Effect of live *Lactocacillus johnsonii* No.1088 (LJ88) on the number of lactobacilli (A), bifidobacteria (B), and chlostoridia (C) in feces of human intestinal microbiota-bearing mice. LJ88 in the measure of 10^9 cfu was orally administered once a day for two weeks, and the number of bacteria in feces was determined. Each bar represents mean with standard deviation ($n = 5$). *$p < 0.05$, and **$p < 0.001$ vs. control by Student's t-test.

2.1.4. Limitation of probiotics against H. pylori

Although many reports including in vitro, in vivo, and clinical studies have suggested the effectiveness of probiotics against *H. pylori* infection, complete eradication cannot be attained by probiotics alone. The standard and more effective way to eradicate *H. pylori* infections is the so-called "triple therapy" consisting of two antibiotics and one proton pump inhibitor (PPI) [20]. But the cost for such a therapy is expensive, and so a lower cost way to control the extent of *H. pylori* at a level under the asymptomatic one is needed. Moreover, since the eradication rate of this triple therapy is not 100%, probiotics effective in increasing the eradication rate of triple therapy might be meaningful. In fact, some strains have been reported to have such a property [21].

2.1.5. *Possible mechanism underlying anti-H. pylori activity of probiotics*

Although the exact mechanisms underlying the anti-*H. pylori* activity of probiotics have not yet been fully elucidated, some putative ones have been proposed, as shown in **Table 2**. We describe them in brief here.

Proposed Mechanisms	**Described in**
Lactic acid production	2.1.5.1
Production of antimicrobial products	2.1.5.2
Competition for adherent sites	2.1.5.3
Immunological mechanisms	2.1.5.4
Co-aggregation with *Helicobacter pylori*	2.1.5.5

Table 2. Putative mechanisms by which probiotics inhibit *H. pylori.*

2.1.5.1. *Lactic acid*

H. pylori can survive in the highly acidic gastric mucosa by producing urease, which degrades urea to ammonia and carbon dioxide, and the resulting ammonia neutralizes the gastric acid to elevate pH of surrounding environment. Lactic acid produced by probiotic bacteria competes with the pH elevation by urease mentioned above, which makes the environment unsuitable for *H. pylori* to survive [22–24]. In addition to acidification, lactic acid inhibits urease activity itself [22], which might be another molecular mechanism for lactic acid to inhibit survival of *H. pylori* in the stomach. But since not all lactic acid bacteria producing the same level of lactic acid can inhibit *H. pylori* to the same extent [3], the production of lactic acid may only be part of the anti-*H. pylori* effect of lactic acid bacteria.

2.1.5.2. *Antimicrobial products*

Some probiotic strains have reported to secrete antimicrobial substances other than lactic acid. The culture supernatants of *L. johnsonii* La1 [3] and *L. acidophilus* Strain LB [12] can inhibit the growth of *H. pylori* in vitro and in vivo in a pH-independent manner, but the molecular structures of these active substances have not yet been determined. Moreover, some strains of *L. delbrueckii supsp. bulgaricus* reportedly inhibit the growth of *H. pylori* in an agar-well diffusion assay under both acidic and neutral pH conditions, suggesting secretion of anti-*H. pylori* substances [15]. Bacteriocins are being widely investigated as proteinaceous antimicrobial substances produced by bacteria [25]. Kim et al. examined the anti-*H. pylori* activity of selected known bacteriocins and found that lacticins A164 and BH5 produced by *Lactococcus lactis subsp. lactis* A164 and BH5, respectively, strongly inhibit the growth of *H. pylori* [26]. Other than lactic acid bacteria, another probiotic strain of bacillus, *B. subtilis* 3, has been reported to produce aminocoumacin A, another anti-*H. pylori* substance [13]. As described here, the molecular nature of almost all of the anti-*H. pylori* substances produced by probiotic bacteria is unknown and remains to be elucidated.

2.1.5.3. Competition

For *H. pylori* to grow in gastric mucosa, it is necessary first for the bacteria to adhere to the inner surface of the stomach. So if probiotics and/or its products can compete with the sites where *H. pylori* adhere, the growth of *H. pylori* might be inhibited. Kabir et al. reported that an anti-*H. pylori* strain of *Lactobacillus salivarius* inhibit the attachment of *H. pylori* to human gastric cell lines (MKN45 and KATO-III) and murine gastric epithelial cells, whereas other lactic acid bacteria not inhibiting *H. pylori* (*Enterococcus faecalis*, and also *Streptococcus aureus*) do not [27]. Furthermore, *L. reuteri* has been reported to compete with the specific binding sites of *H. pylori*, i.e., asialo-GMI and sulfatide [28]. Such competition which is either specific or nonspecific, might be one of the potential mechanisms underlying the anti-*H. pylori* activity of probiotics.

2.1.5.4. Immunological mechanisms

H. pylori infection of the stomach stimulates the production of inflammatory cytokines, such as IL-8, resulting in the activation of monocytes and dendritic cells, which then produce Tumor necrosis factors (TNF)-α, Interleukin (IL)-1, and IL-6, which in turn stimulate Th1 helper T cells [29]. Such reactions promote inflammation in the stomach to combat *H. pylori*, but these inflammatory reactions are unsuccessful to eradicate the bacteria. However, some probiotic strains have reported to reduce the extent of inflammation and to decrease the level of specific Immunoglobulin (IgG) against *H. pylori* in animal models [22, 24, 27].

2.1.5.5. Coaggregation

Coaggregation with pathogenic bacteria has been proposed as a mechanism by which probiotic bacteria can inhibit the growth of pathogenic bacterial. Recently, Holtz et al. reported that nonviable *L. reuteri* DSM17648 coaggregates with *H. pylori* and exerts anti-*H. pylori* activity [30]. So this mechanism can also be thought as one of the possible mechanisms for probiotic bacteria to inhibit *H. pylori*.

2.2. Gastric acid-reducing activity of probiotics

2.2.1. Gastroesophageal reflux disease (GERD)

Gastroesophageal reflux disease (GERD) is a chronic disease caused by backflow of gastric acid to the esophagus and is subjectively recognized mainly as heartburn. Although proton pump inhibitors (PPIs) have been strongly recommended, and their effectiveness against GERD is widely recognized, hypergastrinemia is a concern as a side-effect of long-term usage of PPIs [31]. In relation to *H. pylori*, it had been debated whether *H. pylori* infection is possibly beneficial to the host by moderating the extent of acidity of gastric juice to weaken GERD [32]. However, infection by *H. pylori* itself has not been reported to bring about any difference in subjective or objective measures of GERD [33]. *H. pylori* has another implication in GERD that is related to the adverse effects of drugs used for treat *H. pylori* infection, e.g., PPIs. Mentioned earlier, the recent standard therapy for *H. pylori* is the so-called "triple therapy" including two antibiotics and one PPI. But even after successful eradication of *H. pylori* by triple therapy, cessation of PPI may possibly bring about GERD as a side effect, which might arise because of the hypergastrinemia induced by PPIs via increased gastrin production by gastrin-producing cells (G-cells) and/or an increase in the number of G-cells in the gastric epithelia. So it would be beneficial to have the way to suppress hypergastrinemia possibly caused by PPI administration. Also, in GERD without *H. pylori* infection, a way to avoid a kind of PPI-addiction to control heartburn is desirable.

2.2.2. Probiotics effective in reducing the production of gastric acid

LJ88, as mentioned above, can reduce the number of *H. pylori* in the stomach. Moreover, LJ88 has another interesting property, i.e., that of reducing the production of gastric acid. The mechanism underlying this effect has been investigated, and it was found that LJ88 reduces the number of G-cells. Because gastrin is the hormone secreted by G-cells when stimulated by a variety of stimuli [34, 35]; e.g., distension of gastric antrum, vagal stimulation, presence of partially digested proteins (amino acids, etc.), and hypercalcemia, if the number of G-cells decreases, the maximal level of production of gastrin might be reduced without cessation of the stimuli-induced increase in the production of gastrin itself. Although the standard way to treat GERD and hyperacidity might be drugs directly inhibiting production of gastric acid, e.g., PPI, H2-blocker, and Potassium-Competitive Acid Blocker (P-CAB), probiotics reducing the number of G-cells are thought to be a mild way to treat GERD and hyperacidity. In addition to LJ88, another probiotic bacteria, *L. gasseri* OLL2716 has been reported to reduce the number of gastrin-positive cells in the stomach [36]. The exact mechanism by which these bacteria reduce the number of G-cells has not been elucidated to date, although stimulation of Toll-like receptor 2 by cell-wall components has been proposed as one candidate [7].

2.3. Implications of proton-pump inhibitors for viability of gastric microbiota

The stomach is considered to be a barrier to prevent virulent bacteria from entering the gastrointestinal tract due to its high acidity. However, irrespective of such a harmful condition for bacteria, a significant number of live bacteria exist in the stomach environment.

Namely, in healthy persons, the number of live bacteria in gastric fluid is reportedly about 10^2–10^4 cfu/mL [9, 37]. But in subjects administered PPI, this number is reported to be increased 1000-fold or more over that of the subjects without PPI treatment, i.e., about 10^7 cfu/mL [9]. Since the pH value of gastric fluid in subjects treated or not with PPI is about 3.2 or 1.6, respectively [9], such an increase in live bacteria in the stomach is thought to be caused by the increase in pH due to the PPI administration. Interestingly, the number of bacteria quantified by real-time polymerase chain reaction (PCR) with universal primers to bacterial 16S rRNA is about 10^8 cfu/mL in gastric fluid, irrespective of treatment with PPI [9]. Because the quantitative PCR method counts not only living bacteria but also dead ones, almost all of the bacterial bodies are thought to exist in stomach as their dead form in normal subjects (>99.99% = $(1–10^4/10^8) \times 100$). In PPI-administered subjects, about 10% (= $10^7/10^8 \times 100$) exist alive in the stomach, suggesting that in such a condition, probiotics ingested might affect the stomach partly as their living form. In addition to the total number (both living and dead) of bacteria in gastric fluid, the composition of bacteria at the genus level is not different between PPI-treated and not-treated groups [9], so that a part of the effects of probiotic bacteria will be retained in the stomach even after bacterial death due to high acidity (as biogenics; see below).

3. Prebiotics for the stomach

Prebiotics were defined by Gibson and Roberfroid as "non-digestible food ingredients that beneficially affect the host by selectively stimulating the growth and/or activity of one or a limited number of bacterial species already resident in the colon, and thus attempt to improve host health" [38]. So if indigenous bacteria exist in stomach beneficial to host health, e.g., those corresponding to bifidobacteria in the colon, then the concept "prebiotics for the stomach" will become meaningful. However, since we do not have any evidence showing the existence of such resident bacteria in the stomach, "prebiotics for stomach" remains as a mere hypothesis for now. Of course, some beneficial indigenous bacteria may possibly be found in the stomach in the future. In such a case, "prebiotics for the stomach" will come to have a factual basis for further research and development.

4. Biogenics for the stomach

Biogenics were originally defined by Mitsuoka as "food ingredients that beneficially affect the host by direct immunostimulation, suppression of mutagenesis, tumorigenesis, peroxidation, hyper-cholesterolemia or intestinal putrefaction" [8]. He proposed the following agents as candidates of biogenics: i.e., biological response modifier (BRM), carotenoids, flavonoids, eicosapentaenoic acid, docosahexaenoic acid, lacto-tripeptide, immunopotentiators, etc. [8] Although Mitsuoka's original concept of biogenics seems not to have included beneficial effect to the stomach, we think that agents directly affecting the stomach could be thought as a kind of biogenic as well.

4.1. Heat-killed bacteria as biogenics for the stomach

4.1.1. Gastric acid-reducing activity of heat-killed bacteria

One of the characteristic effects of our LJ88 is the reduced production of gastrin, as mentioned above. We found that such an effect is the property of not only living bacteria but also heat-killed ones [7, 36], allowing LJ88 to be thought as a kind of biogenics for the stomach. We already mentioned about a possible side effect of PPI, i.e., an increase in the number of G-cells, which might cause gastric hyperacidity after cessation of PPI. Especially, such a side effect might be of concern after triple therapy to eradicate a *H. pylori* infection.

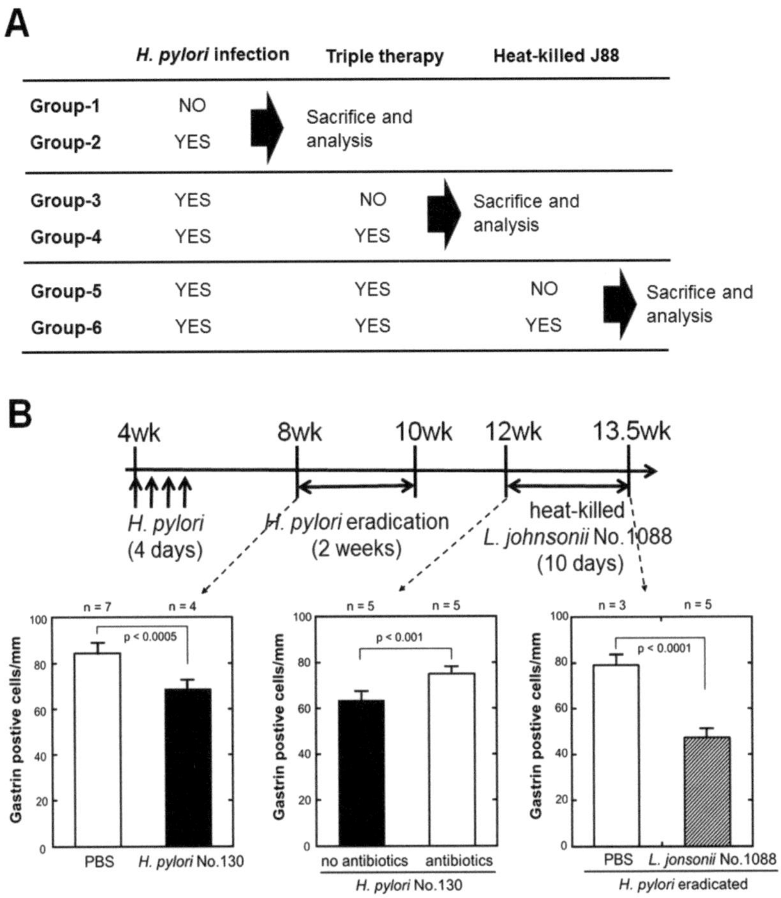

Figure 4. Increase in the number of gastrin-positive cells by *H. pylori* eradication with triple therapy including PPI, and its decrease by treatment with heat-killed *L. johnsonii* No. 1088 (LJ88). (A) Summary of different treatments of six experimental groups. (B) Results of the experiment. *H. pylori* infection of germ-free mice decreased the number of gastrin-positive cells (left-side bar graph), whereas treatment with triple therapy including PPI reverted the number of gastrin-positive cells to a higher level (middle bar graph). However, treatment with heat-killed LJ88 significantly decreased the number of gastrin-positive cells (right-side bar graph). Statistical significance was determined by use of Student's *t*-test.

To determine if LJ88 would ameliorate such a side effect of PPI in the context of triple therapy, we did an animal experiment with germ-free Balb/c mice infected with *H. pylori*. Six groups of germ-free Balb/c mice (four weeks old), each consisting of three to seven mice, were used for this experiment. The different treatments of these six experimental groups (Groups-1 to -6) are summarized in (**Figure 4A**). The mice of five groups (Groups-2 to -6) were orally administered 10^9 cfu of *H. pylori* once a day for four consecutive days, and the remaining group (Group-1) was administered PBS by the same route as a control. Four weeks after the administration of *H. pylori* or PBS, two groups (PBS and *H. pylori* groups; Groups-1 and −2) were sacrificed and examined for the difference in the number of gastrin-positive cells in their stomach as described previously [7, 36]. Three of the remaining four groups (Groups-4 to -6) with *H. pylori* administration were started to be treated with triple therapy [20, 39] (omeprazole, 150 μg/day; amoxicillin 3.75 mg/day; and clarithromycin, 2 mg/day), which was continued for two weeks. The last group (Group-3) was not administered any drugs for the same two weeks. After the triple therapy, two groups (with and without triple therapy; Groups-3 and -4) were sacrificed and analyzed for the number of gastrin-positive cells as above. Finally, the remaining two groups were orally administered (Group-6) or not (Group-5) 10^9 heat-killed LJ88 cells for 10 days; and 24 h after the last administration, these two groups were examined for their number of gastrin-positive cells.

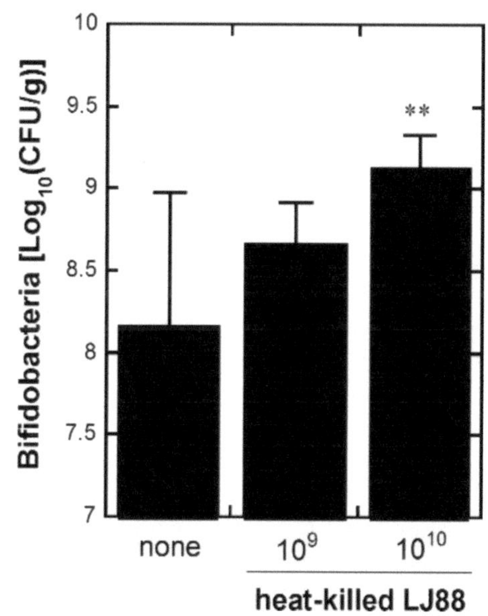

Figure 5. Effect of heat-killed *L. johnsonii* No. 1088 (LJ88) on the number of bifidobacteria in feces of human intestinal microbiota-bearing mice. Heat-killed LJ88 (10^9 and 10^{10} cells) were orally administered once a day for two weeks, and the number of bifidobacteria in the feces was determined. Each bar represents the mean with standard deviation ($n = 5$). $^{**}p < 0.01$ vs. control by Dunnett's *t*-test.

The results are shown in Figure 4B. *H. pylori* infection decreased the number of gastrin-positive cells (left-side bar graph), whereas treatment with antibiotics including PPI reverted the number of gastrin-positive cells to a higher level (middle bar graph). However, treatment with heat-killed LJ88 significantly decreased the number of gastrin-positive cells (right-side bar graph). These results suggest that LJ88, even in its heat-killed form, can prevent the increase in gastric acid after triple therapy by decreasing the number of gastrin-positive cells, the effect of which might be beneficial for prophylaxis of GERD. Since this result was obtained by using a mouse model, it should be examined whether or not the same mechanism works also in humans.

Since live LJ88 were beneficial not only to the stomach but also to intestinal microbiota, as shown in **Figure 3**, we examined the effect of heat-killed LJ88 on intestinal bacteria by determining the number of bifidobacteria in the feces of human intestinal microbiota-bearing mice. As shown in **Figure 5**, heat-killed LJ88 increased the number of bifidobacteria in the feces by the administration of 10^{10} cells for two weeks, suggesting that heat-killed LJ88 might also be beneficial to not only the stomach but also to the intestines as well.

4.1.2 Anti-H. pylori activities of heat-killed bacteria

We already described that some probiotic strains have anti-*H. pylori* activity, and possible mechanisms underlying such an activity were discussed (Section 3 and listed in **Table 2**). Among them, some mechanisms can be expected to belong not only to live bacteria (probiotics) but also to heat-killed ones (biogenics).

One possible mechanism might be competition between *H. pylori* and probiotic bacteria for adherence sites on gastric epithelial cells. So some probiotic strains proposed to compete for adherence sites on gastric surface might have anti-*H. pylori* activity even in their heat-killed forms. However, no such examples have been reported to date.

Another potential mechanism might be coaggregation with *H. pylori*. Examining the anti-*H. pylori* effect of heat-killed *Lactobacius reuteri* DSM17648, Holz et al. found that it coaggregates well with *H. pylori* both in vitro and in vivo, and that it exerts anti-*H. pylori* activity also in the clinical situation [30]. This pioneering result suggests that other probiotic strains having anti-*H. pylori* activity are worth being examined for their ability to coaggregate with *H. pylori.*

4.2 Soybean-related products as biogenics for the stomach

Historically, it has been suggested that soy products prevent the incidence of various cancers including gastric cancer, and several meta-analysis studies concluded that nonfermented and fermented soy foods reduce and increase, respectively, the risk of gastric cancer [40, 41]. However, it has also been suggested that "nonfermented" and "fermented" soy foods are possibly associated with "fruit/vegetable" and "salt intake," respectively [40, 41]. So preventive and stimulatory effects of nonfermented and fermented soy foods should be considered taking these factors in mind. Since isoflavones are one of the proposed molecular candidates for preventing gastric cancer, a large-scale, population-based, prospective, cohort study was conducted to investigate the relationship between isoflavone-intake and risk of gastric cancer in Japan [42]. The results suggested that higher intake of isoflavones does not prevent gastric cancer [42]. So even if nonfermented soy foods can reduce the risk of gastric cancer, the responsible molecules might not be isoflavones in soy foods. However, since genistein, which is one of the soybean isoflavones, reportedly has a protective effect against stress-induced gastric mucosal lesions in rats [43], soy foods might be beneficial to the stomach even if their cancer-preventing effects are not so large.

4.3. Brassicaceae vegetable-related products as biogenics for the stomach

Vegetables of Brassicaceae classification, including cabbage and broccoli, reportedly contain S-methylmethionine, also known as vitamin U. S-methylmethionin is a useful ingredient originally found as anti-ulcerogenic factors in raw cabbage juice [44, 45], and has been used as an ingredient of gastrointestinal drugs in Japan for over 50 years, e.g., Cabagin U. [46]. So Brassicaceae vegetables might be thought as good biogenics for the stomach for treatment and/or prevention of gastric ulcer.

Furthermore, broccoli sprouts especially contain sulforaphane, an isothiocyanate compound reported to have anti-*H. pylori* activity both in vitro [47] and in vivo [48]. Sulforaphone also has been reported to have protective and reparative effects against oxidative stress in gastric mucosa by stimulating nrf2 gene-dependent antioxidant enzyme activities, and also to have anti-inflammatory effects on gastric mucosa during *H. pylori* infections [49]. So among Brassicaceae vegetables, broccoli sprouts are thought to be an especially beneficial biogenic for the stomach.

4.4. Other natural products beneficial to the stomach, including those with anti-H. pylori activity

Because of the wide variety and expected low toxicity of natural products, extracts and essential oils prepared from various plants have been examined their anti-ulcer and anti-*H. pylori* activities. Bonifácio extensively reviewed such products, including 21 different plant extracts and 18 different essential oils [50]. Most of the extracts and essential oils, described in the review mentioned above, were examined only in vitro, although some of them have been evaluated in vivo as well. Bonamin et al. reported that a methanol extract and its enriched alkaloid fraction of a Brazilian plant, *Strychnos pseudoquina* St. Hil. (Loganiaceae), were effective against gastric ulcer induced by acetic acid, and also had anti-*H. pylori* activity in vitro [51]. Extracts of other Brazilian plants, e.g., *Qualea parviflora* Mart. (from bark) [52], *Hancornia speciosa* Gomez (Mangaba; from bark) [53], and *Byrsonima intermedia* A. Juss. (Malpighiaceae; from leaves) [54], have also been reported to have anti-ulcer activity in vivo and anti-*H. pylori* activity in vitro. Ohno et al. reported that 13 different essential oils prepared from a variety of plants inhibited the growth of *H. pylori* in vitro [55]. Among them, essential oils from *Cymbopogon citratus* (lemongrass) and *Lippia citriodora* (lemon verbena) were found to be bactericidal [55]. They also found that essential oil from lemongrass inhibited *H. pylori* in a murine model [55]. Thus, natural sources including herbal and medicinal plants can be thought of as future promising sources of new biogenics for the stomach.

5. Future directions

In this report, we discussed probiotics, prebiotics, and biogenics for the stomach. As shown in **Figure 1**, this research area remains small to date, as only 2% of the total volume of publications concerning "probiotics, prebiotics, or biogenics" as a whole has focused on the stomach. However, the research efforts made related to this interesting research field, as mentioned in this review, are none the less very significant. We think future research in this field will go in the following directions:

Concerning probiotics for the stomach, a search for new probiotic strains beneficial to the stomach is warranted. Although no probiotic bacteria able to reside and grow in the stomach have yet been found, the possible existence of such a kind of so-called "extremophile" [56] type of probiotic bacteria cannot be denied in principle. Indeed, most researchers did not believe in the existence of indigenous bacteria in the stomach until 1984, when *H. pylori* was first described to exist there [57]. Other extremely acid-resistant probiotic strains that can survive in the stomach for a significant time period even if not able to grow there, such as our LJ88, will be a more promising type of bacteria as probiotics for the stomach.

However, since "extremophile" probiotics or indigenous bacteria beneficial to the stomach have not been found to date, prebiotics for such bacteria are also unknown as well. If such bacteria are found in the future, compounds supporting the growth of these bacteria in the stomach may be regarded as "prebiotics for the stomach." Specific substances specifically utilized by supposed stomach bacteria beneficial to the host might be such candidates.

As described in this report, some strains of heat-killed bacteria are thought to be good biogenics for the stomach, as they, like LJ88, might be effective as anti-*H. pylori* agents and also as gastrin-inhibiting ones. Such novel kinds of more effective bacteria may possibly be found in the future. Moreover, the possibility of new biogenics for the stomach, derived from natural sources, e.g., vegetables, fruits, traditional medicinal plants, fungi, products of microorganisms, and marine organisms, should be examined, and promising candidates may well be found in the future.

Practically speaking, appropriate combinations of probiotics, prebiotics (putative), and biogenics might be important for stomach health.

Author details

Yasuhiko Komatsu[1*], Yuji Aiba[1], Yasuhiro Nakano[2] and Yasuhiro Koga[2]

*Address all correspondence to: y_komatsu@snowden.co.jp; gc5y-kmt@asahi-net.or.jp

1 Development Research Department, Snowden, Tokyo, Japan

2 University School of Medicine, Tokai, Kanagawa, Japan

References

[1] Fukushima Y, Yamano T, Kusano A, Takada M, Amano M, Iino H. Effect of fermented milk containing *Lactobacillus johnsonii* La1 (LC1) on defecation in healthy Japanese adults—A double blind placebo controlled study—. *Bioscience Microflora*. 2004;23(4): 139–47.

[2] Felley CP, Corthesy-Theulaz I, Rivero JL, Sipponen P, Kaufmann M, Bauerfeind P, et al. Favourable effect of an acidified milk (LC-1) on *Helicobacter pylori* gastritis in man. *Eur J Gastroenterol Hepatol*. 2001;13(1):25–9.

[3] Michetti P, Dorta G, Wiesel PH, Brassart D, Verdu E, Herranz M, et al. Effect of whey-based culture supernatant of *Lactobacillus acidophilus* (johnsonii) La1 on *Helicobacter pylori* infection in humans. *Digestion*. 1999;60(3):203–9.

[4] Sakamoto I, Igarashi M, Kimura K, Takagi A, Miwa T, Koga Y. Suppressive effect of *L. gasseri* OLL 2716 (LG21) on *Helicobacter pylori* infection in humans. *J Antimicrob Chemother*. 2001;47(5):709–10.

[5] Fujimura S, Kato S, Oda M, Miyahara M, Ito Y, Kimura K, et al. Detection of *Lactobacillus gasseri* OLL2716 strain administered with yogurt drink in gastric mucus layer in humans. *Lett Applied Microbiol*. 2006;43(5):578–81.

[6] Kato-Mori Y, Orihashi T, Kanai Y, Sato M, Sera K, Hagiwara K. Fermentation metabolites from *Lactobacillus gasseri* and *Propionibacterium freudenreichii* exert bacteriocidal effects in mice. *J Med food*. 2010;13(6):1460–7.

[7] Aiba Y, Nakano Y, Koga Y, Takahashi K, Komatsu Y. A highly acid-resistant novel strain of *Lactobacillus johnsonii* No. 1088 has antibacterial activity, including that against *Helicobacter pylori*, and inhibits gastrin-mediated acid production in mice. *MicrobiologyOpen*. 2015;4:465–74.

[8] Mitsuoka T. Development of functional foods. *Biosci Microbiota Food Health*. 2014;33(3): 117–28.

[9] Tsuda A, Suda W, Morita H, Takanashi K, Takagi A, Koga Y, et al. Influence of proton-pump inhibitors on the luminal microbiota in the gastrointestinal tract. *Clin Transl Gastroenterol*. 2015;6:e89.

[10] Guarner F, Schaafsma GJ. Probiotics. *Int J Food Microbiol*. 1998;39(3):237–8.

[11] Peek RM Jr., Blaser MJ. *Helicobacter pylori* and gastrointestinal tract adenocarcinomas. *Nat Rev Cancer*. 2002;2(1):28–37.

[12] Coconnier MH, Lievin V, Hemery E, Servin AL. Antagonistic activity against Helicobacter infection in vitro and in vivo by the human *Lactobacillus acidophilus* strain LB. *Appl Environ Microb*. 1998;64(11):4573–80.

[13] Pinchuk IV, Bressollier P, Verneuil B, Fenet B, Sorokulova IB, Megraud F, et al. In vitro anti-*Helicobacter pylori* activity of the probiotic strain *Bacillus subtilis* 3 is due to secretion of antibiotics. *Antimicrob Agents Chemother*. 2001;45(11):3156–61.

[14] Nam H, Ha M, Bae O, Lee Y. Effect of *Weissella confusa* strain PL9001 on the adherence and growth of *Helicobacter pylori*. *Appl Environ Microb*. 2002;68(9):4642–5.

[15] Boyanova L, Stephanova-Kondratenko M, Mitov I. Anti-*Helicobacter pylori* activity of *Lactobacillus delbrueckii* subsp. bulgaricus strains: preliminary report. *Lett Appl Microbiol*. 2009;48(5):579–84.

[16] Francavilla R, Lionetti E, Castellaneta SP, Magista AM, Maurogiovanni G, Bucci N, et al. Inhibition of *Helicobacter pylori* infection in humans by *Lactobacillus reuteri* ATCC 55730 and effect on eradication therapy: a pilot study. *Helicobacter*. 2008;13(2):127–34.

[17] Tojo R, Suarez A, Clemente MG, de los Reyes-Gavilan CG, Margolles A, Gueimonde M, et al. Intestinal microbiota in health and disease: role of bifidobacteria in gut homeostasis. *World J Gastroenterol*. 2014;20(41):15163–76.

[18] Trifan A, Stanciu C, Stoica O, Girleanu I, Cojocariu C. Impact of *Clostridium difficile* infection on inflammatory bowel disease outcome: a review. *World J Gastroenterol*. 2014;20(33):11736–42.

[19] Shindo Y, Dobashi Y, Sakai T, Monma C, Miyatani H, Yoshida Y. Epidemiological and pathobiological profiles of Clostridium perfringens infections: review of consecutive series of 33 cases over a 13-year period. *Int J Clin Exp Pathol*. 2015;8(1):569–77.

[20] Malfertheiner P, Megraud F, O'Morain C, Bazzoli F, El-Omar E, Graham D, et al. Current concepts in the management of *Helicobacter pylori* infection: the Maastricht III Consensus Report. *Gut*. 2007;56(6):772–81.

[21] Lesbros-Pantoflickova D, Corthesy-Theulaz I, Blum AL. *Helicobacter pylori* and probiotics. *J Nutr*. 2007;137(3 Suppl 2):812S-8S.

[22] Aiba Y, Suzuki N, Kabir AM, Takagi A, Koga Y. Lactic acid-mediated suppression of *Helicobacter pylori* by the oral administration of *Lactobacillus salivarius* as a probiotic in a gnotobiotic murine model. *Am J Gastroenterol*. 1998;93(11):2097–101.

[23] Midolo PD, Lambert JR, Hull R, Luo F, Grayson ML. In vitro inhibition of *Helicobacter pylori* NCTC 11637 by organic acids and lactic acid bacteria. *J Appl Bacteriol*. 1995;79(4): 475–9.

[24] Sgouras D, Maragkoudakis P, Petraki K, Martinez-Gonzalez B, Eriotou E, Michopoulos S, et al. In vitro and in vivo inhibition of *Helicobacter pylori* by *Lactobacillus casei* strain Shirota. *Appl Environ Microbiol*. 2004;70(1):518–26.

[25] Cotter PD, Ross RP, Hill C. Bacteriocins—a viable alternative to antibiotics? *Nat Rev Microbiol*. 2013;11(2):95–105.

[26] Kim TS, Hur JW, Yu MA, Cheigh CI, Kim KN, Hwang JK, et al. Antagonism of *Helicobacter pylori* by bacteriocins of lactic acid bacteria. *J Food Prot*. 2003;66(1):3–12.

[27] Kabir AM, Aiba Y, Takagi A, Kamiya S, Miwa T, Koga Y. Prevention of *Helicobacter pylori* infection by lactobacilli in a gnotobiotic murine model. *Gut*. 1997;41(1):49–55.

[28] Mukai T, Asasaka T, Sato E, Mori K, Matsumoto M, Ohori H. Inhibition of binding of *Helicobacter pylori* to the glycolipid receptors by probiotic *Lactobacillus reuteri*. *FEMS Immunol Med Microbiol*. 2002;32(2):105–10.

[29] Noach LA, Bosma NB, Jansen J, Hoek FJ, van Deventer SJ, Tytgat GN. Mucosal tumor necrosis factor-alpha, interleukin-1 beta, and interleukin-8 production in patients with *Helicobacter pylori* infection. *Scand J Gastroenterol*. 1994;29(5):425–9.

[30] Holz C, Busjahn A, Mehling H, Arya S, Boettner M, Habibi H, et al. Significant reduction in *Helicobacter pylori* load in humans with non-viable *Lactobacillus reuteri* DSM17648: a pilot study. *Probiotics Antimicrob Proteins*. 2015;7(2):91–100.

[31] Kahrilas PJ, Shaheen NJ, Vaezi MF, Hiltz SW, Black E, Modlin IM, et al. American Gastroenterological Association Medical Position Statement on the management of gastroesophageal reflux disease. *Gastroenterology*. 2008;135(4):1383–91.

[32] Richter JE. H pylori: the bug is not all bad. *Gut*. 2001;49(3):319–20.

[33] Fallone CA, Barkun AN, Mayrand S, Wakil G, Friedman G, Szilagyi A, et al. There is no difference in the disease severity of gastro-oesophageal reflux disease between patients infected and not infected with *Helicobacter pylori*. *Aliment Pharmacol Ther*. 2004;20(7):761–8.

[34] Schubert ML, Makhlouf GM. Neural, hormonal, and paracrine regulation of gastrin and acid secretion. *Yale J Biol Med*. 1992;65(6):553–60; Discussion 621–3.

[35] Feng J, Petersen CD, Coy DH, Jiang JK, Thomas CJ, Pollak MR, et al. Calcium-sensing receptor is a physiologic multimodal chemosensor regulating gastric G-cell growth and gastrin secretion. *Proc Natl Acad Sci USA*. 2010;107(41):17791–6.

[36] Takahashi H, Nakano Y, Matsuoka T, Kumaki N, Asami Y, Koga Y. Role of indigenous lactobacilli in gastrin-mediated acid production in the mouse stomach. *Appl Environ Microbiol*. 2011;77(19):6964–71.

[37] Delgado S, Cabrera-Rubio R, Mira A, Suarez A, Mayo B. Microbiological survey of the human gastric ecosystem using culturing and pyrosequencing methods. *Microb Ecol*. 2013;65(3):763–72.

[38] Gibson GR, Roberfroid MB. Dietary modulation of the human colonic microbiota: introducing the concept of prebiotics. *J Nutr*. 1995;125(6):1401–12.

[39] Lind T, Megraud F, Unge P, Bayerdorffer E, O'Morain C, Spiller R, et al. The MACH2 study: role of omeprazole in eradication of *Helicobacter pylori* with 1-week triple therapies. *Gastroenterology*. 1999;116(2):248–53.

[40] Wu AH, Yang D, Pike MC. A meta-analysis of soyfoods and risk of stomach cancer: the problem of potential confounders. *Cancer Epidemiol Biomarkers Prev*. 2000;9(10):1051–8.

[41] Kim J, Kang M, Lee JS, Inoue M, Sasazuki S, Tsugane S. Fermented and non-fermented soy food consumption and gastric cancer in Japanese and Korean populations: a meta-analysis of observational studies. *Cancer Sci*. 2011;102(1):231–44.

[42] Hara A, Sasazuki S, Inoue M, Iwasaki M, Shimazu T, Sawada N, et al. Isoflavone intake and risk of gastric cancer: a population-based prospective cohort study in Japan. *Am J Clin Nutr*. 2012;95(1):147–54.

[43] Takekawa S, Matsui T, Arakawa Y. The protective effect of the soybean polyphenol genistein against stress-induced gastric mucosal lesions in rats, and its hormonal mechanisms. *J Nutr Sci Vitamino*. 2006;52(4):274–80.

[44] Cheney G. Anti-peptic ulcer dietary factor (vitamin "U") in the treatment of peptic ulcer. *J Am Diet Asso*. 1950;26(9):668–72.

[45] Cheney G. Vitamin U therapy of peptic ulcer. *Calif Med*. 1952;77(4):248–52.

[46] Kosaki S, Yoshioka Y, Mitsuba K, Sakai R. Effectiveness of Cabagin U for peptic ulcer (in Japanese). *J New Remedies & Clinics*. 1964;13(11):1288–92.

[47] Fahey JW, Haristoy X, Dolan PM, Kensler TW, Scholtus I, Stephenson KK, et al. Sulforaphane inhibits extracellular, intracellular, and antibiotic-resistant strains of *Helicobacter pylori* and prevents benzo[a]pyrene-induced stomach tumors. *Proc Natl Acad Sci USA*. 2002;99(11):7610–5.

[48] Haristoy X, Angioi-Duprez K, Duprez A, Lozniewski A. Efficacy of sulforaphane in eradicating Helicobacter pylori in human gastric xenografts implanted in nude mice. *Antimicrob Agents Chemother*. 2003;47(12):3982–4.

[49] Yanaka A. Sulforaphane enhances protection and repair of gastric mucosa against oxidative stress in vitro, and demonstrates anti-inflammatory effects on Helicobacter pylori-infected gastric mucosae in mice and human subjects. *Curr Pharma Des*. 2011;17(16):1532–40.

[50] Bonifacio BV, dos Santos Ramos MA, da Silva PB, Bauab TM. Antimicrobial activity of natural products against *Helicobacter pylori*: a review. *Ann Clin Microbiol Antimicrob*. 2014;13:54.

[51] Bonamin F, Moraes TM, Kushima H, Silva MA, Rozza AL, Pellizzon CH, et al. Can a Strychnos species be used as antiulcer agent? Ulcer healing action from alkaloid fraction of *Strychnos pseudoquina* St. Hil. (Loganiaceae). *J Ethnopharmacol*. 2011;138(1):47–52.

[52] Mazzolin LP, Nasser AL, Moraes TM, Santos RC, Nishijima CM, Santos FV, et al. *Qualea parviflora* Mart.: an integrative study to validate the gastroprotective, antidiarrheal, antihemorragic and mutagenic action. *J Ethnopharmacol*. 2010;127(2):508–14.

[53] Moraes Tde M, Rodrigues CM, Kushima H, Bauab TM, Villegas W, Pellizzon CH, et al. *Hancornia speciosa*: indications of gastroprotective, healing and anti-*Helicobacter pylori* actions. *J Ethnopharmacol*. 2008;120(2):161–8.

[54] Santos RC, Kushima H, Rodrigues CM, Sannomiya M, Rocha LR, Bauab TM, et al. *Byrsonima intermedia* A. Juss.: gastric and duodenal anti-ulcer, antimicrobial and antidiarrheal effects in experimental rodent models. *J Ethnopharmacol*. 2012;140(2):203–12.

[55] Ohno T, Kita M, Yamaoka Y, Imamura S, Yamamoto T, Mitsufuji S, et al. Antimicrobial activity of essential oils against *Helicobacter pylori*. *Helicobacter*. 2003;8(3):207–15.

[56] Rothschild LJ, Mancinelli RL. Life in extreme environments. *Nature*. 2001;409(6823): 1092–101.

[57] Marshall BJ, Warren JR. Unidentified curved bacilli in the stomach of patients with gastritis and peptic ulceration. *Lancet*. 1984;1(8390):1311–5.